Managing Anticoagulation Patients in the Hospital

The Inpatient Anticoagulation Service

Michael Gulseth, Pharm.D., BCPS
Assistant Professor
Clinical Pharmacy Specialist
University of Minnesota College of Pharmacy
Saint Mary's Medical Center
Duluth, MN

American Society of Health-System Pharmacists®
Bethesda, Maryland

Any correspondence regarding this publication should be sent to the publisher, American Society of Health-System Pharmacists, 7272 Wisconsin Avenue, Bethesda, MD 20814, attention: Special Publishing.

The information presented herein reflects the opinions of the contributors and advisors. It should not be interpreted as an official policy of ASHP or as an endorsement of any product. The information contained in this program, and the companion workbook, are to be used as guidance.

Because of ongoing research and improvements in technology, the information and its applications contained in this text are constantly evolving and are subject to the professional judgment and interpretation of the practitioner due to the uniqueness of each pharmacy's role in compounding sterile preparations and the handling of hazardous drugs. The editors, contributors, and ASHP have made reasonable efforts to ensure the accuracy and appropriateness of the information presented in this document. However, any user of this information is advised that the editors, contributors, advisors, and ASHP are not responsible for the continued currency of the information, for any errors or omissions, and/or for any consequences arising from the use of the information in the document in any and all practice settings. Any reader of this document is cautioned that ASHP makes no representation, guarantee, or warranty, express or implied, as to the accuracy and appropriateness of the information contained in this document and will bear no responsibility or liability for the results or consequences of its use.

Director, Special Publishing: Jack Bruggeman
Senior Editorial Project Manager: Dana Battaglia
Editorial Resources Manager: Bill Fogle
Cover and Page Design: Carol Barrer

Library of Congress Cataloging-in-Publication Data

Gulseth, Michael.
  Managing anticoagulation patients in the hospital : the inpatient anticoagulation service / Michael Gulseth.
        p. ; cm.
  Includes bibliographical references and index.
  ISBN 978-1-58528-157-2
1. Anticoagulants (Medicine) 2. Hospitals--Drug distribution system. 3. Hospital pharmacies--Administration. I. American Society of Health-System Pharmacists. II. Title.
  [DNLM: 1. Anticoagulants--administration & dosage. 2. Pharmacy Service, Hospital--methods. 3. Inpatients. 4. Medication Systems--organization & administration. 5. Patient Care Planning--organization & administration. QV 193 G973m 2007]

RC684.A6G85 2007
362.11068--dc22

2007017023

©2007, American Society of Health-System Pharmacists, Inc. All rights reserved.

No part of this publication may be reproduced or transmitted in any form or by any means, electronic or mechanical, including photocopying, microfilming, and recording, or by any information storage and retrieval system, without written permission from the American Society of Health-System Pharmacists.

ASHP is a service mark of the American Society of Health-System Pharmacists, Inc.; registered in the U.S. Patent and Trademark Office.

ISBN: 978-1-58528-157-2

Dedication

To Brenda:

Without your love, support, and understanding this would not have been possible. I love you as much today as the day I married you.

Acknowledgments

This book would not have been possible without the support and encouragement of many people. While I cannot possibly name everyone who has had a hand in what led to this work, I would like to mention a few of the major influences:

David Fuhs and Lisa Gersema, who mentored me as a resident to always strive to put pharmacists in a position to provide optimal patient care while training me on how to provide that same care.

Christene Jolowski, who taught me how important is was to invest in good people and be dedicated to resident training.

Steve Meisel, who taught me how to prevent medication errors by fixing systems that lead to errors and then gave me the experience on how to implement those same types of system changes.

Carl Woetzel, who taught me that when it comes to improving patient care provided by pharmacists, it is not *if* you do it, but *how* you do it.

Jim Tomsche, and Debbie Sisson, who were every bit as responsible for the implementation of the St. Mary's Medical Center inpatient anticoagulation service and care improvements that resulted as anyone else.

Bill Dager, whose work in inpatient anticoagulation is unparalleled, and whose dedication to making this book a reality is deeply appreciated. He did much more than write a couple of chapters for this text.

Henry Bussey, and other pioneer pharmacists who established the role of pharmacists working in anticoagulation.

Daniel Gulseth, my father, and the first pharmacist I ever knew.

Michael Gulseth

Preface

The American Society of Health-System Pharmacists (ASHP) asserts "the mission of pharmacists is to help people make the best use of medications."[1] Never has this mission been more important than in the current hospital setting, with the ever-increasing acuity of patients seen and the increasing complexity of medication therapy. Never has the focus on preventing patient-related morbidity and mortality due to medications been greater than now, with organizations such as the Institute for Health-Care Improvement and the Joint Commission using their influence to mandate safer practices in hospitals. Never has a professional been better positioned and trained to meet the challenges of contemporary medication therapy management than the modern pharmacist.

Anticoagulant use inside of hospitals provides a particular challenge to caregivers. The narrow therapeutic indexes of the agents, along with the high patient acuity, are a recipe for adverse drug events (ADEs). Because of this, warfarin, heparin, and low molecular weight heparin are all considered "high-alert" medications by the Institute for Safe Medication Practices (ISMP).[2] A recent report by Winterstein et al. showed that anticoagulant medications were responsible for 32.2% of preventable ADEs in a teaching hospital, and this was double the amount caused by any other medication class.[3] This type of data is leading for more and more hospitals and accreditation bodies to call for pharmacists to lead implementation of systematic anticoagulation management in the inpatient setting, much like what is the standard of care in the outpatient setting.[4]

This book is intended for pharmacists tasked with developing, implementing, and maintaining an inpatient anticoagulation service and for all pharmacists who practice in this type of service. The book contains a comprehensive step-by-step guide for setting up an inpatient anticoagulation service (Part 1). The book also contains a thorough and practical clinical review of the anticoagulant medications managed by pharmacists in the hospital and cases to demonstrate important concepts (Part 2). Part 2 is an excellent resource for any pharmacist who wants to build expertise in caring for inpatients on anticoagulants. It will also serve as an excellent resource for a pharmacist who is tasked with teaching other pharmacists the clinical knowledge they need to manage patients on anticoagulants. This is the first book dedicated to providing systematic anticoagulation management in the inpatient setting.

A unique feature of this book is its practicality. It contains resources such as policies and procedures, clinical dosing tools, and business plans that have been used by other hospitals across America. Many of these resources are included in a usable fashion on the accompanying CD-ROM (Microsoft Word, PowerPoint files, etc.) so that the user can easily adopt them within his or her own setting.

I hope you find this book useful in starting your institution's inpatient anticoagulation service or in providing care within an inpatient anticoagulation service. Very rarely do pharmacists undertake a more important role that will benefit patients as much as the one in which you are now engaged.

Michael Gulseth, Pharm.D., BCPS
February 3, 2007

References

1. Unknown. Mission Statement of the American Society of Health-System Pharmacists. Am Society of Health-Systems Pharmacists. June 4, 2001. Available at: http://www.ashp.org/aboutashp/ASHPmission.cfm?cfid=13106229&CFToken=87464590. Accessed May 26, 2006.
2. Unknown. ISMP's List of High-Alert Medications. Institute for Safe Medication Practices [web page]. Available at: http://www.ismp.org/Tools/highalert-medications.pdf. Accessed May 26, 2006.
3. Winterstein AG, Hatton RC, Gonzalez-Rothi R, Johns TE, Segal R. Identifying clinically significant preventable adverse drug events through a hospital's database of adverse drug reaction reports. *Am J Health-Syst Pharm.* 2002;59(18):1742-9.
4. Ansell J, Hirsh J, Poller L, Bussey H, Jacobson A, Hylek E. The pharmacology and management of the vitamin K antagonists: the Seventh ACCP Conference on Antithrombotic and Thrombolytic Therapy. *Chest.* 2004;126(3 Suppl):204S-33S.

Table of Contents

Dedication iii

Acknowledgments v

Preface vii

Contributors xi

List of CD Resources xiii

Part 1: Program Design and Implementation

Chapter 1: Introduction to the Inpatient Anticoagulation Service 1

Michael Gulseth

Chapter 2: Literature Review Supporting Inpatient Pharmacy Management of Anticoagulation 7

William Dager

Chapter 3: Anticoagulant Safety: Identification of the Gaps 17

Jill Strykowski

Chapter 4: Planning of the Inpatient Anticoagulation Service 23

Michael Gulseth

Chapter 5: Winning Support for the Inpatient Anticoagulation Service 39

Michael Gulseth

Chapter 6: Justifying the Program to Hospital Administration: The Financial Perspective 77

Michael Gulseth

Chapter 7: Pharmacist Education and Training 93

Michael Gulseth

Chapter 8: Patient Education Needs 101
Michael Gulseth

Chapter 9: Monitoring and Maintaining Program Quality 123
Michael Gulseth

Part 2: Anticoagulant Knowledge 101

Chapter 10: Essential Warfarin Knowledge 133
Scott Neel

Chapter 11: Heparin, Low Molecular Weight Heparin, and Fondaparinux 177
Edith Nutescu and William Dager

Chapter 12: Essential Direct Thrombin Inhibitor Knowledge 203
William Dager

Chapter 13: Helpful References and Preparing for the Future 215
Michael Gulseth

Index 221

Contributors

William Dager, Pharm.D., FCHSP
Pharmacist Specialist
UC Davis Medical Center
Sacramento, CA

Michael Gulseth, Pharm.D., BCPS
Assistant Professor
Clinical Pharmacy Specialist
University of Minnesota College of Pharmacy
Saint Mary's Medical Center
Duluth, MN

Scott Neel, Pharm.D.
Clinical Coordinator
Cape Canaveral Hospital, Health-First
Cocoa Beach, FL

Edith A. Nutescu, Pharm.D.
Clinical Associate Professor
Department of Pharmacy Practice
University of Illinois at Chicago
College of Pharmacy
Director, Antithrombosis Center
University of Illinois at Chicago Medical Center

Jill Strykowski, M.S., R.Ph.
Director of Pharmacy
Mercy and Unity Hospitals
Coon Rapids, MN

List of CD Resources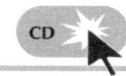

Part 1: Program Design and Implementation

Chapter 1: Introduction to Inpatient Anticoagulation
- No CD resources.

Chapter 2: Literature Review Supporting Inpatient Pharmacy Management of Anticoagulation
- Table 2-1. Selected references supporting pharmacist management of heparin and warfarin in the inpatient setting

Chapter 3: Anticoagulant Safety: Identifying the Gaps
- No CD resources.

Chapter 4: Planning of the Inpatient Anticoagulation Service
- Figure 4-1. Sample modified SOAP note for an initial pharmacist anticoagulation consult.
- Figure 4-2. Standardized evaluation form for initial progress notes
- Figure 4-5. Heparin/Coumadin monitoring form
- Figure 4-6. ARMC pharmacy anticoagulation service flow sheet (CD only)

Chapter 5: Winning Support for the Inpatient Anticoagulation Service
- Figure 5-1. Recombinant factors VIIa orders
- Figure 5-2. Anticoagulation bridging guidelines
- Figure 5-3. Pharmacy policy and procedure: pharmacist-managed warfarin dosing
- Figure 5-4. Conservative warfarin initiation algorithm
- Figure 5-5. Liberal warfarin dose initiation algorithm
- Figure 5-6. Anticoagulation discharge follow-up orders
- Figure 5-7. Warfarin discharge work checklist
- Figure 5-8. Daily INR policy
- Figure 5-9. Vitamin K use policy
- Figure 5-10. Warfarin anticoagulation reversal guidelines
- Figure 5-11. Direct thrombin inhibitor orders
- Figure 5-12. Policy and procedures: pharmacy to dose direct thrombin inhibitors
- Figure 5-13. Dosing guidelines and monitoring plan form argatroban anticoagulation that can be modified to other thrombin inhibitors
- Figure 5-14. Heparin protocol

Chapter 6: Justifying the Program to Hospital Administration: The Financial Perspective
- St. Joseph's Hospital Department of Pharmacy case study and business plan for an inpatient anticoagulation service

Chapter 7: Pharmacist Education and Training
- Figure 7-3. Skills for inpatient anticoagulation pharmacists checklist

Chapter 8: Patient Education Needs
- Appendix 8-1. Patient education information materials: Warfarin
- Appendix 8-2. Patient education information materials: Injectable anticoagulants enoxaparin and dalteparin

Chapter 9: Monitoring and Maintaining Program Quality
- Table 9-1. Process measure data collection form
- Figure 9-1. Percentage of INRs greater than 3.5
- Figure 9-2. Percentage of INRs greater than 6

Part 2: Anticoagulant Knowledge 101

Chapter 10: Essential Warfarin Knowledge
- Table 10-1. Clinically significant interactions with warfarin by level of causation and drug group
- Figure 10-1. Vitamin K cycle. Warfarin blocks the conversion of vitamin K epoxide to vitamin C
- Figure 10-2. Coagulation cascade and vitamin K–dependent clotting factor half-lives
- Carry-around card, "Pocket Reference for Oral Anticoagulation" (CD only)
- PowerPoint presentation, "What Every Pharmacist Needs to Know About Warfarin" (CD only)

Chapter 11: Heparin, Low Molecular Weight Heparin, and Fondaparinux
- Figure 11-1. Mechanism of action of UFH, LMWH, and fondaparinux
- Table 11-1. Pharmacologic and clinical properties of UFH, LMWH, and fondaparinux
- Table 11-2. Sample dosing and monitoring nomogram for adjusted-dose subcutaneous UFH
- Table 11-3. Practical considerations for transitioning between various anticoagulant agents
- Table 11-4. Sample weight-based dosing nomogram for IV UFH in acute thrombosis
- Table 11-5. Sample monitoring nomogram for IV UFH
- Table 11-6. Indications and recommended doses for LMWHs and fondaparinux

- Table 11-7. Sample LMWH dosing nomogram for pediatric patients
- Table 11-8. Recommendations for timing of anticoagulant agents in patients undergoing neuraxial procedures
- Table 11-9. Dosing and monitoring considerations for LMWH and fondaparinux in patients with renal impairment
- Carry-around card, "Heparin, LMWH, Fondaparinux Quick Reference Guide" (CD only)
- PowerPoint presentation, "Heparin, Low Molecular Weight Heparin, and Fondaparinux" (CD only)

Chapter 12: Essential Direct Thrombin Inhibitor Knowledge
- Table 12-1. Pharmacokinetics of available antithrombin agents
- Table 12-2. Steps in the initiation, monitoring, and transition of DTI Therapy
- Table 12-3. Transitioning from a DTI to warfarin
- Carry-around card, "Pocket Reference for DTI therapy" (CD only)
- PowerPoint presentation, "Direct Thrombin Inhibitors" (CD only)

Chapter 13: Helpful References and Preparing for the Future
- Table 13-1. Anticoagulants in the pipeline

Part 1

Program Design and Implementation

Chapter 1: Introduction to the Inpatient Anticoagulation Service
Michael Gulseth

Chapter 2: Literature Review Supporting Inpatient Pharmacy Management of Anticoagulation
William Dager

Chapter 3: Anticoagulant Safety: Identification of the Gaps
Jill Strykowski

Chapter 4: Planning of the Inpatient Anticoagulation Service
Michael Gulseth

Chapter 5: Winning Support for the Inpatient Anticoagulation Service
Michael Gulseth

Chapter 6: Justifying the Program to Hospital Administration: The Financial Perspective
Michael Gulseth

Chapter 7: Pharmacist Education and Training
Michael Gulseth

Chapter 8: Patient Education Needs
Michael Gulseth

Chapter 9: Monitoring and Maintaining Program Quality
Michael Gulseth

Chapter 1

Introduction to the Inpatient Anticoagulation Service

Michael Gulseth

Chapter Outline

- Introduction
- Coordinated, systematic anticoagulation care: outpatient setting
- Coordinated, systematic anticoagulation care: inpatient setting
- Quality of patient care: national focus
- The inpatient anticoagulation service: system improvement in patient care
- Where does the Joint Commission® seem to be going on this issue?
- Conclusion
- Patient case examples

Introduction

Anticoagulant medications have revolutionized the practice of medicine over the past 50 years. They are effective in preventing embolic complications in a wide variety of conditions. Anticoagulants are known to prevent stroke from atrial fibrillation, recurrence of deep vein thrombosis and pulmonary embolism, and clot formation on mechanical heart valves. They have allowed millions of patients to live healthy lives throughout the world after having an embolic event.

Unfortunately, all anticoagulants have a narrow therapeutic index. One of the most basic therapeutics lessons in pharmacy school is that if a patient gets too much of an anticoagulant medication, they are at risk of a major bleeding event. If they get too little, they are at risk of a clot forming, extending, or embolizing. Pharmacists also know that changes in medications and diseases can have a profound effect on a patient's response to anticoagulant medications. Even newer agents such as low molecular weight heparins (LMWHs), which are widely promoted as "safer" alternatives to unfractionated heparin, can cause serious patient harm when used incorrectly. For example, the 1 mg/kg twice daily dose of enoxaparin used regularly for treatment of venous thromboembolism could cause major bleeding in a patient with compromised renal function.

Coordinated, Systematic Care: Outpatient Setting

Classically, these concerns led to the widespread adoption of systematic, coordinated care of warfarin patients in the outpatient setting. According to Dr. Jack Ansell and the Seventh ACCP Conference on Antithrombotic and Thrombolytic Therapy, systematic, coordinated care in regard to warfarin consists of[1,2]:

- Assisting in determining the appropriateness of care
- Providing anticoagulant dosing
- Assuring regular monitoring and patient evaluation

- Provision of repeated patient education
- Communicating with other patient care providers that are involved in the patient's care

To provide this level of care, many pharmacists have been involved with setting up and running outpatient warfarin anticoagulation clinics. Many studies have been generated from these types of clinics showing an improvement in patient outcomes.[2-4]

Coordinated, Systematic Anticoagulation Care: Inpatient Setting

Should systematic, coordinated anticoagulation care also be the practice standard in the inpatient setting? Pharmacists have also been involved for years in the management of anticoagulants in the inpatient setting, but data demonstrating the improvement in care is only recently accumulating.[5-7] Further, very little national emphasis has been given to providing systematic, coordinated anticoagulation care to inpatients. Numerous factors likely led to the almost exclusive outpatient focus for providing systematic, coordinated care. For example, patients spent the vast majority of their time in outpatient setting. During that time, it is difficult to keep track of all anticoagulation outpatients and keep them compliant with needed monitoring. However, many practitioners would argue that systematic, coordinated care of anticoagulants needs to be provided throughout the continuum of care by experienced anticoagulation clinicians, including the inpatient setting. Also, this care should involve multiple agents, not just warfarin which has been mainly the focus of outpatient programs. Finally, this care should extend beyond just the management of individual anticoagulation patients, but also fundamentally address anticoagulation care deliver systems that can lead to unsafe care. Consider the following points:

- Patients are in the hospital because they are ill. Different disease states that cause admission, such as decompensated heart failure, are also known to affect the response of anticoagulant medications like warfarin.[2] This can lead to loss of anticoagulation control necessitating dosing adjustments at least in the short term.
- Patients in the hospital, just as is the case in the outpatient setting, often have anticoagulation interrupted for invasive procedures. This leaves many patients vulnerable to a potentially devastating thrombotic event if an immediate acting "bridge" therapy (heparin, LMWHs) is not utilized or serious bleeding if the "bridge" therapy is not implemented appropriately.
- Heparin administration is frequently the source of potentially devastating medication errors inside of hospitals.[8] Utilizing an inpatient anticoagulation program to change the "systems" in how heparin is delivered could improve care.
- When patients are in the hospital, they have many medications started and stopped. This leads to risk of major drug interactions particularly with warfarin.

Please refer to the patient cases at the end of this chapter for examples of some adverse outcomes, related to the above issues, that can occur to patients in the hospital

Quality of Patient Care: National Focus

The increased focus in recent years on improving the safety of medication delivery systems seemed to flow from the seminal work of the Institute of Medicine (IOM), *To Err is Human*.[9] In that report from 1999, the IOM estimated that 44,000 patient die annually from medical mistakes with 7000 of those due to medication errors. In this report, the IOM says, "Building safety into processes of care is a more effective way to reduce errors than blaming individuals. The focus must shift from blaming individuals for past errors to a focus on preventing future errors by designing safety into the system." They also said that after an appropriate time period "regulators and accreditors should require (proven patient safety systems) as a minimum standard." Interestingly, it does seems that accrediting organizations such as the Joint Commission® have been increasingly requiring implementation of patient safety recommendations from groups such as the Institute for Safe Medication Practices and the Institute for Health-Care Improvement.

The Inpatient Anticoagulation Service: System Improvement in Patient Care

Designing and implementing a systematic, coordinated inpatient anticoagulation service is a prime example of a "system" change that designs safety into the system as suggested by the IOM. For example, having an anticoagulation pharmacist dose warfarin for inpatients assures a medication expert will consider the patients past warfarin needs, current clinical status, current medications, and current labs before a dose is ever chosen. (Ideally, this should always happen, but does it happen 100% of the time in reality? When a physician harms someone, why is more energy spent blaming the physician than determining how to prevent the event from happening again to any physician?) Another example of an anticoagulation service improving the systems of care is the manger of the service could also be reviewing all medication errors due to heparin. Then, after reviewing the cases, the manager would determine what steps could be taken to improve the safety of delivering care and prevent the errors form happening again. (i.e., recommending the organization purchase smart infusion pumps, require double checks, etc.) In other words, the work of an inpatient anticoagulation service is not only delivering care to patients but also improving the safety of the systems as a whole.

Where Does the Joint Commission® Seem to Be Going on This Issue?

The provision of systematic, coordinated anticoagulation care in the inpatient setting also now seems to be a patient safety interest for the Joint Commission®. Early versions of the 2007 draft national patient safety goals called for a pharmacist who "… is involved in inpatient anticoagulation services for both heparin and warfarin to provide input on dosing and monitoring of patients on anticoagulation therapy."[10] Furthermore, the Joint Commission® has draft core measures aimed at systematizing and improving the quality of prevention and treatment of venous thromboembolism (VTE). The proposed core measures do more than simply assure that VTE is being prevented; they also call for systematic and correct use of heparin products and warfarin.[11] As with all standards that are proposed by the Joint Commission®, even the above proposals have already undergone significant revisions. However, it does seem likely that the Joint Commission® is moving closer to mandating the provision of systematic, coordinated anticoagulation care in the inpatient setting. This should provide a powerful argument for pharmacy directors who, after analyzing their current resources, determine they need to add personnel to provide this service.

Conclusion

While anticoagulants have improved the lives of millions of patients, they present a challenge to assure their safe use. The provision of systematic, coordinated anticoagulation care has long been a focus in the outpatient setting, but not as much attention has been paid to assuring the safe use of anticoagulants in the inpatient setting despite the high acuity of the modern patient and the multiple anticoagulants that are utilized. The current climate of fundamentally changing systems to ensure the safety of patients in the healthcare system has led to current proposals to mandate the involvement of pharmacists in the care of patients on anticoagulants in the inpatient setting. Chapter 2 will focus on the published literature supporting these types of services.

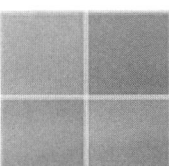

Patient Case Examples

- A patient is admitted with decompensated heart failure and is also on warfarin for stroke prophylaxis due to atrial fibrillation. The INR is not checked at admission or for 2 days. The patient, while out walking, falls and hits his head. The patient has a large intracranial bleed. An INR is finally checked and it is 15.
- A patient is taken off warfarin for a colonoscopy with the possibility of biopsies. The patient undergoes the procedure successfully, but the next day he has a massive stroke. When reviewing the records, it is found the patient had a mechanical mitral valve and did not receive appropriate "bridge" therapy with a heparin product.
- A patient is started on enoxaparin after a total knee replacement for deep vein thrombosis prophylaxis. Two days later, the patient begins losing sensation in his legs. The patient, that same day, had an epidural catheter pulled that had been used post op for pain control. The loss of sensation progresses to permanent paralysis and an epidural hematoma is found to be the cause.
- A patient in the hospital, who is also on warfarin, is started on sulfamethoxazole/trimethoprim for uncomplicated cystitis, and INRs are not checked. Three days later, the patient has gross amounts of blood in his stool and a low blood pressure. The INR is finally drawn and found to be 10.
- A patient with an in range INR with a mitral mechanical heart valve is admitted to the hospital with a new hip fracture. The patient is given 10 mg po of oral vitamin K to lower her INR for surgery the next day. After her procedure, she remains in the hospital 7 days as clinicians attempt to get her INR back into range since she is not an appropriate candidate for outpatient LMWH therapy.
- A nurse in a hospital caring for a patient on IV heparin receives the results of the first aPTT after the heparin is started. She is startled to see the result in > 200 seconds and that the entire

heparin bag has been infused. When investigating the cause, she finds that the pump was set at 900 mL/hour when the order was for 900 units/hour. Luckily, the error is caught before any bleeding occurs.

References

1. Ansell JE. The Value of an Anticoagulation Management Service. In: Ansell JE, Oertel LB, Wittkowsky AK, eds. *Managing Oral Anticoagulation Therapy*. Gaithersburg, MD: Aspen Publishers; 2000.
2. Ansell J, Hirsh J, Poller L, Bussey H, Jacobson A, Hylek E. The pharmacology and management of the vitamin K antagonists: the Seventh ACCP Conference on Antithrombotic and Thrombolytic Therapy. *Chest*. 2004;126(3 Suppl):204S-33S.
3. Chiquette E, Amato MG, Bussey HI. Comparison of an anticoagulation clinic with usual medical care: anticoagulation control, patient outcomes, and health care costs. *Arch Intern Med*. 1998;158(15):1641-7.
4. Witt DM, Sadler MA, Shanahan RL, Mazzoli G, Tillman DJ. Effect of a centralized clinical pharmacy anticoagulation service on the outcomes of anticoagulation therapy. *Chest*. 2005;127(5):1515-22.
5. Dager WE, Branch JM, King JH et al. Optimization of inpatient warfarin therapy: impact of daily consultation by a pharmacist-managed anticoagulation service. *Ann Pharmacother*. 2000;34(5):567-72.
6. Rivey MP, Wood RD, Allington DR, Stratton TP, Erickson CC, Stenson TA. Pharmacy-managed protocol for warfarin use in orthopedic surgery patients. *Am J Health-Syst Pharm*. 1995;52(12):1310-6.
7. Mamdani MM, Racine E, McCreadie S, et al. Clinical and economic effectiveness of an inpatient anticoagulation service. *Pharmacotherapy*. 1999;19(9):1064-74.
8. Winterstein AG, Hatton RC, Gonzalez-Rothi R, Johns TE, Segal R. Identifying clinically significant preventable adverse drug events through a hospital's database of adverse drug reaction reports. *Am J Health-Syst Pharm*. 2002;59(18):1742-9.
9. Unknown. To Err is Human: Building a Safer Health System. *Institute of Medicine*. Available at: http://www.nap.edu/catalog/9728.html#toc. Accessed June 2, 2006.
10. Unknown. Draft Candidate 2007 National Patient Safety Goals, Requirements and Implementation Expectations. *Joint Commission on Accreditation of Healthcare Organizations*. Available at: http://www.jointcommission.org/NR/rdonlyres/4901A094-80A7-4AD6-86CD-4754B896A986/0/07_npsg_hap_cah.pdf. Accessed May 31, 2006.
11. Unknown. *Joint Commission on Accreditation of Healthcare Organizations*. Available at: http://www.JCAHO.org/pms/core+measures/pdf119.pdf. Accessed Feb 15, 2006.

Chapter 2

Literature Review Supporting Inpatient Pharmacy Management of Anticoagulation

William Dager

Chapter Outline

- Introduction/history
- Supporting literature
  - Warfarin
  - Heparin
  - Combined warfarin and heparin
  - Low molecular weight heparin/fondaparinux
- Direct thrombin inhibitors
- Reversal
- Success relies on a multidisciplinary approach
- On the horizon
- Future roles
- Conclusion

Introduction/History

Since the availability of warfarin and unfractionated heparin (UFH) over 50 years ago for the management or prevention of thromboembolism, our understanding on dosing approaches and monitoring of anticoagulant therapy has, and continues to be, constantly revised. Most of the anticoagulants currently in use have fairly narrow therapeutic windows, creating a need to carefully balance either treatment or prevention of thrombosis while minimizing the risk for bleeding. The expansion of information regarding their optimal use along with the availability of additional agents has created numerous choices and management considerations during the implementation of a treatment plan. To address the complex process now associated with anticoagulation therapy in addition to the high incidence of adverse medication-related events associated with these agents, health care systems and physicians have recognized the potential benefits of involving clinical pharmacists with their use. This is not a new concept. Ambulatory care based anticoagulation clinics utilizing pharmacists and nurses were developed to monitor outpatients receiving warfarin have demonstrated improved outcomes when compared to the standard of care.[1] Recent observations have demonstrated that pharmacist involvement in managing inpatient anticoagulation can improve clinical outcomes while reducing the cost of therapy (Table 2-1).[2-11]

Supporting Literature

Warfarin

One of the earliest reports on inpatient pharmacists involved in managing warfarin was a comparison of 57 patients receiving pharmacist-involved care to a pre-involvement control of 97 patients (the majority had a VTE). Pharmacists provided unsolicited consults on all patients receiving warfarin. Activities included interpretation of laboratory values, drug interaction screening, dosing recommendations, and education to both patients and clinicians involved in their care. No difference in time of initiating warfarin from heparin, warfarin dose, or days of anticoagulant therapy was observed. A

Table 2-1.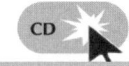
Selected References Supporting Pharmacist Management of Heparin and Warfarin in the Inpatient Setting

Reference	Description	Key Pharmacist Impact	Comments
Pawloski (12)	Pharmacist-dosed heparin using new weight-based protocol ($n = 29$) versus physician ($n = 14$)	Earlier aPTT in target range ($p < 0.001$) with fewer rate changes ($p < 0.001$)	Small community hospital; decreased number of rate changes and days on heparin (NS) in a small study population
Rivey (13)	Pharmacist-adjusted heparin ($n = 42$) compared to physician-directed ($n = 42$)	Pharmacist management achieved first aPTT value <1.5 earlier, shorter time to first aPTT 1.5–2 times normal, and fewer patients with aPTT values <1.5 or >3 times normal; all p values <0.05	
Kershaw (14)	Pharmacy-based, computer-assisted heparin dosing ($n = 131$) compared to random historical cohort ($n = 57$); 1992	Earlier time to target aPTT value ($p < 0.001$)	
Mandami (4)	Usual physician-directed care ($n = 50$) to pharmacist management ($n = 50$) of heparin and warfarin under protocol using independent nomograms for each agent	UFH: increase aPTT values in ($p = 0.05$) or below ($p = 0.03$) the target range; Warfarin: decreased time to initiate therapy ($p = 0.05$); reduction in total hospital costs ($p = 0.05$)	
Dager (5)	Usual physician-directed warfarin dosing ($n = 60$) to pharmacist consultation ($n = 60$) matched for anticoagulation indication	Decrease critical INR values (> 3.5 or > 6.0; $p < 0.001$), length of hospital stay ($p = 0.009$)	University hospital: fewer recurrent thrombosis and bleeding events at 3 months post initiation of anticoagulation; INR more likely in the target range (2–3) at discharge

Continued

reduction in the number of requested laboratory determinations and improved prothrombin time stability at discharge in addition to an increase in referral to the anticoagulation clinic was noted.[2] Their results suggested that a pharmacist involved during the initial phase of initiating anticoagulation for VTE can assist in facilitating long-term outpatient management without compromising current (usual) care.

In an evaluation of a pilot program evaluating pharmacist management of patients being initiated on warfarin ($n = 25$) to a control ($n = 34$), involving pharmacists significantly ($p = 0.0059$) reduced the incidence of INR values over 4 and the need for vitamin K. There was one less thrombotic event in the pharmacist group; however, the comparative cohorts were unequally matched, with more medical reasons for anticoagulation in the pharmacist cohort compared to surgical indications in the control group.[3]

During this same time period, Dager et al. evaluated the impact of inserting a pharmacist consultation into the daily management of warfarin in a matched cohort of 120 patients.[5] A significant reduction in the number of inpatient days on warfarin (9.5 days versus 6.8 days; $p = 0.009$), days of INRs over target (INR > 3.5) values (142 versus 29; $p < 0.001$) or critical (INR > 6.0) values (50 versus 6; $p < 0.001$) were observed. The INR was more likely in the therapeutic range at discharge in the pharmacist group ($p = 0.07$). Long-term outcomes on readmission for bleeding or recurrent thromboembolism measured out to 3 months postdischarge showed a lower incidence of both in

Table 2-1. (cont'd)
Selected References Supporting Pharmacist Management of Heparin and Warfarin in the Inpatient Setting

Reference	Description	Key Pharmacist Impact	Comments
Boddy (6)	Pharmacist-dosed ($n = 74$) warfarin after 4 days versus physician ($n = 64$) having same protocol available	Improved INR control ($p < 0.001$) with reduction in values >6 or <2.0	Protocol refers patients on day 4 or prior to discharge to the outpatient clinic pharmacist for management; fewer INR values requested with improved control associated with pharmacist involvement
Rivey (7)	Protocol-driven dosing by pharmacist ($n = 151$) versus physician independent of protocol ($n = 41$) in orthopedic surgery patients		Similar duration of inpatient therapy, no difference in complication rates
Ellis (2)	Pharmacist-involved warfarin dosing consultation ($n = 52$) to pre-pharmacist involvement ($n = 97$)	Decreased number of aPTT or PT assays requested per day ($p = 0.02$); increased PT values in target range at first outpatient follow-up ($p = 0.001$)	No difference in time to initiate UFH to warfarin, days of warfarin or heparin therapy
To (3)	Pharmacist-assisted warfarin dosing protocol ($n = 41$) compared to physician-directed dosing ($n = 46$)	Decreased INR values > 4 per patient ($p = 0.0059$)	Non-significant reduction in days to target INR or increase in INR values in target range favoring the pharmacist dose cohort; cohorts unequally matched for anticoagulation indication
Bridges (18)	Inpatient pharmacist involved in collaborative process as part of discharge on low molecular weight heparin bridge therapy ($n = 108$) compared to historical control ($n = 69$) matched for injury severity in trauma	Reduced length in stay ($p < 0.002$) and inpatient days on warfarin ($p < 0.0001$)	Anticoagulation indication was DVT prophylaxis

Source: Reprinted from Dager W, Gulseth M. Implementing anticoagulation management by pharmacists in the inpatient setting. *Am J Health-Syst Pharm.* In press.

the cohort receiving pharmacist consultations. For every $1 spent on pharmacist staffing, $8 in direct hospital cost savings were realized.[5]

Health systems with established outpatient anticoagulation clinics have the potential to expand the role of their pharmacists into the inpatient setting. In one such health system, an internal audit had observed delays in initiating warfarin therapy, failure to maintain INRs in the target range, frequent INR measurements, and poor continuity between medical teams managing patients. Subsequently, an open comparison between pharmacist and physician warfarin dosing using the same newly implemented management protocol was undertaken to investigate if a pharmacist could provide improved inpatient outcomes as had previously been established with the health system's outpatients. Pharmacist dosing led to significantly better INR control ($p < 0.001$), including a reduction in the number of INR values over 6 and overall INR lab draws. An additional benefit observed was an increase in continuity of care in managing the patient after discharge.[6]

A positive role can be observed in small hospital settings as well. Rivey et al. described the impact of a warfarin dosing protocol managed by pharmacists ($n = 151$) compared to physician determined dosing ($n = 41$) in a small community hospital setting. No difference in symptomatic thromboembolism or major bleeding was observed. An increase in the use of oral anticoagulation observed with pharmacist involvement suggests the program enabled more patients to receive an oral anticoagulant.[7] In a initiative undertaken by a health system, pharmacists were key in reducing the incidence of adverse related events from warfarin by 45% utilizing a lab based system to identify patients at risk who then underwent chart review.[9]

Heparin

The value of a pharmacist monitoring continuous infusion UFH therapy compared to existing management approaches has also been reported.[4,10,12-14] Observations with pharmacist dosed UFH using an established protocol, nomogram, or computer assisted dosing showed a reduction in measured anticoagulation intensity tests outside target ranges, fewer infusion rate adjustments, improved documentation of infusion rates, and shorter time to achieve anticoagulation goals.[4,10,12-14] Pawloski et al. reported that pharmacists in a small community hospital involved in monitoring therapeutic UFH ($n = 29$) compared to a physician cohort ($n = 14$) could achieve therapeutic aPTT values earlier ($16.5 +/- 10.9$ hours versus $46.5 +/- 34.1$ hours; $p < 0.001$) and, although not significant, reduce the number of rate changes and days on heparin. The impact of the program on hard outcomes, such as recurrent thrombotic complications was not measured.[12] Rivey reported that pharmacists utilizing a UFH dosing protocol reduced the number of aPTT results above or below the target range, improved adherence to the protocol including documentation of the rate, and earlier attainment of target goals.[13] Similar reductions in aPTT values outside the target range and earlier achievement of target values have been observed with pharmacist based computer assisted heparin dosing.[14] Achieving aPTT values in the target range for patients with either DVT or PE within the first 24–48 hours has been demonstrated in multiple trials to reduce the incidence of recurrent events.[11,15-17] Achieving earlier target aPTT values with pharmacist assisted heparin dosing and monitoring of UFH infusion could potentially reduce the incidence of recurrent VTE.

Combined Warfarin and Heparin

In a prospective, observational cohort study conducted at two teaching hospitals, Mandami et al. compared usual care to pharmacist managed care for the treatment of DVT or PE with both UFH and warfarin.[4] For UFH, the occurrence of therapeutic aPTT values within the target range was higher ($p = 0.05$), and the median time to a dosing rate adjustment shortened ($p < 0.001$), when pharmacists were involved in managing the infusions. Pharmacists managing warfarin reduced the duration of inpatient therapy from 7 to 5 days ($p = 0.05$), with a higher percentage having a therapeutic INR by day 5 (47 versus 40%; $p = 0.51$) and at discharge (71 versus 58%; $p = 0.21$). A significant cost savings (21%) for hospitalization in favor of pharmacist management ($1594 versus $2014; $p = 0.04$) was observed.[4]

Bond and Raehl investigated the potential impact of pharmacist involvement in managing either unfractionated heparin or warfarin by analyzing the 1995 Medicare and the National Clinical Pharmacy Services Databases.[8] Hospitals with pharmacists providing management of either warfarin or UFH were observed to have significantly (all $p < 0.001$) lower anticoagulation-related mortality, length of hospital stay, bleeding complications, blood transfusion requirements, and cost of therapy (Table 2-2). In hospitals with pharmacists monitoring UFH or warfarin, death rates were lower (11.4% and 6.2% respectively), length of stay longer (10.5% and 5.7% respectively), and Medicare charges higher (6.6% and 2.2% respectively) compared to hospitals without pharmacist provided management.[8] Noting that UFH and enoxaparin are commonly prescribed anticoagulants frequently associated with harmful prescribing errors, the authors concluded "pharmacy directors and clinical coordinators should develop pharmacist-provided anticoagulation management as an integral component of their core service mix."

Low Molecular Weight Heparin/ Fondaparinux

The addition of the low-molecular weight heparins (LMWH) and fondaparinux has opened new challenges in selecting and managing anticoagulation. Although initial inpatient pharmacists' anticoagulation roles focused on warfarin and UFH, additional responsibilities have emerged as newer anticoagulants combined with recognizing needs for unique dosing in selected situations. Unique dosing populations and challenging clinical situations along with proposed monitoring of anti-Xa activity has created a need for clinicians who with expertise in the area to assist in optimizing management. Pharmacists involved in the recommending LMWH dosing regimens have reported a high degree of acceptance by physicians.[19]

The subcutaneous administered LMWH and fondaparinux have provided a means for either treatment or continued prevention of thrombotic disorders to be managed at home during periods

Table 2-2.
Major Health Care Outcomes for Medicare Patients with ICD-9 Code Diagnoses Indicating the Need for Anticoagulation

Variable	Pharmacist-Provided Heparin Management			Pharmacist-Provided Warfarin Management		
	Hospitals With This Service	Hospitals Without This Service	Significance	Hospitals With This Service	Hospitals Without This Service	Significance
Hospitals, no. (%)	197 (20.62)	758 (79.4)		97 (10.16)	858 (89.89)	
Patients, no. (%)	148,597 (20.71)	568,799 (79.29)		84,219 (11.74)	633,177 (88.26)	
Deaths, no. (%)[a]	9460 (6.37)	40,906 (7.19)	$X^2 = 122.84$, df = 1, $p < 0.0001$	5607 (6.66)	44,759 (7.10)	$X^2 = 19.20$, df = 1, $p < 0.0001$
Excess deaths, no. (% increase)[b]		4664 (11.41)			2786 (6.20)	
Length of stay, mean ± SD days	7.79 ± 9.41	8.66 ± 11.17	$U = 40039529342$, $p < 0.0001$	8.04 ± 9.60	8.54 ± 10.98	$U = 25730993838$, $p < 0.0001$
Total patient-days, no.	1,158,039	4,924,381		677,043	5,405,376	
Excess patient-days, no. (% increase)[c]		494,855 (10.05)			316,589 (5.86)	
Total Medicare charges, mean ± SD $	16,216 ± 24,258	17,361 ± 26,172	$U = 41004749266$, $p < 0.0001$	16,797 ± 26,119	17,167 ± 25,746	$U = 25995512970$, $p < 0.0001$
Increases in Medicare charges/patient, $		1145 ± 1462			370 ± 721	
Excess Medicare charges, $ (% increase)[d]		651,274,844 (6.60)			234,275,490 (2.16)	
Patients with bleeding complications, no. (%)[e]	13,138 (8.84)	51,867 (9.12)	$X^2 = 10.996$, df = 1, $p = 0.0009$	7082 (8.41)	57,923 (9.15)	$X^2 = 49.259$, df = 1, $p < 0.0001$
Excess patients with bleeding complications, no. (% increase)[f]		145 (3.1)			429 (8.09)	
Deaths in patients with bleeding complications, no. (%)	2282 (17.37)	9224 (17.78)	NS	1213 (17.12)	10,193 (17.60)	NS
Patients receiving blood transfusions, no. (%)	1816 (13.82)	7774 (14.99)	$X^2 = 11.24$, df = 1, $p = 0.0008$	830 (11.72)	8760 (15.12)	$X^2 = 78.68$, df = 1, $p < 0.0001$

Continued

Table 2-2. (cont'd)
Major Health Care Outcomes for Medicare Patients with ICD-9 Code Diagnoses Indicating the Need for Anticoagulation

Variable	Pharmacist-Provided Heparin Management			Pharmacist-Provided Warfarin Management		
	Hospitals With This Service	Hospitals Without This Service	Significance	Hospitals With This Service	Hospitals Without This Service	Significance
Units of blood/patient used during transfusion, mean ± SD	4.68 ± 7.77	5.90 ± 22.40	U = 6965094, p = 0.0302	4.89 ± 8.11	5.75 ± 21.41	NS
Excess units of blood, no.		9784			8991	

ICD-9 = International Classification of Diseases, Ninth Revision; U = Mann-Whitney U test, NS = not significant.

[a] Death rates were 63.7 and 71.9 deaths/1000 patients, respectively, in hospitals with and without pharmacist-provided heparin management (odds ratio [OR] 1.140, 95% confidence interval [CI] 1.114–1.166); death rates were 66.6 and 71.0 deaths/1000 patients, respectively, in hospitals with and without pharmacist-provided warfarin management (OR 1.066, 95% CI 1.036–1.098).

[b] Percentage difference in death rate × number of patients in hospitals without pharmacist-managed protocols and the percentage increase in deaths over hospitals with pharmacist-provided anticoagulation management.

[c] Percentage difference in mean patient-days × number of patients in hospitals without pharmacist-provided protocols × length of stay and the percentage increase in patient-days over hospitals that have pharmacist-provided anticoagulation management.

[d] Percentage difference in Medicare charges × number of patients in hospitals without pharmacist-provided protocols and the percentage of Medicare charges over hospitals that have pharmacist-provided anticoagulation management.

[e] Bleeding complication rates were 88.4 and 91.2 bleeding complications/1000 patients, respectively, with and without pharmacist-managed heparin anticoagulation (OR 1.031, CI 1.011–1.052); bleeding complication rates were 84.1 and 91.5 bleeding complications/1000 patients, respectively, with and without pharmacist-managed warfarin anticoagulation (OR 1.088, CI 1.060–1.116).

[f] Percentage difference in bleeding complications × number of patients in hospitals without pharmacist-managed protocols and the percentage increase in bleeding complications over hospitals with pharmacist-provided anticoagulation management.

Source: Reprinted with permission from Bond CA, Raehl CL. Pharmacist-provided anticoagulation management in United States hospitals: death rates, length of stay, Medicare charges, bleeding complications, and transfusions. *Pharmacotherapy.* 2004;24:953-63.

of sub-therapeutic warfarin effects. Such programs have utilized pharmacists in key roles to develop and maintain successful outpatient treatment programs.[20-22] Despite the higher medication costs, some of these agents have the capability of lowering the overall costs of care. The impact of utilizing both inpatient and outpatient pharmacists to facilitate transition of care to home therapy with LMWH while initiating warfarin to reducing the length of hospital stay and related costs of therapy has been shown is several reports.[18,20-22]

Direct Thrombin Inhibitors

Literature describing the direct impact of pharmacist in the management of direct thrombin inhibitors (DTIs) is limited. The infrequent use of the DTIs, their unique pharmacokinetic profile with considerable variability between acutely ill patients and lack of reversibility has created a need for centralized expertise on approaches to their use. Pharmacists have demonstrated their ability to fill the role of managing the use of DTIs, authoring numerous manuscripts that describe or clarify their use in clinical practice.[23] Pharmacists actively involved in the management of DTIs have published their measured observations and insights with their use, some of which have driven current management approaches. Examples include continued DTI therapy in heparin-induced thrombocytopenia (HIT) until the platelet count is under substantial recovery, effects of DTI on clot-based assays, dosing of agent in the presence of renal or hepatic function, anticoagulation in extracorpreal membrane oxygenation (ECMO) or assessing the probability of HIT and the need to initiate or continue DTI therapy (Chapter 13). Given that heparin and development of HIT can occur in patients cared for by numerous patient care specialties, the pharmacist background in pharmacology and centralized role in patient care can be an asset in DTI pharmacotherapy. Each case provides an opportunity to gain such experiences in addition to allowing pharmacists to create and provide a vital role in initiating, monitoring and meeting additional anticoagulation needs when DTIs are in use.

Reversal

Having proactive pharmacist involvement in managing thrombosis can also create an opportunity to assist in the management of bleeding as well.[24] Reducing the frequency of INR values over target can decrease the risk and incidence of hemorrhagic events. This can be accomplished by identifying factors in the patients' clinical presentation or changes in the presence of interacting medications that might alter the pharmacologic response to a particular anticoagulant. An understanding of pharmacokinetic and pharmacodynamic principles as they related to a response in a particular anticoagulation regimen can be vital component in interpreting the response to a given therapy. Examples might include adjusting for changes in hepatic, renal, or cardiac function, or validating the actual amount of anticoagulant administered instead of reliance on what was ordered. Further application of these concepts are frequently required to develop a alternative plan that may increase to chance of achieving the desired effect without overshooting the target, which then increases the risk for a hemorrhagic event. In several of the trials mentioned above, the observed reduction in excessive aPTT, INR values and reported hemorrhagic events including need for transfusions support the potential benefits of pharmacists involvement. In the report by Dager et al., pharmacists were able to reduce the time the INR above the therapeutic range, and the incidence of hemorrhagic or thromboembolic events.[1] In the report by Bond et al., hospitals with pharmacist managing warfarin or separately heparin observed less bleeding complications or use of blood transfusions.[8]

For patients who are over anticoagulated and at risk of bleeding, management choices to reverse anticoagulant effects can make a difference in potential morbidity, mortality or length of hospital stay. Determining the necessary dose of a reversal agent to avoid over or under reversal can be vital in controlling or reducing the risk of bleeding as well as reduce challenges in re-establishing anticoagulation. Creating a centralized expertise in developing reversal approaches, which can be variable between patients, and the degree of reversal desired, can improve chances for meeting the goal of therapy without the need for longer than necessary hospital stays or use of costly bridge therapies. For example, although vitamin K is relatively inexpensive, over aggressive dosing may lead to prolonged inability to re-establish warfarin anticoagulation. This can create a notable financial burden to the health care system by prolonging hospital stay, or a need for expensive parenteral bridge therapy in the outpatient setting until warfarin effects are seen. Some forms of vitamin K commonly used for reversal of warfarin, such as subcutaneous administration, have been replaced by oral of intravenous administration because of greater predictability and response onset.[1] The degree of reversal may also depend on the amount of warfarin consumed, or how far of a reversal is desired.[25] Having a strategy to limit the amount of vitamin K available outside the pharmacy (i.e., stocking only 1-mg ampoules in the emergency room), and a process advise physicians on approaches to reverse therapy, can facilitate reversal goals in addition to addressing long-term anticoagulation needs.

Another agent used for the acute management of bleeding and reversal of warfarin effects is recombinant activated factor VII, an extremely expensive agent for which many pharmacy departments have drafted appropriate usage criteria. Due to associated costs and risk for encouraging thrombosis formation combined with lack of sufficient phase II clinical trials, the use of rFVIIa may require careful consideration for use. Use of rFVIIa should include a carefully assessment of the situation, and include an overall reversal and bleeding management plan that could include additional reversal agents having a more sustained effect.

Success Relies on a Multidisciplinary Approach

Keys to success in optimizing anticoagulation therapy in the inpatient setting is a multidisciplinary approach. Physicians, nursing, laboratory and pharmacy in addition to other health professionals each have unique training and perspectives that can improve anticoagulation therapy. The nurse at the bedside is usually responsible for administrating the anticoagulant, draw related coagulation studies at the correct time in relation to a dose or infusion rate change, and adjust the rate based on the results. Pharmacists can provide a separate perspective on interpretation of laboratory results and assist the nurse in accomplishing their charge in drug administration. Cooperation between pharmacists and nursing has been shown to provide a positive impart on anticoagulation therapy.[26,27] Outside the outpatient setting, data measuring the impact of non-physician personal in the absence of pharmacist involvement for management of anticoagulation is not currently available. Health-systems that understand the big picture to optimize multidisciplinary management of anticoagulation therapy, especially if regulatory entities such as the Joint Commission, National Quality Forum, and Centers for Medicare and Medicaid Services place emphasis on achieving this.[28,29] This may lead to benchmarking or pay for performance comparisons that each health system would want to show optimal performance. On example in achieving this is supported by a report showing that a pharmacy driven education programs on the importance of VTE prophylaxis in medical patients increased the utilization of suitable prophylaxis regimens.[30]

On the Horizon

The increasing number of anticoagulation indications and treatment options, in addition to increased associated costs, has created new challenges in providing optimal, cost-effective therapy. In many situations, patients receiving these therapies would have been excluded from the clinical trials. Experience gained with the use of newer anticoagulants, such as the LMWHs or DTIs, continues to identify unique patient populations requiring different dosing regimens. As more special patient populations are identified, the pharmacist may be able to provide insights on how to approach anticoagulation therapy. Advancement in technology in situations where anticoagulation is one example of new challenges for adjusting anticoagulation regimens. Examples include new approaches to hemodialysis, approaches to prevent embolic stroke in the setting of atrial arrhythmias, or other mechanical devices that influence risks for potential for thrombus formation, bleeding, or drug removal. Availability of new anticoagulation agents and how to sort out their use in patients also creates additional challenges in management that can benefit from pharmacists' insights.

Newer assay methods, expanding lists of interacting drugs or herbs, in addition to managing undesirable adverse effects, are just a few examples of additional management considerations. Issues in anticoagulation can go beyond monitoring and adjusting anticoagulation therapies to include management of combined anticoagulation therapy during transition from the initial parenteral anticoagulant to long-term warfarin. Preventing undesirable effects such as major bleeding, identifying and initiating therapy for heparin-induced thrombocytopenia (HIT), or facilitating continuity of care during transition to long-term ambulatory care management should be considered. Options for long-term treatment success may be contingent upon assuring the patient is able to administer, has close follow-up, and is able to afford and receive the chosen therapy.

Future Roles

The complexities of the newer anticoagulants and expansion of indicated uses constantly creates new challenges in finding the most optimal dose in a given patient. The numerous potential anticoagulants (see Table 13-1, Chapter 13) in development will continue to create ongoing challenges on deciding which anticoagulation approach to use, including transitioning between agents, in addition to the cost of the therapy to the health care system. Another challenge with newer agents is to consider identifying patients that may or may not be best suited for a given agent by assessing potential risks and benefits, especially for those patients being considered to receive the agent who may not have been candidates for the therapy in the clinical trials conducted. As more agents become available, the costs associated with their use may also be a factor to consider in agent selection. The pharmacist is in a key position to implement the policies of the health systems' pharmacy and therapeutics committee, or other governing committee responsible for determining which agent is used, and in what setting. This may not only apply to approaches to prevention and treatment of thromboembolic disease, but also the approach to managing bleeding complications.

Conclusion

The reports currently available exploring the use of pharmacists in managing inpatient anticoagulation consistently observes a positive impact. The benefits are not isolated to dosing warfarin alone, but include other anticoagulants such as heparin, transitional therapy with LMWH, or the approaches to reversing the pharmacologic effects of anticoagulants. The pharmacist, who receives extensive training in pharmacokinetic and pharmacodynamic principles, can provide a critical component to optimizing the use of anticoagulation therapy. Utilizing pharmacist as a resource to the management of anticoagulation therapy can reduce complications or incidence of over-anticoagulation, shorten hospital stay, etc., overall improving patient care while reducing the cost of therapy.

References

1. Ansell J, Hirsh J, Poller L, et. al. The pharmacology and management of the vitamin K antagonists. *Chest.* 2004;126:204S-33S.
2. Ellis RF, Stephens MA, Sharp GB. Evaluation of a pharmacy-managed warfarin-monitoring service to co-ordinate inpatient and outpatient therapy. Am J Hosp Pharm. 1992;49:387-94.
3. To EK, Pearson GJ. Implementation and evaluation of a pharmacist-assisted warfarin dosing program. *Can J Hosp Pharm.* 1997;50:169-75.
4. Mamdani MM, Racine E, McCreadie S, et al. Clinical and economic effectiveness of an inpatient anticoagulation service. *Pharmacotherapy.* 1999;19:1064-74.
5. Dager WE, Branch JM, King JH, et al. Optimization of inpatient warfarin therapy; impact of daily consultation by a pharmacist-managed anticoagulation service. *Ann Pharmacother.* 2000;34:567-72.
6. Boddy C. Pharmacist involvement with warfarin dosing for inpatients. *Pharm World Sci.* 2001;23:31-5.
7. Rivey MP, Wood RD, Allington DR, et al. Pharmacy-managed protocol for warfarin use in orthopedic surgery patients. *Am J Health-Syst Pharm.* 1995 Jun 15;52(12):1310-6.
8. Bond CA, Raehl CL. Pharmacist-provided anticoagulation management in United States hospitals: death rates, length of stay, Medicare charges, bleeding complications, and transfusions. *Pharmacotherapy.* 2004;24:953-63.
9. Lederer J, Best D. Reduction in anticoagulation-related adverse drug events using a trigger-based methodology. *J Comm J Qual Patients Saf.* 2005:31:313-8.
10. Saya FG, Coleman LT, Martinoff JT. Pharmacist-directed heparin therapy using a standard dosing and monitoring protocol. *Am J Hosp Pharm.* 1985;42:1965-9.
11. Hull R, Raskob GE, Brant RF, et al. Relation between the time to achieve the lower limit of the APTT therapeutic range and recurrent venous thromboembolism during heparin treatment for deep vein thrombosis. *Arch Intern Med.* 1997;157:2562-8.
12. Pawloski SJ, Kersh PL. Therapeutic heparin monitoring service in a small community hospital. *Hosp Pharm.* 1992;27:703-6.
13. Rivey MP, Peterson JP. Pharmacy-managed, weight-based heparin protocol. *Am J Hosp Pharm.* 1993;50:279-84.
14. Kershaw B, White RH, Mungall D, et al. Computer-assisted dosing of heparin. Management with a pharmacy-based anticoagulation service. *Arch Intern Med.* 1994;154:1005-11.
15. Anand S, Ginsberg JS, Kearon C, et al. The relation between the activated partial thromboplastin time response and recurrence in patients with venous thrombosis treated with continuous intravenous heparin. *Arch Intern Med.* 1996;156:1677-81.
16. Anand SS, Bates S, Ginsberg JS, et al. Recurrent venous thrombosis and heparin therapy: an evaluation of the importance of early activated partial thromboplastin times. *Arch Intern Med.* 1999;159:2029-32.
17. Raschke RA, Reilly BM, Guidry JR, et al. The weight-based heparin dosing nomogram compared with a "standard care" nomogram. A randomized controlled trial. *Ann Intern Med.* 1993;119:874-81.
18. Bridges GC, Lee MD, Jenkins JK, et al. Expedited discharge in trauma patients requiring anticoagulation for deep venous thrombosis prophylaxis: the LEAP program. *J Trauma.* 2003;54:232-5.
19. Devlin JW, Tyburski JG, Moed B. Implementation and evaluation of guidelines for use of enoxaparin as deep vein thrombosis prophylaxis after major trauma. *Pharmacotherapy.* 2001;21:740-7.
20. ASHP therapeutic position statement on the use of low-molecular-weight heparin for adult outpatient treatment of acute deep-vein thrombosis. *Am J Health-Syst Pharm.* 2004;61:1950-5.
21. Boucher M, Rodger M, Johnson JA, Tierney M. Shifting from inpatient to outpatient treatment of deep vein thrombosis in a tertiary care center: a cost-minimization analysis. *Pharmacotherapy.* 2003;23:301-9.
22. Dager WE, King JH, Chow S, et al. Outpatient tinzaparin in patients with pulmonary embolism or deep vein thrombosis. *Ann Pharmacother.* 2005;39:1182-7.
23. Dager WE, Dougherty JA, Nguyen PH, Militello MA, Smythe MA. Heparin-induced thrombocytopenia: a review of treatment options and special considerations. *Pharmacotherapy.* 2007;27(4):564-87.
24. Dager W, Regalia R, Williamson D, et al. Low dose (< 60 mcg/kg) recombinant factor VIIa in trauma or

coagulopathy. *J Thromb Haemost.* 2005;3(suppl 1): P1955
25. White RH, Minton SM, Andya MD, Hutchinson R. Temporary reversal of anticoagulation using oral vitamin K. *J Thromb Thrombolysis.* 2000;10:149-53.
26. Porter B. The role of the advanced practice nurse in anticoagulation. *AACN Clinical Issues.* 2002;13:221-3.
27. Oertel LB; Heparin Consensus Group. Unfractionated heparin: a nursing dilemma. *Pharmacotherapy.* 2004;24(suppl):156S-60S.
28. Joint Commission on Accreditation of Healthcare Organizations. Draft candidate 2007 national patient safety goals, requirements and implementation expectations. Available at: http://www.jcaho.org/NR/rdonlyres/4901A094-80A7-4AD6-86CD-4754B896A986/0/07_npsg_hap_cah.pdf. Accessed March 8, 2006.
29. Joint Commission on Accreditation of Healthcare Organizations. Available at: http://www.jcaho.org/pms/core+measures/pdf119.pdf. Accessed February 15, 2006.
30. Dobesh PP, Stacy ZA. Effect of a clinical pharmacy education program on improvement in the quantity and quality of venous thromboembolism prophylaxis for medically ill patients. *J Manag Care Pharm.* 2005;11(9):755-62.

Chapter 3

Anticoagulant Safety: Identification of the Gaps

Jill Strykowski

Chapter Outline

- Introduction
- Just culture
- High reliability organizations
- The role of professional regulatory and advisory organizations
  - Joint Commission® Medication Management Standards
  - Joint Commission® National Patient Safety Standards
  - Institute for Safe Medication Practices
- Failure mode and effects analysis and the antithrombotic gap analysis tool
- Root cause analysis
- Conclusion

Introduction

Fostering cultures of safety in a hospital is critical to sound medication management of anticoagulant therapy. At the time of this writing, three infants have died in an Indiana Hospital due to a heparin error; human error was speculated to be at the root cause of the deaths.[1] A pharmacy technician with more than 25 years of experience mistakenly took the wrong dose from inventory to stock the automatic dispensing cabinet. The nurses, who had grown accustomed to one strength in their cabinet, administered the wrong dose without attention to the "five rights" of medication administration. Although we have moved into an era of "just cultures" and "high reliability organizations," the recent events remind us that we still have process work to do to assure no patients are harmed. A look at how anticoagulant therapy fits into the organization's safety framework requires an exploration of what is meant by just culture and high reliability.

Just Culture

In 1999, the term *just culture* was popularized to describe a culture where members could maintain their professional accountability and feel comfortable disclosing errors. In a just culture, individuals are not held accountable for system failings when human error is involved. A just culture does not tolerate reckless behavior, nor is there tolerance for gross negligence or blatant misconduct. The organization has an insistence on justice for outright disregard of safe behaviors yet recognizes that even the most seasoned, vigilant workers can be subject to human failings. In a just culture, individuals that typically practice safely are not held to "blame and shame" when an error occurs. Instead, the system is the focus for improvement. Errors that are due to human failing are distinguished from intentional, conscious disregard for risky behavior. Risk behavior is seen as unjust. According to the Institute for Safe Medication Practices (ISMP)[2,3] in a just culture, workers seek to get the work done reliably and know that safety is valued, while managers seek to continually look for system improvements.

Given the narrow safety margins for anticoagulation therapy, development and maintenance of a just culture allows for safe disclosure of medication mishaps so processes and systems are funneled to zero potential for error while professional accountability is maintained.

High Reliability Organizations

High reliability organizations (HRO) work in higher than average risk areas, yet have fewer than average adverse outcomes. Antithrombotic therapy is certainly a high risk health care area owing to the adverse event profiles and narrow therapeutic indices of the medications. HROs have a preoccupation with failure. Systems are changed such that under periods of high demand and high intensity, safety does not falter. Examples of such organizations are aircraft carriers, nuclear power plants and air traffic controllers; all of these teams share commonalities with health care organizations[4] as the work carries higher than average risk. HRO provide a culture in which workers can feel value in bringing potentially unsafe areas to the attention of managers without fear of censure from leadership. Creating a highly reliable, just culture is the cornerstone of achieving and maintaining an environment of safe delivery of anticoagulation medications.

The Role of Professional Regulatory and Advisory Organizations

Professional regulatory and advisory organizations have missions that support development of high reliability just cultures with tools that are available to assist pharmacy administrators in evaluation and mitigation of risk. Although standards and tools can often be seen as onerous to implement, organizations that produce the standards are committed to the protection of patients with continual evaluation of medication events happening in the field. Given the risks that antithrombotic medications carry, the tools and learnings from these organizations infiltrate daily practice as both a mandate and guiding light to safety.

Joint Commission® Medication Management Standards

In 2004 the Joint Commission on Accreditation of Healthcare Organizations issued new medication management standards to improve the safety of medication use in hospitals. The inception of the standards was in response to the Institute of Medicine (IOM) Report, "To Err is Human: Building a Safer Health System."[3] The report highlighted medication errors and the request went to the Joint Commission® to change the medication standards as they were often seen as unclear and the first priority for the standards was to provide clarity. A second reason for the standards was that the Joint Commission® had not incorporated best practices into their standards in entirety; for example, the National Quality Forum had issued some best practices that the Joint Commission® had not addressed.[5]

Key to the safe use of antithrombotic therapy are several of the 2004 Medication Management Standards (MM). The standards had a shift to a prescriptive mandate for safe medication use. The following standards are reviewed for relevance to antithrombotic therapy:

MM 1.10: Patient information is readily accessible to those involved in the medication management system.

- Key to anticoagulant therapy is the recognition that pharmacists should have access to laboratory values, height, and weight at the point of medication management duties. The Joint Commission® has clarified that it is not enough to have the information on the floor in a hard copy chart, it must be available at the point the medication order is reviewed.

MM 2.20: Medications are properly and safely stored throughout the organization.

- In this standard the Joint Commission® calls for standardization of medications that are infused and that the rate of the infusion should vary, not the concentration. Organizations are asked to standardize heparin infusions. In addition, the Joint Commission® requires that organizations limit the number of drug concentrations as part of the National Patient Safety Goals. This is of particular importance to heparin given the wide ranging indications for use.

MM 4.10: All prescriptions or medication orders are reviewed for appropriateness.

- A pharmacist must review all medication orders unless an urgent/emergent situation dictates otherwise or a licensed independent practitioner is present to order, prepare, and administer the medication.

MM 4.20: Medications are prepared safely.

- In this standard, if an i.v. pharmacy is available, sterile medications must be mixed in the pharmacy when feasible. The exceptions to this standard are in emergencies or when the practice is not feasible as in the case of a short stability medication. For anticoagulant therapy- all heparin infusions must be prepared by the pharmacy department unless commercially available.

MM 4.40: Medications are dispensed safely.

- Medications must be dispensed in the most readily available forms available from the manufacturer (unit dose) or repackaged by the pharmacy or another organization licensed to repackage. The standard applies to warfarin as the drug is commonly repackaged in practice. the Joint Commission® also mandates that if repackaging is to occur, proper education be provided to staff.

MM 5.10: Medications are safely and accurately administered.

- The organization is required to have policies for persons that administer medications to: verify that the medication is correct by looking at the label, verify that the medication is stable, that medications have not expired, and that there is no contraindication to use. In addition, the organization must have policies that require patient or family member notification of side effects of the medication. The standard is particularly relevant to narrow therapeutic index anticoagulant medications; the patient and/or family must be informed of the bleeding risks associated with the therapy.

MM 6.10: The effects of medications on patients are monitored.

- The Joint Commission® requires that organizations have a process for monitoring the effect of the first dose of medications that are new to the patient while under the direct care of the accredited organization.

MM 6.20: The organization responds appropriately to actual or potential adverse drug events and medication errors.

- The Joint Commission® requires that there is an appropriate reporting response when an adverse event occurs and this response must be both internal and external.

7.10: The organization develops processes for managing high-risk or high-alert medications.

- The Joint Commission® called on organizations to develop processes and then policies, for selecting, procuring, storing, ordering, transcribing, preparing, dispensing, administering, and monitoring high-risk and high-alert medications. Organizations were asked to identify these medications and then address the processes for managing these medications. The Joint Commission® allows for either national lists or organization-specific data to identify which medications would have focused processes for management. One national list is supplied by the ISMP and includes several anticoagulant therapies. Included in the 2003 list published by ISMP are: heparin, low molecular weight heparin, and warfarin. These medications carry a high risk for error or adverse outcomes and have been involved in a high percentage of medication errors and other adverse outcomes. Hospitals that develop comprehensive inpatient anticoagulation programs that address all of these agents will have an easier time complying with this standard than hospitals that do not.

The Joint Commission® also surveys for sound-alike look-alike medications under the National Patient Safety Goals. Organizations must identify and at a minimum, annually review a list of look-alike/sound-alike drugs used in the organization, and take action to prevent errors involving the interchange of these drugs. One such pairing identified by the the Joint Commission® is heparin-hespan; organizations are asked to assure that processes are separate for each of these medications.

The Joint Commission® National Patient Safety Goals

The Joint Commission® National Patient Safety Goals' (NPSG) mission is to promote specific improvements in patient safety. The goals arise in part, from sentinel events and the solutions are focused on broad-based system design. Organizations are evaluated for continuous compliance with the goals. Several goals apply to anticoagulant therapy and organizations are asked to build policies and processes that support mitigation of risk through use of the standards.

Goal 2B: Standardize a list of abbreviations, acronyms, symbols, and dose designations that are not to be used throughout the organization.

- The Joint Commission® publishes an official list of "do not use" abbreviations which includes U (unit) and IU (International Units). The U symbol should be written as "unit" the Joint Commission® has had errors of U being interpreted as "cc", "0," or "4," and in the case of heparin or low molecular weight heparin, can cause significant harm. The IU symbol should be written as "international unit" as the Joint Commission® has had reports of misinterpretation to "IV" or the number "10." In the case of dalteparin, which is dosed with IU, patient harm could occur.

Goal 3B: Standardize and limit the number of drug concentrations used by the organization.

- The Joint Commission® specifically calls out that this standard applies to "high-alert" medications including heparin therapy. Of particular concern with this goal is pediatrics: the order must state drug dose, not volume, and the dose calculation should be written out.

Goal 8A and 8B: Medication reconciliation.

8A: Implement a process for obtaining and documenting a complete list of the patient's current medications upon the patient's admission to the organization and with the involvement of the patient. This process includes a comparison of the medications the organization provides to those on the list.

8B: A complete list of the patient's medications is communicated to the next provider of service when a patient is referred or transferred to another setting, service, practitioner, or level of care within or outside of the organization.

- This NPSG is difficult to implement yet relevant to sound anticoagulation management. More than half of all medication errors occur at the interfaces of care.[6] Warfarin, enoxaparin/LMWHs, and fondaparinux are all medications where safety of management is particular vulnerable at transitions between the hospital and clinic setting. The NPSG requires organizations implement a process to collect the home list with the involvement of the patient, and compare that list to the medications to be administered. The list is then communicated to the next provider of care and to the patient. The process relies on purposeful gathering of the list on entry into the health system, and intentional communication at transitions within the organization and at discharge. Many states have also empowered the patient to know medications through use of state-wide medication cards. With intentional communication across the continuum of care, and patient empowerment to know detailed medication lists, the Joint Commission® is setting the stage for safe longitudinal medication management. Seamless transitions of warfarin and other injectable anticoagulant dosing information will improve safe anticoagulation care.

Institute for Safe Medication Practices and the Antithrombotic Gap Analysis Tool

ISMP is the only nonprofit organization dedicated exclusively to safe medication use and prevention of medication errors. The organization's mission is to "understand the causes of medication errors and to provide time-critical error reduction strategies to the healthcare community, policy makers, and the public." ISMP is multidisciplinary and made up of nurses, pharmacists, and physicians dedicated to understanding system-based causes of medication errors. Through the voluntary Medication Error Reporting Program (MERP), ISMP is able to learn about errors, understand their causes, and provide information back to the public to promote safety. In 2005, the ISMP published a new tool to assist organizations in identifying gaps in their antithrombotic practices, "The 2005 Medication Safety Self-Assessment for Antithrombotic Therapy in Hospitals." The tool is designed to assist organizations with identifying safety gaps in antithrombotic therapy through comparison with like organizations. Many of the antithrombotic care areas in the tool came to ISMP through the MERP reviews.[6] Organizations were called to voluntarily submit data by March 1, 2006, on antithrombotic practices. The aggregated report is to be used for both self-assessment by the organization and for research and education by ISMP. To successfully complete the tool, ISMP asked each organization to establish a multidisciplinary team for assessment of the current use of antithrombotic agents. Data was submitted and ISMP assigned a numerical, weighted score to assess each of the items for comparison to like organizations. The baseline values are then tracked and trended as organizations work on different care areas in antithrombotic management. Further, ISMP will use the data as a means of supporting and assisting curricula development in enhancing safety of antithrombotic therapy. The tool is organized into eight key elements with safe medication practice at the core of the element. The key elements assessed are: patient information, drug information, communication of drug orders and other drug information, drug storage stock standardization and distribution, medication device acquisition use and monitoring, competency and staff education, patient education, quality processes, and risk management. The weighted scores are given the highest value when there is a focus on the system not the workforce, and when it is difficult for healthcare workers to do the job wrong due to error-proof systems. Although the reporting period is complete, the tool is still a useful exercise for organizations to conduct to identify at risk areas and target opportunity for process improvement. The tool can still be found at: http://www.ismp.org/selfassessments/asa2006/ASAISMPAssessmentsm.pdf

Failure Mode and Effects Analysis

Failure mode and effects analysis (FMEA) is a prospective, quantitative technique for predicting the error potential in a process before the error occurs. In an FMEA, the likelihood of a given failure is linked with the consequence of the error to produce a "criticality index." Failure modes or discrete process steps are identified for cause and effect and a numerical value is assigned based on the likelihood of occurrence, the likelihood of detection, and the severity of the occurrence. The three numerical values are multiplied to determine a "risk priority number" for rank ordering to target improvement efforts. In this method, the most unsafe failure mode has the highest numerical value assigned and will have the greatest impact on preventing an unsafe practice.

A FMEA can be best illustrated by example. Heparin is a high-risk drug, and the error potential can be dissected from the point of a physician order to administration of the drug. Each part of the process can be broken down into discrete steps or "failure modes": examples of these discrete steps that could lead to error involving heparin would be a pharmacist dispensing the wrong dose of heparin, incorrect aPTT lab values being reported, and the physician ordering the wrong rate of heparin infusion. Each failure mode is evaluated for cause and effect. For example, the cause of wrong heparin dose could be a wrong weight and effect is underdose or overdose. The likelihood of occurrence and detection of the error is given a numerical value within a pre-specified range as is the severity of the failure mode. In the case of a 1–10 scale, the likelihood of detection is 8, the likelihood of occurrence is 3, and the severity is 8 for a risk value of ($8 \times 3 \times 8 = 192$) for the particular failure mode. All failure modes are assessed in this manner, rank ordered, and the top modes are targeted for process improvement as they likely have the highest impact on safety. The Institute for Healthcare Improvement (www.ihi.org) and the FMEAInfoCentre (www.fmeainfocentre.com) both have examples of FMEA analysis templates that can be used for heparin and warfarin respectively.

Root Cause Analysis

Root cause analysis (RCA) is a process to identify the underlying causes or contributing factors to an error after it occurs. The root cause analysis follows a pre-defined script to evaluate causal factors in various categories: personnel, equipment, training and education, staffing, etc. The evaluation is centered on a detailed description of the events that led up to and included the error and not an evaluation of "who should have done what, when." The Joint Commission® mandated the use of RCA in 1997 to evaluate sentinel events in accredited hospitals. In general, RCA is a case study that is most useful in uncovering system errors.[6] RCA is capable of uncovering system causes for a series of events that are occurring due to poor process design such as errors occurring at a certain time of day. Wald et al. have reported limitations of RCA: hindsight bias, qualitative versus quantitative review of the event, heavy reliance on labor for the RCA that is costly and time-consuming, and influence by the issues of the day that may have no relationship to the RCA.[7] If the RCA falls prey to these limitations, the outcomes may not have an impact on medication safety and may hinder future improvements using the same technique; repeat participants may feel that their efforts will not have significant value.

A common matrix that is used to conduct the RCA or FMEA is the "fishbone diagram." The categories of contributing factors to the error are on the tips of "fishbone" with causes for the error within the category detailed on the arms; the analysis leads ultimately to the end effect. Caudill-Slosberg and Weeks recently reported on the use of the fishbone diagram in evaluating warfarin errors in the context of physician order entry[7,8]; the example is a useful description of use of the matrix (Figure 3-1).

Both the RCA and FMEA are suited to evaluation of errors for complex therapies such as warfarin and heparin. One must bear in mind that both methods have limitations and that the analysis alone may be an oversimplification of cause while being costly to conduct. In the absence of other more rigorous evaluations of medical error, however, FMEA and RCA are standards that organizations continue to find helpful in mitigating risk.

Conclusion

Safety of anticoagulation therapy must focus first on creating a culture that is "just" and highly reliable. Regulatory and quality organizations exist to promote safe medication management in the hospital environment. Tools are available to study

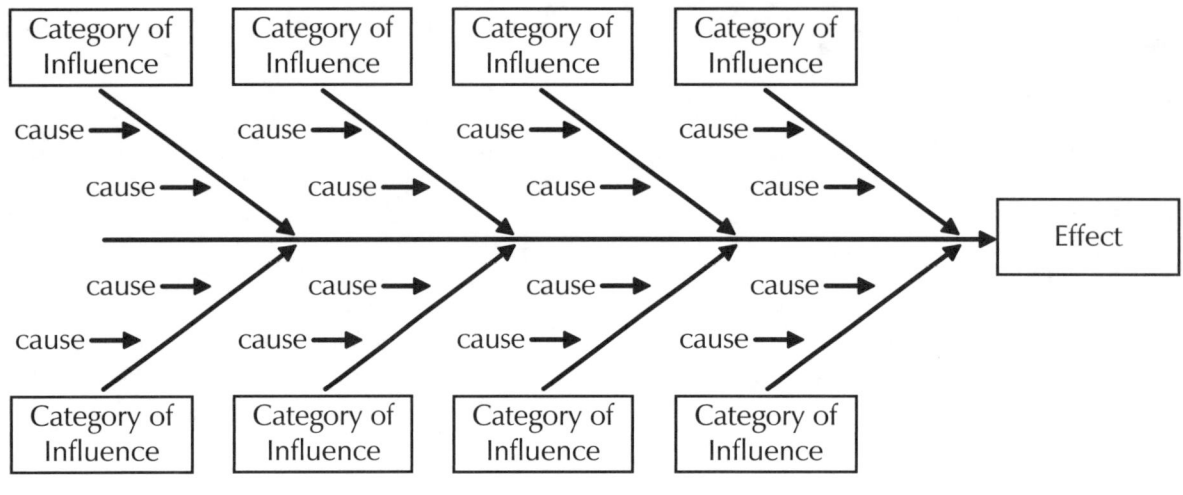

Figure 3-1. Fishbone diagram: dissecting complexity of an adverse event.

error both prospectively (FMEA) and retrospectively (RCA) with goals of improving processes and focusing on system failings. The recent events in Indiana remind us of the trust and responsibility our profession carries in providing safe medication care.

References

1. Unknown. Third Preemie Dies From Drug Overdose at Indiana Hospital. Fox News. September 20, 2006. Available at: http://www.foxnews.com/story/0,2933,214729,00.html. Accessed November 23, 2006.
2. Unknown. ISMP Medication Safety Alert. 2006;11(18).
3. Unknown. ISMP Medication Safety Alert. 2006;11(19).
4. Kohn LT, Corrigan JM, Donaldson MS. To Err is Human: Building a Safer Health System. Institute of Medicine. Available at: http://www.nap.edu/catalog/9728.html#toc. Accessed June 2, 2006.
5. Rich DS. New JCAHO medication management standards for 2004. *Am J Health-Syst Pharm.* 2004;61(13):1349-58.
6. Unknown. The 2005 medication safety self-assessment for antithrombotic therapy in hospitals. Institute for Safe Medication Practices. Available at: http://www.ismp.org/selfassessments/asa/ASA-ISMPAssessmentsm.pdf. Accessed November 23, 2006.
7. Wald H, Shojania KG. Root cause analysis. In: Shojania KG, Duncan BW, eds. Making Health Care Safer: A Critical Analysis of Patient Safety Practices. Evidence Report/Technology Assessment No. 43. Vol AHRQ Publication No. 01-E058.: Agency for Healthcare Research and Quality; 2001.
8. Caudill-Slosberg M, Weeks WB. Case study: identifying potential problems at the human/technical interface in complex clinical systems. *Am J Med Qual.* 2005;20(6):353-7.

Chapter 4

Planning of the Inpatient Anticoagulation Service

Michael Gulseth

Chapter Outline

- Introduction
- Identification of program manager
- Identification of medical staff champion
- Planning the change
  - Creating a flowchart of the service design
- Barriers and possible solutions
- Input into patient care plans and chart documentation
- Addressing anticoagulation transitional care issues
- Data tracking/organization/software needs
- Policies, procedures, and guidelines
- Pharmacist training
- Conclusion
- References
- Appendix 4-1: Case study

Introduction

How does one go about planning and designing an inpatient anticoagulation service that will provide systematic, coordinated care? At this point, this book has shown the general reasons systematic, coordinated anticoagulation care is necessary in the inpatient setting, reviewed the literature supporting this type of service, and helped identify unsafe anticoagulation practices a new service could help address. Still, understanding why a service is important and being knowledgeable about the data supporting such a service is not the same as knowing *how* to plan the service. This chapter will discuss critical elements to consider when planning an inpatient anticoagulation program.

Identification of Program Manager

Implementing systematic, coordinated anticoagulation care in the inpatient setting is a difficult and serious issue to address. Pharmacy departments cannot make half-hearted attempts to implement this type of service; on the contrary, it must be well thought out and meticulously planned. First when considering implementing a change of this magnitude experts recommend freeing resources committed to maintaining programs and services that no longer contribute to the performance of a department. Second, the change, once implemented, needs to be improved systematically and continuously. Third, the program must focus on opportunities and allocate enough resources to make it successful. To assure the change succeeds in the long run, it must have a sound philosophical basis, appropriate leadership, supporting justification, and effective communications.[1]

For the above reasons, it is imperative that the director of pharmacy appoint a pharmacist as program manager to design and launch this service (in a small department, this may be a dual hat the director wears). When selecting the program manager, someone with good management skills should be selected, however, it is also important that they posses strong leadership skills. The manager should have the experience and wisdom to design comprehensive action plans, the ability to delegate parts of the task to others, and willingness to hold others accountable for their delegated tasks. This manager should be given clear organizational authority to make change or the firm backing from those with that authority. The manager should be a pharmacist who is dedicated to patient care and has sound clinical experience. This manager, when working on this project, should be focused on improving patient care even though the profession, the hospital, and physicians will also benefit from the service.

An important job of the program manager is to carefully consider the roles currently being filled in the pharmacy department. Does the department already have strong clinical programs? Do the pharmacists consider their primary responsibility direct patient care over product distribution? Does the hospital environment already consider the pharmacist part of the patient care team? If the answer is yes to these questions, the tasks in launching a service may be much easier.[2] If the answers were no, the program manager must consider many other factors. For example, job descriptions may need to be changed if they do not address the clinical aspects of patient care. The manager may need to work both with those in the department and outside the department to explain the value of patient centered as opposed to product centered pharmacy services. This may be a major paradigm shift both for the department and the hospital. The pharmacists providing this service should strive to develop an expertise that gives them the confidence to consider themselves as a peer with physicians.

The responsibilities of the program manager do not end when the program is up and running. Remember, for change to succeed (see discussion above) the program should be improved systematically and continuously. Also, new opportunities should be explored and exploited whenever possible. That means the program manager should continuously monitor program quality and prepare data that clearly show how the program has improved care (this is a major focus of Chapter 9). It is common occurrence in today's healthcare setting to encounter consultants who are often partly paid on how many human resources they can cut. Cutting the high salary of a pharmacist is an attractive option for these consultants, but a strong program manager could help prevent this if they can show clear data how they have improved care and explain the service would need to be dropped if pharmacist positions are eliminated.

Identification of Medical Staff Champion

Early in the planning of an inpatient anticoagulation service, a medical staff champion should be identified. This physician should have expertise in the care of inpatient anticoagulation patients. Examples of physicians well suited for this role are hematologists, cardiologists, hospitalists, and general internists. This medical staff champion should ideally be involved with all planning of the program. But, if that is not possible, his or her opinion should be sought on all issues that involve care delivered to the patient and how the program relates with the medical staff. Ideally, the champion should also be a member of the pharmacy and therapeutics committee so he or she can speak in favor of the program when approval is requested. Further, he or she should remain as a resource after the program is launched and be available for clinical questions from the pharmacists. Depending on the design of the program, he or she may also be appointed medical director of the program and perform specialty consults on more complicated patients.

Planning the Change

Program managers should not plan the service completely on their own; instead, a team approach is suggested with the program manager serving as team leader. The following members of the team are recommended:

- Anticoagulation program manager (team leader)
- Patient-centered pharmacists, who would be providing the service on a day-to-day basis
- Director of pharmacy
- Pharmacy technician (in case more distributive duties need to be handled by technicians)
- Medical staff champion
- Nursing representative where the service will likely be heavily utilized

A team of this makeup will provide valuable input to the program manager on necessary details to address and on how the service should look when up and running. It will also help with buy-in from other pharmacists, physicians, and nurses. This will help assure support at the pharmacy and therapeutics committee.

When the team begins to plan what service will look like, a good place to start is to envision the end product. In other words, what will the service look like? What will be the responsibilities of the pharmacists? What anticoagulants will they directly manage? A helpful tool for planning change is the RAID analysis (Results desired, Actions necessary, Indicators to watch, and Decisions that remain). See Part 1 of Appendix 4-1 (case study) for an example of team utilizing this approach.[3]

After RAID, conducting a SWOT analysis (strengths, weaknesses, opportunities, and threats) can help the team reach final decisions. It helps add more form and substance to the ideas generated by the RAID analysis. This process forces the team to look at the real world implications of what they are working on and how it will be perceived by others. See Part 2 of Appendix 4-1 for the SWOT analysis conducted by the same team after the RAID analysis.[3]

After the manager performs the RAID and SWOT analysis, they should assure the following have also been addressed:

- Is the anticoagulation service only a direct patient care activity, or will it also have organizational authority to:
  - evaluate new anticoagulation medications as they emerge?
  - standardize the use of vitamin K, recombinant factor VIIa, or other reversal agents?
  - evaluate new opportunities for program expansion?
- How will this practice be incorporated into daily pharmacist activities?
- Does the department already incorporate the delivery of clinical care into pharmacist job descriptions? If not, the job descriptions should be changed to reflect this aspect of practice so the pharmacists clearly know the expectations of the department to which the will be held accountable.
- Who is responsible for addressing performance concerns for the program as a whole and individual pharmacists as they arise?[2]
- Will the pharmacists have face-to-face interactions with the patients they are serving? (This is highly recommended and supports the ASHP 2015 initiative.)[4]
- Which pharmacists will provide the service?

When addressing this last question, at least for the launch of the program, consider utilizing pharmacists with strong moral reasoning skills. What pharmacists have strong moral reasoning skills? They are often the top clinical performers as they consider delivering inadequate care morally reprehensible, and this drives them to pursue excellence in practice. Recently, a pharmacist who many consider to have strong moral reasoning explained what he thinks to himself when tempted to cut corners to save time. He said that when faced with this temptation, he thinks, "What if it was my mother? Is this the care I would want my mother to receive?" This is an example of an excellent pharmacist who takes personal responsibility for medication therapy outcomes as envisioned by the pharmaceutical care movement and would be ideal to help launch an anticoagulation service.[5]

A major question for every new inpatient anticoagulation service is deciding where the service will initially be targeted/piloted. A good rule of thumb is to target the service in patient areas where the need is perceived the greatest. Ideas of patient populations that may make sense to pilot the program are:

- Patient groups who were identified as receiving unsafe care in Chapter 3.
- Patients who personally request a pharmacist or anticoagulation clinic to be involved in their care.
- Pediatric and geriatric patients.
- Any critical care patient receiving anticoagulation therapy.
- Patients where the physician has specifically consulted a pharmacist to assist in anticoagulation management.
- Specific units where the physicians have a strong desire for pharmacist help in management (i.e., the orthopedic unit in the case study).
- Patients with disease states considered to increase the risk of adverse drug events due to anticoagulants (see Part 2 of Appendix 4-1).
- Patients that are on a high number of concurrent medications.
- Patients who are suspected of not adhering to anticoagulation therapy.[5]

Creating a Flowchart of the Service Design

Once the team feels they have answered all foreseeable questions as to the design of the service, it is a good idea to create a flowchart as to how the service will work. This will help identify any system problems that have not yet been identified. Part 3 of Appendix 4-1 contains a flowchart of the planned service. The ovals in the figure show concerns that the manager had not yet recognized/addressed.

Barriers and Possible Solutions

It is inevitable that the program manager tasked with launching an inpatient anticoagulation program will encounter many barriers. It is essential that the program manager asserts leadership skills when these situations arise. From the very beginning of planning, the manager must remember that an inpatient anticoagulation program can have a profound effect on improving care as covered in Chapter 2. Since improved patient care is at stake, the question when planning the service should never be "if" the service can get off the ground but instead all discussion should center on "how" to get the service off the ground. The program manager cannot let those on his or her planning team dwell on how they have always done things in the past. They will likely need to "think out of the box" to overcome the barriers encountered in planning. The following are examples of some of the barriers that may be encountered and ways to overcome them.

The program manager may find resistance to change in the pharmacy department itself. Three common issues that arise is the need for additional staffing, the pharmacists don't feel qualified to provide the service, or it is not the pharmacist role to provide the service. The staffing issue is covered below and Chapter 6, so let's focus on pharmacists who do not feel qualified to provide the service or it is not their role. A first question that may need to be asked is, What has your department done to ensure your pharmacists are focused on patient-centered care? While a detailed discussion of this is beyond the scope of this text, here are some suggestions that help assure a patient-centered pharmacy department:

- The department should have clear mission and vision statement that clearly shows its primary job is providing patient-centered care.
- Review the pharmacist job descriptions and assure they include tasks related to delivering pharmaceutical care to patients.
- New pharmacists, when orientated to the department, should undergo clinical competency assessment and the orientation should include clinical care training.
- The department should place a strong emphasis on hiring those with a patient-centered approach to care and with strong moral reasoning skills. Hiring ASHP-accredited residency program graduates is a strong qualification to consider.
- The department should utilize technology and pharmacy technicians to limit the hands-on dispensing work that pharmacists need to conduct.
- The department should make every effort to assure pharmacists have a regular presence on the patient care units.
- Educational programs should regularly be provided on clinical pharmacy patient care issues on a regular basis. Utilizing pharmacy students on rotations or residents to provide these presentations can be helpful.

It is important to note that the program manager cannot force other pharmacists to change paradigms, but working with the department management to assure the above measures are in place helps set the stage that the department is dedicated to patient centered care. The pharmacists should also be assured that adequate training will occur before anyone is expected to provide the service.

Finally, the pharmacists should be told how, strategically, this will benefit the pharmacy. If an inpatient anticoagulation program is successfully implemented and demonstrates improvement in patient care, the organization will be thankful and consider utilizing pharmacy to rectify future patient care issues.

The medical staff may also resist the change. It is important to note that physicians are data driven scientists just like pharmacists. Consider utilizing the peer reviewed data presented in Chapter 2 to show the possible improvements. For physicians who are still resistant to change after being presented with this scientific data, ask the program medical staff champion to speak with them to address their concerns. If the program is going to work with physicians who are surgeons, perhaps the department can arrange for pharmacist to observe their patients during surgery to better understand physician concerns for bleeding. This will show the department is striving to understand their view of patient care. Be sure to never criticize the care already being provided by physicians and appreciate the scope and gravity of the patient care they provide and how difficult it is to provide that care. If you frame the program as "helping them do their difficult job better" rather than "caring for anticoagulation patients better than you do" you will likely experience greater success.

How to provide adequate staffing for the program may be the single most important barrier that needs to be addressed. At this time, one point must be made abundantly clear; it will take more pharmacist time to provide this service. At St. Mary's Medical Center in Duluth, MN, each warfarin anticoagulation patient day on the service takes approximately 10–15 minutes on average. This fact must be confronted and realized or a program manager will lose the support and respect of the pharmacists of the department who likely consider themselves overworked already. Three good options exist to provide enough time for pharmacists to provide the service:

1. Hire more pharmacists. It is easy to jump to this conclusion immediately, but this solution may not always be feasible. How would an administrator over pharmacy react to that message if other options have not yet been investigated? In other words, the program manager must make a reasonable attempt to identify how a change can occur with the existing resources of the department. This may take reorganization and increased delegation of dispensing duties

as discussed below.¹ If it is determined that additional pharmacist resources need to be added, see Chapter 6 on making the justification to administration. Even if new pharmacist positions are approved, hiring qualified candidates may not be easy considering the tight job market.

2. Remove current duties from the pharmacists. Are the pharmacists checking fills for patient carts or automated distribution systems? If so, investigating a tech check tech system may be a good option to pursue if allowed by the state board of pharmacy. Are pharmacists continually chasing down missing doses of medications or answering the phones? Again, these are duties that can usually be handled by pharmacy technicians. Does the wholesale distributor offer prepackaging to facilitate easy loading of automated dispensing systems? This may be cheaper than utilizing department personnel to package medications. It may be helpful to have the pharmacists list all the duties they perform each day and then consider which of those duties could be delegated to other support personnel or addressed by other means. Remember, even adding a pharmacy technician is a lot cheaper option than adding a pharmacist.

3. Make your pharmacists more efficient in performing their work. Many of the clinical activities pharmacists already performed cannot be delegated to others, but that does not mean others cannot help perform those functions. For example, with the large number of pharmacy students needing rotation sites, could setting up a rotation site help the pharmacists get their work done and still meet the students' needs? Could these same students be hired as interns and used to help with clinical data collection, performing medication reconciliation, making patient medication lists, etc.?

Many pharmacists who want to implement an inpatient anticoagulation program may be practicing in a rural setting where they are the only pharmacist. Pharmacists in this setting are asked to consider the following:

1. Can they relocate much of their time to the patient care unit, as do pharmacists at larger institutions? It will likely not be possible to spend all day on the unit, but could order entry be done on the unit? Could pharmacists be evaluating patients on the unit while the technician fills the cart and makes IVs? Could pharmacists periodically return to check the technicians work? This option may require a variance from their state board of pharmacy if they require pharmacists to be in a pharmacy at all times when in operation.

2. Even if pharmacists cannot relocate much of their time to the patient-care unit, could they follow coagulation labs on ordered anticoagulants and investigate further when they see potential problems? Could they design systems that assure coagulation labs are addressed by the medical staff prior to ordering anticoagulants (i.e., requiring daily INRs and daily warfarin orders)?

Much of the above discussion regarding freeing up pharmacists to provide the service also pertains to rural areas if the resources mentioned are available/possible. One further option to consider would be starting a residency program at the rural hospital. ASHP is in need of more residencies in rural settings and this could help provide economical resources to get the program off the ground (the residency idea may also help a larger institution if they do not already have a program).

Input into Patient Care Plans and Chart Documentation

Different anticoagulation programs approach the issue of chart documentation of the pharmacist's care plan in different ways. Some document in the patient's chart daily and others perform this function only when unusual circumstances are encountered. It is important to remember that when a physician consults a pharmacist, the physician is expecting the pharmacist's help and expects to be kept informed regarding important issues regarding the patient's care just as he or she would expect from a physician consultant. For this reason, optimally, the pharmacist care plan should be documented in the chart. Further, when pharmacists gain full provider status, this will be necessary for billing. If pharmacist documenting in the progress notes has not yet been accepted in the organization, this is an issue that should be addressed prior to launch of the inpatient anticoagulation program.

When formulating the care plan, sources of information needed to make decisions can be gathered from patient interview, the medical record, other health professionals caring for the patient, and from friends and family members of the patient.⁵ SOAP notes, or variations of SOAP notes can work well for documenting the pharmacist care plan in the chart. An example of an initial consult modified SOAP note is provided in Figure 4-1. Figure 4-2 represents and alternative approach to standardize written progress notes after initial consultation. This form is filled out by the pharmacist and placed in the chart for all initial consultations.

S/O: Pt is 81-yo female (wt = 63.4 kg, ht = 61 in) admitted for SOB, mild orthopnea, and dyspnea on exertion. Received consult to dose warfarin for treatment of PE. Target INR of 2–3. No h/o bleeding, easy bruising. PMH = PVD, smoking, COPD, HTN, s/p stent placement (1/05). Meds = enoxaparin (dose is appropriate), levofloxacin, HCTZ, metoprolol XL, pantoprazole, prednisone, nicotine cartridge, albuterol neb.

Labs: Hgb 14.3, Hct 42.0, Albumin 4.1, Plts 246, AST/ALT 15/14, Alk Phos 58, Baseline INR 0.9

A: Initiate per dosing guidelines. Titration will be performed to attain an INR of 2–3. Slight chance of levofloxacin will increase the response to warfarin.

Plan:
1. Daily INR
2. Monitor for signs of bleeding
3. Warfarin 5 mg po today

Pharmacy will continue to follow. Thank you for the consult.

John Anderson, R.Ph.

Figure 4-1. Sample modified SOAP note for an initial pharmacist anticoagulation consult: pharmacy anticoagulation consult, warfarin dosing.
Source: Adapted with permission from Mercy Hospital, Coon Rapids, MN.

As mentioned above, the inpatient anticoagulation pharmacist serves in a consultant capacity and the physicians will only be expecting documentation in that role. It is very common when practicing as an anticoagulation pharmacist to find serious medication problems not directly related to the patient's anticoagulation care. When this happens, the obligation of pharmacists is to patients, so they must address the situation to resolve the medication problem. However, before documenting in the patient's chart the assessment and plan to resolve this non-anticoagulation related issue, it is strongly recommended that the pharmacist discuss this with the attending physician. Both pharmacist and physician should both be in agreement with the plan to address the issue. Further, the note should reflect the pharmacist has discussed the issue with the physician and both agree on the plan. This approach will help avoid politically charged situations or accusations that the anticoagulation pharmacist is "overstepping his or her bounds."

Situations may arise when performing chart documentation that could have legal ramifications. Please note that the chart is not a forum for offering opinions on the care that has, or is, being provided by others. Instead, the note should only offer objective information and the pharmacist's observations that are important for others caring for a patient. For example, a pharmacist is asked to consult on restarting warfarin on a patient who has had serious gastrointestinal bleeding who is about to be discharged. Upon review of the case, he finds the patient was chronically anticoagulated for atrial fibrillation by her cardiologist (also managed the warfarin) and had stable outpatient INRs for the past 2 years. One year ago, her primary physician started the patient on naproxen 500 mg by mouth twice daily for osteoarthritis. Two days prior to admission, the patient was started on trimethoprim-sulfamethoxazole for uncomplicated cystitis by the same primary physician (trimethoprim-sulfamethoxazole can cause serious elevations of the INR). On admit, the patient was dizzy and had noticed gross amounts of blood in her stool and had an INR of 10. The blood loss was found to be due to a duodenal ulcer.

In this case, the pharmacist knows that neither the naproxen nor trimethroprim-sulfamethoxazole was appropriate for the patient. Further, it is also likely the oversight could be due to lack of communication between providers or poor maintenance of medication lists. In this case, it would be appropriate to document that the INR of 10 was likely due to a drug interaction with the trimethoprim-sulfamethoxazole, but it would not be appropriate to make comments that this was a "poor choice" to treat the cystitis. Likewise, it would be okay if the pharmacist's plan strongly recommends future avoidance of naproxen or similar drugs with warfarin, but it is inappropriate to speculate this was due to lack of communication between providers or not maintaining current medication lists. The key when documenting in the chart is "stick to the facts" that are important to be communicated to other providers to assure optimal care of the patient.[5]

Addressing Anticoagulation Transitional Care Issues

Anticoagulation issues pose some of the greatest challenges in transitional care. Patients coming in to the hospital can be very ill and have diseases or newly prescribed medications that directly conflict with their chronic warfarin therapy. Further, the pharmacist may have difficulty obtaining outpatient medical records even if the primary physician is employed by the same health system. On the flip

Chapter 4 ■ Planning of the Inpatient Anticoagulation Service

PHARMACIST INITIAL PROGRESS NOTE

Please keep this sheet in the progress note section of chart.

PHARMACY SERVICES—CONSULTS. Anticoagulation Service.
= =

Total Body Weight: _____ BUN: _____ Serum Creatinine: _____ mg/dL. Creatinine Clearance: _____ mL/min.
Recent LFT (AST/ALT/Alk Phos): _____
Baseline labs - PTT:_____PT: _____ INR: _____ WBC: _____RBC: _____ Hgb: _____Hct: _____ Plt: _____
Significant SH: _____
PMH: _____

Treatment Indication:_____. Did patient receive thrombolytics or IIb/IIIa? ____ YES____ NO
- Hemodialysis • Continuous Peritoneal dialysis

Requesting Physician: _____Requested Drug: _____ Date/ Time of Request: _____

The following parameters were noted: Other medications that can affect anticoagulation.
_____ Start Date: _____
_____ Start Date: _____
_____ Start Date: _____

Dose of Warfarin prior to admit: _____ OR Not applicable.
= =
INITIAL PROGRESS NOTE. Day # 1.

PHARMACY ANTICOAGULATION SERVICE SUGGESTS THE FOLLOWING

1. Medication
   - Heparin IV _____ Units as bolus.
   - Heparin IV _____ Units/ hour = _____ mL/ hour.
   - Warfarin _____ mg PO once for today.

2. Lab
   - CBC _____
   - Obtain PTT therapeutic at a minimum of 6 hours after the initiation. Approximately at _____ on _____.
   - Obtain INR in the AM

   (**Instructions for blood draw:** Obtain PTT at a minimum of 6 hours after the initiation of heparin and/or rate change.)

3. Target Therapeutic Range—PTT: 60 – 90 seconds.
   GOAL INR: _____

4. Will follow.

Comments

Pharmacist: _____Date: _____ Time: _____

Figure 4-2. Standardized evaluation form for initial progress notes documentation.
Source: Courtesy of AtlantiCare Regional Medical Center, Atlantic City, NJ.

side, what has occurred and recommended for the patient at discharge must be clearly communicated to the primary care physician or anticoagulation care provider. This is increasingly important with the further implementation of the hospitalist model making it less likely the outpatient primary provider will be intimately aware of the patient's acute medical issues.

To improve transitional care at admission, investigate which clinics employ an outpatient anticoagulation service. Set up a means of obtaining current dosing information from those programs if at all possible. If the health system has an anticoagulation clinic and has electronic medical records, assure the pharmacists have access to the anticoagulation record. Figure 4-3 is an example of an electronic outpatient anticoagulation flow-sheet that is available to an inpatient anticoagulation service. The pharmacist should also review the nursing admission medication history (or the pharmacist medication history if done by pharmacy) and the physician's history and physical to assure the records are consistent. Finally, the pharmacist should confirm the actual doses of warfarin or other anticoagulants currently being utilized with the patient, if necessary.

Just as the anticoagulation pharmacist needs the outpatient information at admission, the outpatient providers need the inpatient information at discharge. Critical information includes pertinent laboratory data (i.e., INRs, platelets, etc.), all doses and routes of anticoagulants given, the plan for anticoagulation from discharge to outpatient follow-up, and when follow-up will occur. Increasingly, inpatient anticoagulation programs are relying on automated mechanisms to facilitate this transition.[6,7] Figure 4-4 is an example of a communication form that is generated from an electronic database that can be faxed to the outpatient care provider.

Data Tracking/Organization/ Software Needs

It is imperative that the anticoagulation program develop a system to document the patient evaluation aside from the official patient chart documentation as much of this information is not critical for providers outside of pharmacy. This is typically performed with some type of anticoagulation monitoring form or electronic program that performs the same function.[6,7] An example of these have already been presented in Figure 4-4. This type

Anticoagulation	Diagnosis	INR Goal	Result Date	INR	INR/Lab	Tab Size	Wkly Dose	Dose Text mg
7/29/2005	atrial fibrillation	2.0-3.0	07/29/2005	2.7		5	17.5	2.5 daily (mg)
7/7/2005	atrial fibrillation	2.0-3.0	07/07/2005	2.2		5	17.5	2.5 daily (mg)
6/20/2005	atrial fibrillation	2.0-3.0	06/20/2005	1.1		5	17.5	2.5 daily (mg)
5/26/2005	atrial fibrillation	2.0-3.0	05/26/2005	2.2		5	17.5	2.5 daily (mg)
5/5/2005	atrial fibrillation	2.0-3.0	05/05/2005	3.9		5	17.5	2.5 daily (mg)
4/14/2005	atrial fibrillation	2.0-3.0	04/14/2005	3.7		5	20	5 W & 2.5 ROW (mg)
3/9/2005	atrial fibrillation	2.0-3.0	03/09/2005	1.0		5	22.5	5 MF & 2.5 ROW (mg)
2/3/2005	atrial fibrillation	2.0-3.0	02/03/2005	2.2		5	22.5	5 MF & 2.5 ROW (mg)
1/3/2005	atrial fibrillation	2.0-3.0	01/03/2005	2.3		5	22.5	5 MF & 2.5 ROW (mg)
12/10/2004	atrial fibrillation	2.0-3.0	12/10/2004	1.6		5	22.5	5 MF & 2.5 ROW (mg)
11/18/2004	atrial fibrillation	2.0-3.0	11/18/2004	1.5		5	20	5 W & 2.5 ROW (mg)
10/27/2004	atrial fibrillation	2.0-3.0	10/27/2004	2.1		5	20	5 W & 2.5 ROW (mg)
10/7/2004	atrial fibrillation	2.0-3.0	10/07/2004	2.4		5	20	
9/30/2004	atrial fibrillation	2.0-3.0	09/30/2004	1.8		5	20	
9/16/2004	atrial fibrillation	2.0-3.0	09/16/2004	2.2		5	20	
9/10/2004	atrial fibrillation	2.0-3.0						
9/9/2004	atrial fibrillation	2.0-3.0	09/09/2004	3.2	3.2 (H)	5	20	
8/26/2004	atrial fibrillation	2.0-3.0	08/26/2004	3.4		5	22.5	
8/19/2004	atrial fibrillation	2.0-3.0	08/19/2004	2.9		5	25	

Figure 4-3. Outpatient electronic anticoagulation flow sheet available to inpatient pharmacists at St. Mary's Medical Center, Duluth, MN.

Chapter 4 ■ Planning of the Inpatient Anticoagulation Service

Anticoagulation Patient Profile

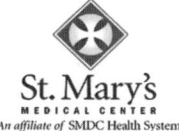

SMMC Pharmacy Department
407 East 3rd Street
Duluth, MN 55805
(218) 786-4502   Fax: 786-7375

MRN	Last Name	First Name	DOB	Age
				70

Admit	Account	Bed	Ht (in)	Wt (kg)	Diagnosis	Physician	Target INR Range
7/19/2005			0 in	0 kgs	HEMATOMA OF RIGHT TK	FOSTER	2 To 3

HISTORY — **Drug Interactions** — **Warfarin Indication**

COPD. HTN, DJD. OSTEOPOROSIS, AAA, RECENT TKA 6/28/05, COMPRESSION FRACTURES
ADMITTED WITH HEMATOMA OF RIGHT TKA (PUT IN ON 6/28/05). MD CLEARED TO RESTART WARFARIN ON 7/8/05
WAS ON 1.5MG PO QD AT NH

Drug Interactions: PAMELOR? PREDNISONE (7/10)
Warfarin Indication: KNEE REPLACEMENT

Therapy	RPh	INR	HGB	Plts	Rec Dose	COMMENTS
7/8/2005	JT	1.6	9.1	593	0 mg	WAS ADMITTED LATE AND APPARENTLY LAST TOOK DOSE ON 7/7/05
7/9/2005	JT	1.4			2.5 mg	RECEIVED 2MG AT 0200 AND I ADDED 0.5MG PO AT 1700 ON THIS DAY =2.5MG TOTAL TODAY
7/10/2005	JT	1.4			2.5 mg	SHOULD START TO GO BACK UP
7/11/2005	JH	1.3			4 mg	STARTED ON PREDNISONE
7/12/2005	JH	1.6			3 mg	DISCHARGE TOMORROW
7/13/2005	JH	2.3			1.5 mg	DISCHARGE CANCELLED TODAY D/T PAIN AND ANXIETY
7/14/2005	JH	2.3			3 mg	TO ELY SWING BED TODAY

DISCHARGE SUMMARY

Discharge Dose	3 MG TODAY, THEN PER ORTHO COUMADIN.		
DC Order Written	✓	Rx Written	☐
INR Follow Up Plan	7/15/2005	Bleeding Events	☐
Fax Anticoag Clinic	✓	Thrombosis Event	☐
Interagency Form Completed	✓	Fax Other Facilities ☐	Faxed To:
Comments			

Admit	Account	Bed	Ht (in)	Wt (kg)	Diagnosis	Physician	Target INR Range
6/28/2005			54 in	106 kgs	TOTAL RIGHT KNEE	PATNOE	2 To 3

History — **Warfarin Indication**

COPD
HTN
AORTIC ANEURISM
OBESITY
CHRONIC LOW BACK PAIN

Warfarin Indication: KNEE REPLACEMENT

Therapy	RPh	INR	HGB	Plts	Rec Dose	COMMENTS
6/28/2005	JH	1.0			5 mg	SURG DAY DOSE
6/29/2005	MZ	1.2	9.4		5 mg	TRAfNSFER TO 4 EAST TODAY, NO PROBLEMS
6/30/2005	MZ	1.4	8.9		5 mg	D/C FRIDAY TO ELY SWING BED
7/1/2005	MZ	3.0			0 mg	HOLD DOSE TODAY AND SATURDAY

DISCHARGE SUMMARY

Discharge Dose	START 2 MG PO DAILY ON 7/3/05 UNTIL NEXT INR		
DC Order Written	✓	Rx Written	☐
INR Follow Up Plan	7/5/2005	Bleeding Events	☐
Fax Anticoag Clinic	✓	Thrombosis Event	☐
Interagency Form Completed	✓	Fax Other Facilities ☐	Faxed To: COPY SEND TO ELY SWINGBED UNIT
Comments	FAX INR RESULTS TO ORTHO COUMADIN CUNIC		

Figure 4-4. Electronic anticoagulation summary report at St. Mary's Medical Center, Duluth, MN from the inpatient anticoagulation program to the outpatient anticoagulation program or anticoagulation care provider.

Managing Anticoagulation Patients in the Hospital: The Inpatient Anticoagulation Service

of system helps assure adequate communication between pharmacists. Two additional forms that work well for heparin or warfarin are presented in Figure 4-5.

HEPARIN/COUMADIN MONITORING FORM

Indication: ___ DVT ___ PE ___ Unstable angina/ACS ___ CVA ___ A. fib. Other: _____

Demographics: Age: ___ Gender: ___ Ht: _____ **Wt:** *TBW*____ kg *IBW*____ kg *ABW (50% between TBW and IBW)* ____ kg

Prescribing physician: _____ Pager/phone: _____ Date initiated: _____

❑ **Heparin per Pharmacy**
Goal PTT (range): _____
Must be at least 20 point range

❑ **Warfarin per Pharmacy**
Goal INR (range): _____ Warfarin dose PTA: _____
Must be at least 1.0 point range *(if known)*

Any conditions that might increase risk of bleeding (list): _____
Any possible warfarin interactions (list/delete): _____

❑ Initial documentation in Interdisciplinary Plan of Care (IPC)   ❑ No ASA >162mg/day (except in cardiac cases)   ❑ No IM injections while on hepar

Goal aPTT: **78 to 115 seconds** (revised 12/05)
STANDARD BLEEDING RISK

aPTT (sec)	HOLD INFUSION	RATE ADJUSTMENT (use adjusted BW)*	Next aPTT
< 60	= = = =	↑ 2.5 u/kg/hr	4 hrs
61-77	= = = =	↑ 1 u/kg/hr	4 hrs
78-115	= = = =	no change	next am
116-132	60 min.	↓ 1 u/kg/hr	4 hrs
> 132	60 min.	↓ 2.5 u/kg/hr	4 hrs

Goal aPTT: **70 to 101 seconds** (revised 12/05))
HIGHER BLEEDING RISK or ACS

aPTT (sec)	HOLD INFUSION	RATE ADJUSTMENT (use adjusted BW)*	Next aPTT
< 57	= = = =	↑ 3 u/kg/hr	4 hrs
57-69	= = = =	↑ 1.5 u/kg/hr	4 hrs
70-101	= = = =	no change	next am
102-114	60 min.	↓ 1.5 u/kg/hr	4 hrs
> 114	60 min.	↓ 3 u/kg/hr	4 hrs

* Round off any infusion rate to nearest 50 unit/hr increment.

DATE	TIME	Rx name/ Rx initials	Documented in IPC? (only for significant events, pt education)	Progress note written?	HEPARIN DOSE	PTT (sec)	PT (sec)	INR	COUMADIN DOSE	H/H (CBC QOD; cardiac CBC QD)	Platelets count #	Notes (include any potentially interacting medicatio possible bleeding complications)

Call MD to suggest possibility of HIT if platelet count decreases by >30% (diagnosed at >50% decline) or to <100,000

Updated 0406
MS

Continued

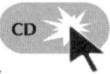

Figure 4-5. Heparin/Coumadin monitoring form example.
Source: Courtesy Cedars-Sinai Medical Center, Los Angeles, CA.

Chapter 4 ■ Planning of the Inpatient Anticoagulation Service

Goal aPTT: **78 to 115 seconds** (revised 12/05)
STANDARD BLEEDING RISK

aPTT (sec)	HOLD INFUSION	RATE ADJUSTMENT (use adjusted BW)*	Next aPTT
< 60	= = = =	↑ 2.5 u/kg/hr	4 hrs
61-77	= = = =	↑ 1 u/kg/hr	4 hrs
78-115	= = = =	no change	next am
116-132	60 min.	↓ 1 u/kg/hr	4 hrs
> 132	60 min.	↓ 2.5 u/kg/hr	4 hrs

Goal aPTT: **70 to 101 seconds** (revised 12/05)
HIGHER BLEEDING RISK or ACS

aPTT (sec)	HOLD INFUSION	RATE ADJUSTMENT (use adjusted BW)*	Next aPTT
< 57	= = = =	↑ 3 u/kg/hr	4 hrs
57-69	= = = =	↑ 1.5 u/kg/hr	4 hrs
70-101	= = = =	no change	next am
102-114	60 min.	↓ 1.5 u/kg/hr	4 hrs
> 114	60 min.	↓ 3 u/kg/hr	4 hrs

* Round off any infusion rate to nearest 50 unit/hr increment.

DATE	TIME	Rx name/ Rx initials	Documented in IPC? (only for significant events, pt education)	Progress note written?	HEPARIN DOSE	PTT (sec)	PT (sec)	INR	COUMADIN DOSE	H/H (CBC QOD; cardiac CBC QD)	Platelets count #	Notes (include any potentially interacting medication, possible bleeding complications)

Call MD to suggest possibility of HIT if platelet count decreases by >30% (diagnosed at >50% decline) or to <100,000

Updated 0406
MS

Figure 4-5. Heparin/Coumadin monitoring form example.
Source: Courtesy Cedars-Sinai Medical Center, Los Angeles, CA.

Policies, Procedures, and Guidelines

Specific suggestions for needed policies, procedures, and guidelines are covered in Chapter 5, but it is important to mention at this time how important these are to the success of the program. Not only are they necessary to be able to perform the service, they are critical to ensure the service is supported not only by the medical staff, but also by the pharmacists. These help assure the pharmacists, who will be performing the service, that the program is well organized and planned. They also specifically detail what they have authority to do and where they need to involve the attending physician. Finally, they help assure evidence-based practice as much as that is possible.

Pharmacist Training

An in-depth discussion on the how to conduct pharmacist training will be covered in Chapter 7, but when designing the service, this is a critical step to assure success. Plan on this being one of the most time consuming steps when implementation begins. A solid, well-planned training program will help assure:

- the competence of the pharmacists providing the service. This should be the primary goal of any pharmacist training utilized. The institution should also consider professional meeting support, etc., for those who strive for the expert level.
- the support of departmental pharmacists. Many pharmacists who are asked to perform this service may not have as strong of a clinical background as some of their colleagues. They, naturally, may have some trepidation about providing this service; however, they are more likely to be supportive if they see the department making a concerted effort to provide them with the needed training to perform the function safely.
- the support of your medical staff. Even for institutions already with strong clinical pharmacy programs, physicians may be worried about the liability of delegating the important function of managing anticoagulants to pharmacists. Being able to show that a strong training program will be implemented will help assure their support.

Conclusion

It is a daunting task to design and implement an inpatient anticoagulation program. Program managers must be diligent and thorough with their planning. They must exercise leadership by focusing on "how" they will implement the program rather than "if" they can start the program. They must assure all needed parties have been adequately engaged. The good news is that the payoff in improving patient care is worth all of the planning effort.

References

1. Greene SA. Planning to change practice. In: Nimmo CM, ed. *Staff Development for Pharmacy Practice*. Bethesda, MD: American Society of Health-System Pharmacists; 2000:39-48.
2. Guerrero RM, Hepler CD. Defining the scope of your pharmacy department's practice. In: Nimmo CM, ed. *Staff Development for Pharmacy Practice*. Bethesda, MD: American Society of Health-System Pharmacists; 2000:7-13.
3. Pate LE, Chesteen SA. Decision-making and work motivation: reframing the role of the pharmacist from intervention to direct patient care. In: Nimmo CM, ed. *Staff Development for Pharmacy Practice*. Bethesda, MD: American Society of Health-System Pharmacists; 2000:49-64.
4. Unknown. Increase the extent to which pharmacists help individual hospital inpatients achieve the best use of medications. *American Society of Health-System Pharmacists*. Available at: http://www.ashp.org/2015/Obj1.cfm?cfid=13787224&CFToken=37005052. Accessed July 26, 2006.
5. Galt K. *Developing Clinical Practice Skills for Pharmacists*. Bethesda, MD: American Society of Health-System Pharmacists; 2006.
6. Schneider BL, Gulseth MP, Cusick MA, Sisson DC, Tomsche JJ. Computer program to assist pharmacy management of an inpatient warfarin dosing service. *Am J Health-Syst Pharm*. 2005;62(22):2393-6.
7. Paradiso-Hardy F, Seto A, Ong S, Bucci C, Madorin P. Use of a personal digital assistant in a pharmacy-directed warfarin dosing program. *Am J Health-Syst Pharm*. 2003;60(19):1943-6.

Appendix 4-1

Case Study: Planning a Warfarin Dosing Service: RAID, SWOT Analysis, and Creating a Flowchart of the Service Design

Part 1: RAID Analysis in Planning Change[3]

A new clinical coordinator at a 320-bed hospital is tasked by his director of pharmacy to aid the orthopedic surgeons in warfarin dosing. The orthopedic surgeons have requested this service. The clinical coordinator convenes a multidisciplinary team including pharmacists, pharmacy technicians, a physician, and a nurse. To decide what the service will look like, he decides to use the RAID strategic planning process.

1. What do we want to accomplish? (**R**esults desired)

    - The team throws out many ideas of what the new anticoagulation service should look like. Ideas range from having pharmacists automatically dose and monitor all anticoagulants in the hospital to creating a formal new medical team of which the pharmacist is a member that rounds on all anticoagulation patients. In the end, the team decides to focus on the specific request from the orthopedic surgeons. They decide that the pharmacists should automatically dose and manage the warfarin used for DVT prophylaxis for orthopedic patients. They also want the pharmacists to be very knowledgeable on other anticoagulants but want them to discuss recommendations regarding those agents with the attending physician prior to making changes in care. They also want the service to assure a seamless transition to the outpatient setting. If this service works well, they will recommend rolling out the service further to other areas of the hospital.

2. What needs to be done to accomplish this? (**A**ctions necessary)

    - The standing orders for orthopedic surgery need to be changed to reflect the new pharmacist service.
    - The orthopedic nurses need to be educated on the change and how it may alter their practice.
    - Policies, procedures, and guidelines that give the needed authority to pharmacists to perform this service need to be developed, reviewed with key physicians, and approved for use by the pharmacy and therapeutics committee.
    - The pharmacists who will be providing the service need competency training.
    - A system to keep the data organized needs to be developed.
    - The technicians will need to take over more of the distributive duties to give the pharmacists the time needed to perform this service.

3. How do we know if we have done what it takes? (**I**ndicators to watch)

    - The pharmacy and therapeutics committee will pass all needed policies, procedures, and guidelines and encourage the medical staff in other areas (outside of orthopedics) to utilize the service.
    - Pharmacists will enjoy providing the service and want to work in areas where it is heavily utilized.
    - Pharmacists will not feel other care is suffering due to the service.
    - Physicians will utilize the service.
    - Consistency of the service will be objectively demonstrated in quality indicators used by the department to monitor the service.
    - Outpatient anticoagulation care providers will not need to track down dosing information when a pharmacy managed patient comes back to them.

4. What decisions do we now need to make? (**D**ecisions that remain)

    - The staffing model of the pharmacy department needs to be changed to free up the pharmacists planned to provide this service.
    - The department must explore new options like tech check tech to free up the pharmacist resources needed to launch the service.
    - The department must decide if all pharmacists need to be trained to provide the service, or only a select few.
    - The program manager must come up with a way to provide a competency program including hands-on training to all pharmacists who will provide the service.
    - The plan must be shared directly with the orthopedic group to ensure their full support.
    - Important thought leaders on the pharmacy and therapeutics committee need to be engaged and asked for input prior to the plan coming to the committee to ensure swift approval.

- The data collection system must be developed and implemented.
- A system to ensure continuity of care must be developed.
- Quality indicators to monitor service excellence need to be developed.
- The revised standing orders must be distributed.
- The nurses must be educated on how the service will change their workflow.
- The needed policies, procedures, and guidelines to support the service must be drafted and approved by the pharmacy and therapeutics committee.
- The didactic education sessions for competency training must be held and assessment criteria developed.

Part 2: SWOT Analysis in Planning Change[3]

The same clinical coordinator reconvenes his team after the RAID analysis and conducts a SWOT analysis before specific plans are implemented. He wants to see if there are outstanding issues that must be addressed not yet identified prior to making final decisions. The following four questions are what he asks his team about the planned program after reviewing with them the results of their RAID analysis:

1. What are the **S**trengths of the planned anticoagulation program?

    - Small initial focus of the program makes success likely.
    - After bouncing the ideas generated for the program off of many orthopedic surgeons and prominent physicians on the pharmacy and therapeutics committee, the program appears to have strong support.
    - Administration feels the program fits with their focus on medication safety since anticoagulants are some of the highest risk medications utilized in the health system.
    - The pharmacists are pleased that training is planned prior to implementation.
    - The technicians are excited about performing what many thought of as "pharmacist's work."

2. What are the **W**eaknesses of the planned anticoagulation program?

    - The program seems mainly focused on warfarin dosing in a narrow patient population, but care problems are encountered with all anticoagulants in all care settings.
    - The pharmacists may neglect other anticoagulation needs of patients as they do not have independent authority to make decisions.
    - Since the pharmacists are serving in a consultant role, they could easily miss drug therapy problems not directly related to anticoagulation.
    - Since the pharmacist is not providing outpatient anticoagulation management of the patients, continuity of care may suffer.
    - The program does not have any specific plans for improving the use of agents associated with anticoagulation like vitamin K or recombinant factor VIIa.
    - The program does not have any planned role in evaluating the place in therapy of future anticoagulants.
    - The program leaves it possible for physicians not skilled in anticoagulant management to continue to manage anticoagulation.
    - No formal process has been put in place to assure all INRs are reviewed before warfarin in dosed.

3. What **O**pportunities exist for anticoagulation program?

    - If the program is successful, the team feels it will be easy to roll out in other areas.
    - If the program is successful, the team feels the program would have support to take over the management of intravenous unfractionated heparin, argatroban, and lepirudin.
    - The director of pharmacy is worried about expensive anticoagulant drugs in the pipeline. The team feels it should continue to exist after implementation to evaluate new therapies or address issues related to the service provided. It should become a formal subcommittee of the pharmacy and therapeutics committee.

4. What **T**hreats exist to the new anticoagulation program?

    - The lack of provider status for pharmacists makes additional staffing hard to justify. Hospital administration has already told the director of pharmacy that he is expected to perform this service with the same number of pharmacists that he already has.
    - The cardiology department wants to continue to manage their own patients without the help of a pharmacist. They use nurse

practitioners to provide this service.
- Some of the pharmacists are nervous about providing the service. They do not feel they are qualified.
- Many of the pharmacists lack extensive clinical experience, making the training very challenging.
- The department does not have a formal technician training program necessary for the technicians to take on more pharmacist duties.

The clinical coordinator is surprised at how many important issues they missed with the RAID analysis. He resolves to address the above issues prior to program launch.

Part 3: Flowchart of an Initial Pilot Anticoagulation Service

Circles represent concerns of the program manager when reviewing the system.

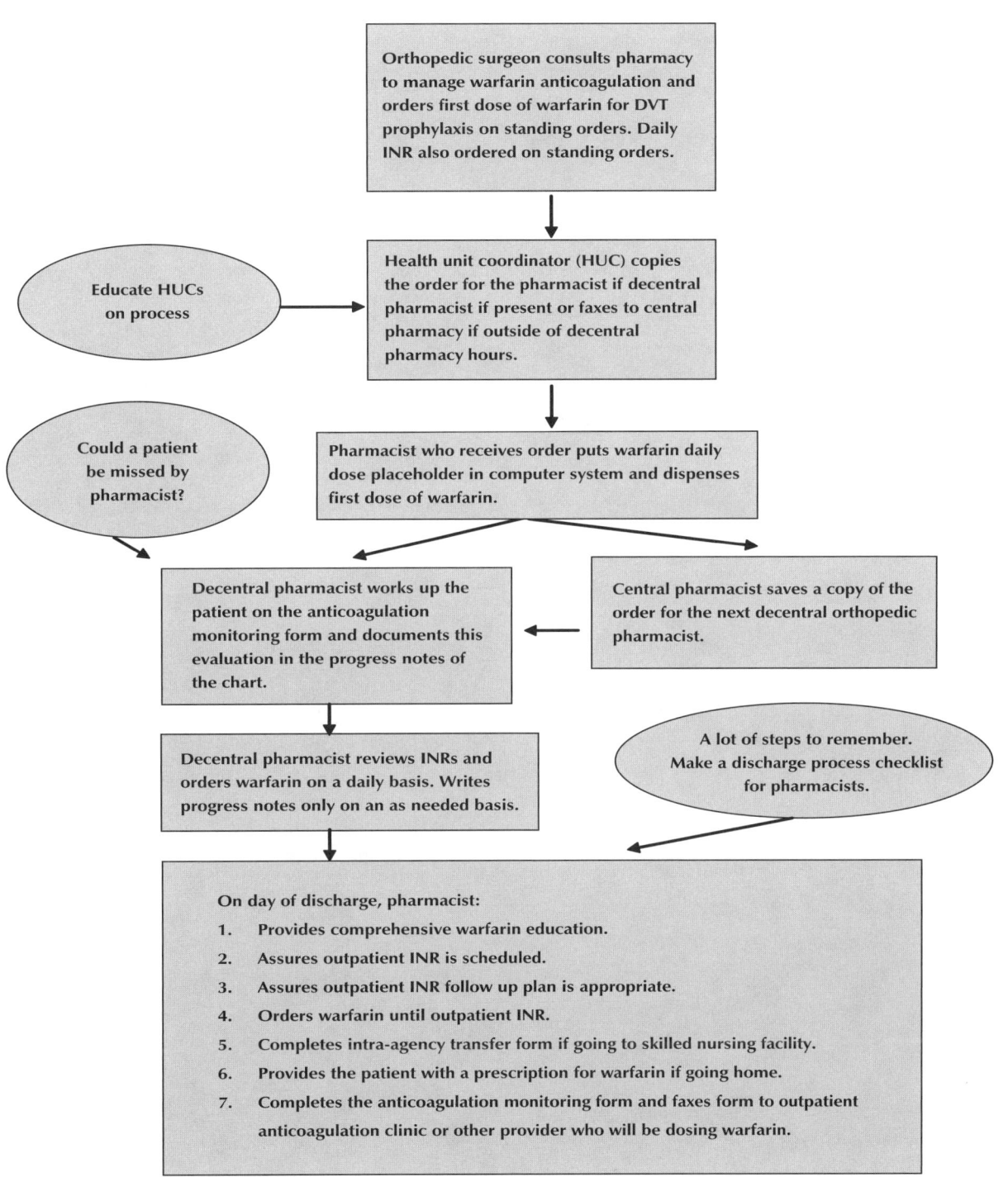

Chapter 5

Winning Support for the Inpatient Anticoagulation Service

Michael Gulseth

Chapter Outline

- Introduction
- Assuring a sound philosophical basis
- Leadership essentials
- Supporting justification
- Communication essentials
- Consensus guidelines for outpatient anticoagulation management
- Pharmacy and therapeutics committee role
- Making the proposal to administration
- Conclusion
- References

Introduction

Now that the program manager has a clear vision of what the anticoagulation service will look like (Chapter 4), it is time to discuss how to make this vision a reality. As anyone who has successfully created change in practice can tell you, it is just as important to "sell" the planned change as planning the change itself. Many practice improvements are never implemented in healthcare due to lack of adequate buy-in from stakeholders. In orders to win support for this important practice change, the program manager must provide a sound philosophical basis for the change, exert leadership, give supporting justification, and effectively communicate with stakeholders.[1]

Assuring a Sound Philosophical Basis

When examining the philosophical basis of the program, the program manger should consider how this program fits with the organizations mission and vision. If an organization has as its number one priority ensuring the safe and effective provision of patient care, the program manager is more likely to be successful. A powerful selling technique when promoting the program to others is showing how it ties into the organization's mission and vision.

Leadership Essentials

Leadership must be displayed by the program manager and director of pharmacy to assure all pharmacy mangers support the new program. If the program manager and director of pharmacy do not successfully educate the pharmacy managerial staff as to the reason for the change and their roles during the change, they risk a lack of buy-in and support that could filter throughout the department. This must be avoided, as a change of this magnitude is not likely to succeed if individual pharmacists do not have the direct support of their manager.[1]

Another key leadership quality needed by the program manager is perseverance. As with any major undertaking of this magnitude, bumps in the road will be experienced but must be overcome. While careful planning prior to implementation is important, the planning process can sometimes lead to excuses to delay implementation of the program. In other words, the manager must realize that every bump in the road cannot be anticipated, and a point will come when the program simply needs to be implemented. The leader has to remember that many of the problems that others are concerned about are likely not as important as the bigger problem of not having an anticoagulation program in place! As mentioned in Chapter 4, it is not a matter of *if* the program will be implemented, but *how*.

Supporting Justification

When winning support for the anticoagulation program, the program manager needs some supporting justification for the change. First, consider reviewing the adverse drug events (ADEs) and/or instances of medication errors involving anticoagulants. When reviewing these, pay close attention to medications the department wishes to target with the new anticoagulation service. Could utilizing inpatient anticoagulation pharmacists improve patient care? For example, are patients on heparin infusions having their doses calculated correctly? Are physicians reviewing INR results before picking warfarin doses? For both examples, could implementation of an inpatient anticoagulation program fix these issues? Second, since most hospital ADEs and medication error reporting systems are based on voluntary reporting, it is a good idea to conduct a medication use evaluation (MUE) of the anticoagulants that are of most concern to the program manager and the organization as a whole. Is the medication in question being used appropriately? Are the doses used in line with nationally published standards and the scientific evidence? Are appropriate target laboratory ranges being used? Third, after finding the key areas where problems in medication use are evident, the program manager should review the peer reviewed literature from Chapter 2 to gain into insights how others have successfully fixed these problems with an inpatient anticoagulation service. Finally, if still more data is needed to support making the change, the program manager could design and conduct a research study on a pilot program to demonstrate the benefit (covered in more detail in Chapter 6). This is an excellent project for a pharmacy resident at the institution to conduct. Throughout all of this data collection and justification, the key is to remember that the stakeholders need a clear, data driven reason as to *why* the change is needed before they are likely to support it.

Perhaps the most powerful justification that an anticoagulation program can make is what may be coming from accreditation agencies, particularly, the Joint Commission®. If future national patient safety goals make pharmacist involvement in the dosing of heparin and warfarin mandatory,[2] the justification will likely be very easy as accredited organizations will have no choice but to comply. However, if these goals are not enacted, opportunities may still exist. As mentioned in Chapter 1, core measures for the systematic prophylaxis and treatment of venous thromboembolism (VTE) could open up numerous opportunities for pharmacy to help the organization comply with the measures.[3] Utilizing some of the same techniques mentioned in the previous paragraph, but applied to VTE, could provide a powerful justification for an inpatient anticoagulation service.

Communication Essentials

Chapter 4 already reviewed critical stakeholders to involve when planning the anticoagulation service. It is important to mention that these are not the *only* stakeholders in the process, and the plans generated by the team will need to be communicated and feedback received from other stakeholders. Additional key stakeholders to consider include:

- Physician groups heavily involved with anticoagulation management who do not have a representative on the planning team. Groups to consider are hospitalists, general internists, family practice, trauma, intensivists, cardiothoracic surgeons, cardiologists, orthopedic surgeons, and hematologists/oncologists.
- The chair of the pharmacy and therapeutics committee should be involved as he will be chairing the committee that will formally approve the program.
- The pathologist who is in charge of the coagulation laboratory. He must be involved in all changes/protocols that involve the interpretation of coagulation labs.
- Nurses that regularly care for many of the anticoagulation patients to be targeted by the program who are not already on the planning team.
- Key pharmacists, pharmacy managers, and technicians not already on the planning team.
- Administrators that oversee the pharmacy department budget.

When engaging these stakeholders and others, the manager should consider how might the anticoagulation service affect this stakeholder? How much support can be counted on from them, and why?

What strategies should be used in dealing with this stakeholder? Be sure to clearly communicate the goals and objectives of the program. The manager must try to anticipate the response they will receive from stakeholders, listen to the feedback received, and address concerns that do not compromise the planned effectiveness of the program. Some resistance is likely to be encountered, but listening and addressing presented concerns will go a long way to gain support from those who express concerns.[1]

Consensus Guidelines for Outpatient Anticoagulation Management

Another key article to review when attempting to win support for an inpatient anticoagulation program is the "Consensus Guidelines for Coordinated Outpatient Oral Anticoagulation Therapy Management," generated by the Anticoagulation Guidelines Task Force.[4] These guidelines provided a framework for the development of an outpatient warfarin anticoagulation management service that provides systematic, coordinated care. While the document is not intended for inpatient anticoagulation programs, is only focused on warfarin management, and is 10 years old, many of the recommendations can also be applied to the current inpatient setting. By meeting the stated practice standards, the inpatient anticoagulation program will provide excellent care and will help win support for the program with physicians who are familiar with these standards.

The following numbered points are the actual recommendations (in italics) in their entirety.[4] Following each point are comments about how they may or may not apply to inpatient anticoagulation management.

1. *Anticoagulation providers should meet minimum competencies and hold a license in a patient-oriented health-related field.*

   Comment: A detailed discussion of the competence requirements for pharmacists to provide this service is in Chapter 7. Chapter 2 presented that pharmacists are the only non-physician healthcare providers who have shown benefit of their services in the management of inpatient anticoagulation patients in the peer-reviewed literature.

2. *The physician or healthcare provider with ultimate responsibility for therapeutic decisions should develop an agreed-upon policy and procedure for personnel supervision and oversight of those healthcare providers actually managing the anticoagulation therapy.*

   Comment: Policies and procedures that clearly delineate the role of the pharmacist and the role of the attending physician when delegating anticoagulation management to the pharmacist must be developed. These policies need to be approved by the P & T committee and should apply to all medical groups who wish to utilize the service. The "physician or health care provider with ultimate responsibility for therapeutic decisions" is usually the individual physician who consults the pharmacy department to manage a patient's anticoagulation therapy.

3. *Written protocols for the management of anticoagulation should be established.*

   Comment: Protocols and guidelines to support the service need to be developed and approved by the P & T committee. The document offers suggestions for needed policies and procedures.[4] The ones that may apply to inpatient management are presented in Table 5-1. More details on these suggested policies, procedures, and guidelines are provided later in the chapter.

4. *The anticoagulation provider should have a systematic process to identify patients who need to be scheduled for a blood sample and/or medical assessment, to schedule the necessary appointments, to retrieve laboratory results, and to provide patient instruction and follow-up.*

   Comment: Since the patient is in the hospital, most of the above is not applicable. The exception is the program must have a standard on how often coagulation laboratory measures will be drawn for different agents. Further, the program must have policies in place to assure a smooth transition of care back to the ambulatory setting.

5. *The anticoagulation provider should have policies and procedures regarding communications with the patient, primary care physician or health care providers, laboratory, and designated pharmacies. Documentation of these interactions, as well as documentation of outcomes assessment, should be recorded in the database of the patient.*

   Comment: In the inpatient setting, the main area of application of this recommendation is that it is essential the pharmacist communicate both verbally and in writing with the referring physician and other physicians regarding important anticoagulation issues. These interactions should be documented both in the patient chart

Table 5-1.
Recommended Policies and Procedures for Anticoagulation Management that Apply to Inpatient Management[4]

- Patient assessment
- Patient education
- Intensity of anticoagulation therapy
- Systematic method for interpretation of INR results and management of nontherapeutic laboratory values
- Adverse events protocol with definitions of minor and major bleeding and disease recurrence with appropriate actions
- Method for dosage adjustment based on INR results; patient assessment; and evaluation of dietary, disease state, and lifestyle changes
- Systematic method for therapy initiation
- Intervals for monitoring INR and other laboratory parameters pertinent to anticoagulation therapy

and the patient repository the pharmacist is using (i.e., monitoring form, computer program).

6. *The anticoagulation provider should use the INR to assess patient anticoagulation control.*

   Comment: As this has long been the standard of care for monitoring warfarin, this should not be an issue.

7. *The referring physician or healthcare provider recommending anticoagulation therapy shall determine the appropriateness of anticoagulation therapy for a particular patient. The actual anticoagulation provider or director of the service, in order to manage the care, must agree with the appropriateness of therapy.*

   Comment: Anticoagulation therapy providers must continually weigh the risks versus benefits of the therapy. The inpatient anticoagulation pharmacist should not agree to manage patients where they feel the risks of therapy outweigh the benefit. When this type of case arises, the pharmacist should directly share his or her concerns with the referring physician. Often, this conversation will result in the pharmacist convincing the physician to pursue alternative therapy for the time being, or the physician provides facts the pharmacist hadn't considered and convinces the pharmacist that the benefits of therapy outweigh the risk. If physician and pharmacist continue to not agree on the appropriateness of therapy, the organization's conflict resolution policy should be utilized. At this point, both the pharmacist's and physician's supervisors would become involved with the case. Again, it is essential that pharmacists involved in anticoagulation management remember that their primary obligation is to the patient. If this maxim is kept in mind and tactful, yet assertive, communication is utilized, these issues typically do not escalate.

8. *The anticoagulation provider should assess the patient's current medical, medication, dietary, and lifestyle history; level of understanding and literacy; health beliefs and attitudes; motivation for self-care behavior; and other environmental or behavioral barriers to learning and adherence when therapy is instituted.*

   Comment: This assessment should be rolled into the warfarin education program enacted by the hospital. This will be covered in more detail in Chapter 9.

9. *A patient-specific INR range, based on the medical literature and other patient-specific information, should be established.*

   Comment: The policies and procedures the program operates under should allow the referring physician to specify a therapeutic range. If they do not specify a therapeutic range, the pharmacist should have default ranges that are based on the most current literature.

10. *The anticoagulation provider should base dosage adjustments on INR and other pertinent laboratory results, individual assessment, patient-specific response, and guidelines approved by the anticoagulation service as part of its policies and procedures.*

    Comment: While many articles have evaluated different warfarin initiation nomograms, few have focused on the inpatient setting.[5-13] Further, considering the numerous issues that can affect warfarin responsiveness (e.g., diet, concurrent disease, medications, lifestyle, genetics, weight, etc.),[14] no model or nomogram is adequate in picking initiation warfarin doses. An excellent review on this topic can be found in *Annals of Pharmacotherapy*.[15]

For patients on chronic warfarin therapy, the pharmacy should treat them much like outpatients. In the rare cases that their INR is stable, the home dose should be continued. In cases where they are unstable, the guidelines the pharmacist operates under should give guidance on when to increase the dose, decrease the dose, and when to hold the dose.

One key point on these issues cannot be stressed enough; any enacted policies, procedures, and guidelines must give the ability for the pharmacist to vary from the approved guidelines based on his or her clinical judgment. Note that this text continually mentions the word "guidelines," and less often "protocols" or "nomograms." Pharmacists performing this service must be allowed to utilize their clinical skills and not be tied to a rigid protocol or nomogram.

11. *Initial monitoring should occur every week or more frequently following initiation of therapy or hospital discharge, depending of the stability of the patient. After the patient's anticoagulation has been stabilized, follow-up evaluation should occur at least every 4 weeks.*

   Comment: For warfarin, many hospital pharmacy departments required daily INRs while a patient is an inpatient. If not, INRs should be drawn every 2–3 days during initiation at a minimum. Since inpatients are inherently medically unstable, it may be difficult to ever allow INRs less frequently than every 2–3 days even in seemingly stable patients. The key is the department should have a policy and procedure on the frequency of needed INRs.

12. *The anticoagulation provider should have a systematic process for follow-up evaluations focused on patient assessment for potential side effects of therapy; recurrent disease; hemorrhagic complications, drug-drug/drug-disease state and drug-food interactions; lifestyle changes, review of laboratory results; adherence issues; and patient education.*

   Comment: The inpatient anticoagulation pharmacist must assess their patients for the above issues on a daily basis and take appropriate steps to address issues encountered. So how does an inpatient pharmacist assess these issues? At St. Mary's Medical Center in Duluth, MN, the pharmacists review the medication administration record (MAR), all new physician orders and progress notes not yet seen by pharmacy, and all pertinent labs. Further, the pharmacist interviews other professionals (physicians, nurses) and the patient on an as needed basis when dosing warfarin.

13. *The anticoagulation provider should have a policy on the interval for follow-up blood testing after a dosage adjustment has been made. The determination should consider the magnitude of the nontherapeutic INR and dosage change, as well as other variables influencing patient responsiveness and stability.*

   Comment: This was already commented on above for #11.

14. *Anticoagulation providers should develop guidelines regarding management of anticipated changes in anticoagulant response that result from a change in patient status, medication use, diet, or other factors.*

   Comment: This is important, however, it is difficult and time consuming to write guidelines for every possible scenario a pharmacist will see in practice. Time would be better spent focusing on setting up an excellent pharmacist education program so pharmacists completing the program have seen many different types of situations and have the ability to use judgment to address each individual situation.

15. *The anticoagulation provider should have a policy and procedure pertaining to the desired goals and objectives of its educational program. Patient education should be individualized according to the initial assessment, based on the patient's level of understanding; be accompanied by written information as a reinforcement; and be reviewed on a regular basis.*

   Comment: This is an extremely important objective that must also be accomplished in the inpatient setting. This education does not necessarily have to be provided by a pharmacist, but it would be preferred as they would be the most familiar with each patients individual anticoagulation needs. The patient education topic will be covered in much more detail in Chapter 9.

16. *Anticoagulation providers should have a policy and procedure for the management of major and minor bleeding episodes, signs and symp-*

toms of thromboembolism, other potential anticoagulation side effects, or other medical problems not related to anticoagulation therapy. This should include the use of vitamin K or fresh-frozen plasma to correct an excessively prolonged INR or to treat serious hemorrhage.

Comment: The Seventh American College of Chest Physicians Conference on Antithrombotic and Thrombolytic Therapy provides excellent recommendations regarding the appropriate use of warfarin reversal agents. An important recent development is the use of recombinant factor VIIa in the treatment of refractory bleeding. This agent can have serious vascular morbidity and is quite expensive. Guidelines regarding its use are only recently accumulating[16] and an example of an order set is shown in Appendix 5-1, Figure 5-1.

17. *Anticoagulation providers should have a policy and procedure for the management of anticoagulation when the patient requires and invasive procedure.*

    Comment: This is also an issue in the inpatient setting. An example of anticoagulation bridging guidelines to address this issue is illustrated in Appendix 5-1, Figure 5-2.

18. *Anticoagulation providers should have a policy and procedure for the management of patients who are nonadherent with therapy, appointments, or other aspects of anticoagulation treatment. This policy should include guidelines for termination of anticoagulation management by the anticoagulation service.*

    Comment: This is not pertinent to inpatient management.

19. *The anticoagulation provider should perform a program evaluation of organizational components on an annual basis or more often as deemed necessary. Anticoagulation providers should analyze the contribution of various processes to patient outcomes.*

    Comment: The processes set up in Chapter 4 should be reviewed on a yearly basis. The same team that set up the program could perform this analysis. This topic will be covered in Chapter 9.

20. *The anticoagulation provider should perform an outcomes evaluation on an annual basis or more often as deemed necessary. This outcome assessment should include, as a minimum, information pertaining to degree of therapeutic effectiveness as determined by the INR, hemorrhagic complication rates, thromboembolism rates, and other complications resulting from anticoagulant therapy.*

    Comment: Traditionally, in the outpatient setting, anticoagulation programs have monitored indicators of program quality such as therapeutic failure rates, bleeding rates, time in the therapeutic range, and patient overdue for INRs. Less work in this arena has been done for inpatient management, but Chapter 9 will discuss ideas on how to accomplish this recommendation.

Pharmacy and Therapeutics Committee Role

All hospital pharmacy departments who are attempting to launch an inpatient anticoagulation service will need to get the approval of their P & T committee or the equivalent body in that hospital/health-system. The P & T committee traditionally has jurisdiction over all clinical matters that involve the pharmacy department. To be prepared to present the program, the program manager should already have done the political homework suggested above. If not, the program stands little chance of being approved. If the political homework has been completed, the program manager should be prepared to share the vision and scope of the program with the committee. Again, some of the committee members should have been engaged already, so that the actual presentation of the program can be tailored to those who may not know about the program. All policies, procedures, consults forms, and guidelines the program will operate under should have been included in a P & T meeting packet that goes out prior to the meeting, so all members have time to review these documents prior to the meeting and are prepared to offer suggestions for improvement.

To assure the presentation with the P & T committee ends with full approval of the program, the program manager should keep a few things in mind. First, although the manager will have already put many hours of thought and energy into starting the program at this point, they must not get frustrated when a committee member requests further changes. Remember, the committee member is not attacking the work already done, rather they are trying to make suggestions that will further improve patient care. Next, the program manager must be able to present a clear vision of the size and scope of the program with the aim of answering questions physicians may have about the program (in other words, the manager must think like the physicians; what would they be worried about?). A clear plan should be shared on how the pharmacists will be educated to provide the service and how it will be organized. Finally, they should also be told how the quality of the service will monitored in the long term.

So, what policies, procedures, consult forms, guidelines, etc., are needed for a new service? This will largely depend in the scope and size of the planned anticoagulation service. Appendix 5-1, Figures 5-1–5-14 provide numerous examples of these documents that could be adapted by a newly planned inpatient anticoagulation service. These documents are also on the CD resource to provide easy adaptation.

Making the Proposal to Administration

Too often, one will encounter pharmacists saying the hospital administrators don't understand what pharmacists do and frustration in not adding pharmacist resources to expand clinical services to improve patient care. While this frustration may or may not be justified, it would be interesting to ask those same pharmacists if they know what hospital administrators do and if they think it is easy to decide when and where to invest institutional resources. Further, if the administrator over pharmacy does not understand what pharmacy does, has pharmacy taken steps to provide that education? Suggestions to improve relationships with the pharmacy administrators are:

- Invite the administrator to shadow floor-based pharmacists to see up close their integral role in patient care.
- Promote the great work the department does for the organization by celebrating National Health-System Pharmacy Week, sponsored by the American Society of Health-System Pharmacists.
- Establish pharmacist and technician of the year awards to be given during pharmacy week. Invite the administrator to attend the award ceremony and clearly describe how the individual won the award for improving patient care.
- Promote any milestones achieved by the department in organizational newsletters and personally tell the administrators about the accomplishments.

The point of the above ideas is that while it may be true the administrator over pharmacy may have limited knowledge of what pharmacists do to provide clinical care to patients, blaming the administrator for this lack of knowledge is unjustified if the pharmacy department has not tried to provide this education. By regularly engaging the administrator in the critical role pharmacists play in providing safe and effective care of patients and providing data to demonstrate that improvement in care, it will likely make future pharmacy requests to expand services more likely to be granted.

When the proposal to implement a service is made to hospital administration, it may be best to have the Director of Pharmacy make the presentation due to a closer relationship to the administrators, but the director will likely need extensive help from the program manager. The person making the presentation needs to remember to speak in lay terminology as many administrators do not have training as a medical professional. The specific content of what should be presented to hospital administration will be covered in Chapter 6.

Conclusion

Winning support for an inpatient anticoagulation service is not easy, but the hard work and leadership of the program manager will be rewarded. The manager must not neglect the work mentioned in this chapter, or the program will likely not be supported by the medical staff, administration, or both. Managers striving to provide systematic, coordinated anticoagulation care in the inpatient setting should consider the outpatient national guidelines when setting up the service. Numerous policies, procedures, and guidelines will likely need to be approved by the P & T Committee prior to program launch. Proactively educating hospital administration about the important patient care role pharmacists play is also critical to the successful implementation of an inpatient anticoagulation service.

References

1. Greene SA. Planning to change practice. In: Nimmo CM, ed. *Staff Development for Pharmacy Practice.* Bethesda, MD: American Society of Health-System Pharmacists; 2000:39-48.
2. Unknown. Draft Candidate 2007 National Patient Safety Goals, Requirements and Implementation Expectations. *Joint Commission on Accreditation of Healthcare Organizations.* Available at: http://www.jointcommission.org/NR/rdonlyres/4901A094-80A7-4AD6-86CD-4754B896A986/0/07_npsg_hap_cah.pdf. Accessed May 31, 2006.
3. Unknown. *Joint Commission on Accreditation of Healthcare Organizations.* Available at: http://www.jcaho.org/pms/core+measures/pdf119.pdf. Accessed Feb 15, 2006.
4. Ansell JE, Buttaro ML, Thomas OV, Knowlton CH. Consensus guidelines for coordinated outpatient oral anticoagulation therapy management. Anticoagula-

tion Guidelines Task Force. *Ann Pharmacother.* May 1997;31(5):604-15.
5. Harrison L, Johnston M, Massicotte MP, Crowther M, Moffat K, Hirsh J. Comparison of 5-mg and 10-mg loading doses in initiation of warfarin therapy. *Ann Intern Med.* 1997;126(2):133-6.
6. Tait RC, Sefcick A. A warfarin induction regimen for out-patient anticoagulation in patients with atrial fibrillation. *Br J Haematol.* 1998;101(3):450-4.
7. Kovacs MJ, Cruickshank M, Wells PS, et al. Randomized assessment of a warfarin nomogram for initial oral anticoagulation after venous thromboembolic disease. *Haemostasis.* 1998;28(2):62-9.
8. Crowther MA, Ginsberg JB, Kearon C, et al. A randomized trial comparing 5-mg and 10-mg warfarin loading doses. *Arch Intern Med.* 1999;159(1):46-8.
9. Anderson DR, Wilson SJ, Blundell J, et al. Comparison of a nomogram and physician-adjusted dosage of warfarin for prophylaxis against deep-vein thrombosis after arthroplasty. *J Bone Joint Surg Am.* 2002;84-A(11):1992-7.
10. Kovacs MJ, Anderson DA, Wells PS. Prospective assessment of a nomogram for the initiation of oral anticoagulation therapy for outpatient treatment of venous thromboembolism. *Pathophysiol Haemost Thromb.* 2002;32(3):131-3.
11. Wilkinson TJ, Sainsbury R. Evaluation of a warfarin initiation protocol for older people. *Intern Med J.* 2003;33(9-10):465-7.
12. Roberts GW, Helboe T, Nielsen CB, et al. Assessment of an age-adjusted warfarin initiation protocol. *Ann Pharmacother.* 2003;37(6):799-803.
13. Kovacs MJ, Rodger M, Anderson DR, et al. Comparison of 10-mg and 5-mg warfarin initiation nomograms together with low-molecular-weight heparin for outpatient treatment of acute venous thromboembolism. A randomized, double-blind, controlled trial. *Ann Intern Med.* 2003;138(9):714-9.
14. Ansell J, Hirsh J, Poller L, Bussey H, Jacobson A, Hylek E. The pharmacology and management of the vitamin K antagonists: the Seventh ACCP Conference on Antithrombotic and Thrombolytic Therapy. *Chest.* 2004;126(3 Suppl):204S-33S.
15. Dager WE. Initiating warfarin therapy. *Ann Pharmacother.* 2003;37(6):905-8.
16. Goodnough LT, Lublin DM, Zhang L, Despotis G, Eby C. Transfusion medicine service policies for recombinant factor VIIa administration. *Transfusion.* 2004;44(9):1325-31.

Appendix 5-1: Forms for Adoption by a Newly-Planned Inpatient Coagulation Service

Recombinant Factor VIIa Orders

APPROPRIATE USE GUIDELINES
1. Give clotting factor replacement FIRST (unless intracerebral hemorrhage or traumatic head injury with expansion—skip clotting factor replacement and give rFVIIa 80 mcg/kg IV × 1)
   a. Fresh Frozen Plasma (FFP) if INR, aPTT or anti-Xa level elevated → 20 mL/kg *or* 6 units
   b. Platelets (if less than 50,000 or platelet dysfunction) → 6 pack × 2
   c. Cryoprecipitate (if low fibrinogen) → 10 units × 2
2. Draw INR, aPTT, Thrombin Time, Fibrinogen, D-Dimer prior to each dose of rFVIIa
3. Check platelet count if not done within the past 24 hours

Use of rFVIIa is NOT APPROPRIATE in the following conditions:
1. No clotting factor replacement has been attempted (except in patients with intracerebral hemorrhage or traumatic head injury with expansion)
2. Prophylactic use before major surgery in patients without pre-existing coagulopathy
3. Patients who have an abnormal coagulation profile (e.g., elevated INR, aPTT, anti-Xa level) but are not actively bleeding
4. Patients with a known hypersensitivity to mouse, hamster or bovine proteins

	Patient <u>Actual</u> Body Weight = _____ kg (Pharmacist to calculate dose) <u>Indication</u> – Please check appropriate box below.		Significant Clotting Factor Replacement Required?	Dosing†
☐	Closed Space Bleeding	▪ Intracerebral hemorrhage within 3 hours of symptom onset ▪ Isolated traumatic head injury with evidence of expansion	NO	80 mcg/kg IV × 1
☐	Closed Space Bleeding	▪ Retroperitoneal bleed	YES	40 mcg/kg IV × 1
☐	Bleeding Rescue in Surgical Patients	▪ Cardiac or thoracic aorta surgery ▪ Hepatic resection or transplant ▪ Nontraumatic high blood loss spinal surgery	YES	40 mcg/kg IV × 1
☐	Other Uses	▪ Bleeding rescue post-partum or post-hysterectomy ▪ Severe trauma with ongoing bleeding despite surgery and rate of blood loss ≥ 10 units of PRBCs over 6 hours ▪ Blunt trauma < 12 hours after admit and 8 units PRBCs already transfused ▪ Hepatic failure with GI bleeding or pending invasive procedure	YES	40 mcg/kg IV × 1

†All indications *except* ICH or traumatic head injury: May repeat same dose in 1 hour. May be given sooner per physician discretion but no sooner than 20 minutes after first dose.

Notes
▪ Dose will be rounded to nearest 1200-mcg increment.
▪ For IV bolus administration only (give over 2–5 minutes). Should not be mixed with infusion solutions or be given in an IV drip. Must be used within 3 hours of reconstitution.

Physician/Credentialed Practitioner Signature _____

Date ____/____/____ Time_____

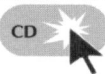

Figure 5-1. Courtesy of St. Mary's Medical Center, Duluth, MN.

Managing Anticoagulation Patients in the Hospital: The Inpatient Anticoagulation Service

Anticoagulation Bridging Guidelines

Background

It is a frequent occurrence that patients who are on long-term warfarin therapy will need a temporary discontinuation of therapy to facilitate invasive procedures. Literature recently published on this subject give us some new guidance on how this should be done.

Which Patients Should Receive Bridging Therapy?

A frequent misconception is that all patients who have sub-therapeutic INRs need anticoagulation bridge therapy. On the other hand, it is also common for clinicians not to bridge any patients who take warfarin to prevent strokes from atrial fibrillation. Neither of these types of "cookbook" approaches are appropriate when deciding whether to use or not to use bridge therapy. On the contrary, clinicians must weigh the risk of bridge therapy (bleeding) versus the risk of thrombosis and its potentially devastating consequences for each patient. In other words, the patient must be treated as an individual, not as a population.

The following tables are meant to offer some guidance to clinicians to accomplish this difficult task. The charts help identify which patient should be bridged and how they should be bridged. They are derived from other health-system recommendations that have been published in the literature. **Please note these are guidelines only and it is quite possible and likely that deviation from these guidelines may be necessary and appropriate when caring for an individual patient.**

Figure 5-2. Table 1.

Guidelines for Perioperative Management of Patients with Noncardiac Disease Who Receive Oral Anticoagulation

Acute Episode	Before Surgery	After Surgery[g]
Venous Thromboembolism[a]		
Within 2 weeks	Consider retrievable IVC filter[b] + IV UFH[c]	Consider retrievable IVC filter[b] + IV UFH[c]
Within 1 month	IV UFH[c]	IV UFH[c]
Within 2–3 months		
High risk[d]	IV UFH[c]	IV UFH[c]
Moderate risk[e]	IV UFH[c] or enoxaparin 1 mg/kg sc bid or enoxaparin 1.5 mg/kg sc daily	IV UFH[c] or enoxaparin 1 mg/kg sc bid or enoxaparin 1.5 mg/kg sc daily
Low risk[f]	None	IV UFH[c] or enoxaparin 1 mg/kg sc bid or enoxaparin 1.5 mg/kg sc daily
> 3 months	None	sc UFH 5000 units q 8 or 12 hours or enoxaparin 40 mg sc daily or 30 mg sc bid ± GPS or IPS
Arterial Thromboembolism[a]		
Within 1 month	IV UFH	IV UFH,[c] only if low bleeding risk
> 1 month	None	sc UFH 5000 units q 8 or 12 hours or enoxaparin 40 mg sc daily or 30 mg sc bid ± GPS or IPS

IVC = inferior vena cava; UFH = unfractionated heparin; GPS = graduated compression stockings; IPS = intermittent pneumatic compression.

[a]Elective surgery should be avoided in the first month after a venous or arterial thromboembolic event.

Continued

Figure 5-2. Courtesy of St. Mary's Medical Center, Duluth, MN.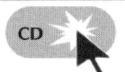

[b]Consider IVC filter also if risk of perioperative bleeding with IV UFH is high during the first month of acute thromboembolic episode; call radiology for all IVC filter questions.
[c]IV heparin per standard SMDC inpatient infusion orders.
[d]High risk indicates patients with multiple episodes of venous thromboembolism, a hereditary or acquired hypercoagulable state, or active cancer.
[e]Moderate risk indicates patients with other risk factors for thromboembolism (e.g., chronic heart failure, renal failure, acute illness).
[f]Low risk indicates all other patients.
[g]Postoperative anticoagulation should not be started until 12–24 hours after the procedure when hemostasis is achieved when bleeding risk if low. **In contrast, if the bleeding risk of the procedure is felt to be high (e.g., craniotomy, spinal surgery, partial organ removals, etc.), consideration should be given to administering reduced doses of LMWH or UFH or holding therapy until the bleeding risk subsides.** It is strongly recommended to discuss the appropriate time to restart therapy with the surgeon.

Figure 5-2. Table 2.
Guidelines for Perioperative Management of Patients with Cardiac Disease Who Receive Oral Anticoagulation

Disease	Before Surgery	After Surgery[c]
Atrial Fibrillation		
High Risk[a]	IV UFH or enoxaparin 1 mg/kg sc bid	IV UFH or enoxaparin 1 mg/kg sc bid
Low Risk[b]	None	sc UFH 5000 units q 8 or 12 hours or enoxaparin 40 mg sc daily or 30 mg sc bid ± GPS or IPS
Heart Valves		
Mechanical prosthesis		
Caged-ball, any position	IV UFH or enoxaparin 1 mg/kg sc bid	IV UFH or enoxaparin 1 mg/kg sc bid
Mitral valve position	IV UFH or enoxaparin 1 mg/kg sc bid	IV UFH or enoxaparin 1 mg/kg sc bid
Mitral and aortic valves	IV UFH or enoxaparin 1 mg/kg sc bid	IV UFH or enoxaparin 1 mg/kg sc bid
Aortic position with LVD	IV UFH or enoxaparin 1 mg/kg sc bid	IV UFH or enoxaparin 1 mg/kg sc bid
Aortic position with atrial fibrillation	IV UFH or enoxaparin 1 mg/kg sc bid	IV UFH or enoxaparin 1 mg/kg sc bid
Aortic position in NSR, no LVD, and left atrium is of normal size	None or IV UFH or enoxaparin 1 mg/kg sc bid	None or IV UFH or enoxaparin 1 mg/kg sc bid
Bioprosthesis (either position)	None	sc UFH 5000 units q 8 or 12 hours or enoxaparin 40 mg sc daily or 30 mg sc bid ± GPS or IPS
With associated atrial fibrillation	IV UFH or enoxaparin 1 mg/kg sc bid	IV UFH or enoxaparin 1 mg/kg sc bid

UFH = unfractionated heparin; GPS = graduated compression stockings; IPS = intermittent pneumatic compression; LVD = left ventricular dysfunction.
[a]High risk indicates patients with severe LVD (ejection fraction < 25%), clinically significant rheumatic heart disease, previous thromboembolic events within 6 months, status post cardioversion, or severe left atrial enlargement.
[b]Low risk includes all other patients.
[c] Post-operative anticoagulation should not be started until 12–24 hours after the procedure when hemostasis is achieved when bleeding risk is low. **In contrast, if the bleeding risk of the procedure is felt to be high (e.g., craniotomy, spinal surgery, partial organ removals, etc.), consideration should be given to administering reduced doses of LMWH or UFH or holding therapy until the bleeding risk subsides.** It is strongly recommended to discuss the appropriate time to restart therapy with the surgeon.

Figure 5-2. Table 3.
Anticoagulation Bridging Procedures

Anticoagulation Bridging Procedures
Enoxaparin needs to be dose-adjusted for estimated creatinine clearance (CrCl) < 30 mL/min to 1 mg/kg sc daily or unfractionated heparin should be used. To estimate CrCl from serum creatinine (SrCr): 1. Estimate lean body weight (LBW). Men→50 + 2.3 (inches > in height than 60)=LBW; Women →45.5 + 2.3 (inches > in height than 60) = LBW 2. Estimate clearance. Men→[(140-age)LBW]/[(72)(SrCr*)] = CrCl; Women→(Men's result)(0.85) = CrCl 3. Call a pharmacist at St. Mary's Medical Center if you need assistance with this calculation

*In patients older than 65, use 1 for SrCr if it is < 1 to avoid overestimating clearance.

Heparin may also be used subcutaneous in therapeutic doses, but aPTTs need to be drawn and the dose adjusted based on these results. A typical dose would be 500 units/kilogram/day in two to three divided doses with aPPT checked 4–6 hours after each dose and then daily when in range. The therapeutic aPPT range depends on the lab; check with the lab for their recommended range. Please call hematology/oncology for assistance with these patients.

Heparin and low molecular weight heparin should **NOT** be used for bridging patients with a history of heparin-induced thrombocytopenia. Please call hematology/oncology for specific recommendations in these patients.

According to the American Society of Regional Anesthesia, "Indwelling (spinal) catheters should be removed prior to initiation of LMWH thromboprophylaxis." Prophylactic doses of heparin are considered compatible with neuraxial analgesia.

Figure 5-2. Table 4.
Dosing Schedules Relative to Surgery

- Once patient is classified into a risk group and their bridging therapy of choice is decided, it is time to determine the dosing schedule.
- If a patient is on aspirin therapy, it should be discontinued 7 days before the surgery, and warfarin should then be discontinued 4–5 days prior. An INR should be checked 24–48 hours after the warfarin is stopped, and prior to starting the LMWH or UFH. From this INR, clinicians will be able to estimate when the INR will start to be subtherapeutic. This will likely be 2–3 days prior to surgery, and the LMWH or UFH should be started at that time, according to the appropriate therapeutic doses listed in the table above. If it is difficult to predict when the INR will be low, a daily INR should be checked to determine the start date of LMWH or UFH.
- One day prior to surgery, the INR should be checked. If it is still >1.5, vitamin K may need to be administered to reverse the anticoagulant effects. Please refer to the Warfarin Reversal Guidelines on the SMDC intranet for dosing guidelines of vitamin K.
- If patient is receiving enoxaparin as an outpatient, the patient should administer the last dose 12–24 hours (24 hours for 1.5 mg/kg enoxaparin dose) prior to surgery. If the surgery is scheduled for early morning, the evening dose the day prior should be held. If patient is receiving UFH as an inpatient, the heparin should be discontinued 5 hours prior to surgery.
- After surgery, if patient has achieved adequate hemostasis, warfarin should be restarted the evening after surgery at the patient's previously determined maintenance dose. If the bleeding risk is low, LMWH or UFH should be restarted at the dose provided above at 12–24 hours after surgery if hemostasis is achieved. **However, if the bleeding risk of the procedure is high, consideration should be given to administering reduced doses of LMWH or UFH or holding therapy until the bleeding risk subsides. LMWH or UFH should be discontinued when INR is >2.0 for at least 2 days.**

Figure 5-2. Table 5.
Timeline for Dosing of Warfarin and Enoxaparin in Relationship to Surgery

Timeline	Treatment Action
7 days prior to surgery	Stop aspirin or other antiplatelets (clopidogrel, ticlopidine, etc.)
4–5 days prior to surgery	Stop warfarin
24 to 48 hours after stopping warfarin	Check INR
2–3 days prior to surgery (or when INR is sub-therapeutic)	Start enoxaparin or UFH at appropriate dose
1 day prior to surgery	Give last pre-op enoxaparin dose 12–24 (24 hours for 1.5 mg/kg enoxaparin dose) hours prior to surgery (patients with morning surgeries will need to hold their evening dose the night before), or stop UFH at least 5 hours prior to surgery. INR should be checked to determine if vitamin K will need to be given
Surgery day	INR should be re-checked if it was above surgery goal the day prior. Start warfarin in the evening at maintenance dose, if hemodynamically stable.
1 day after surgery	Start enoxaparin or UFH dosing 12–24 hours after surgery, if bleeding risk is low. **In contrast, if the bleeding risk of the procedure is felt to be high (e.g., craniotomy, spinal surgery, partial organ removals, etc.), consideration should be given to administering reduced doses of LMWH or UFH or holding therapy until the bleeding risk subsides.** It is strongly recommended to discuss the appropriate time to restart therapy with the surgeon.
5–6 days after surgery	Stop enoxaparin or UFH after INR is >2 for 2 days.

Spyropoulos AC, Jenkins P, Bornikova L. A disease management protocol for outpatients perioperative bridge therapy with enoxaparin in patients requiring temporary interruption of long-term oral anticoagulation. *Pharmacotherapy.* 2004;24(5):649-58.

Douketis JD, Johnson JA, Turpie AG. Low-molecular-weight heparin as bridging anticoagulation during interruption of warfarin. *Arch Intern Med.* 2004;164:1319-26.

Pharmacy Policy and Procedure Example for Pharmacist-Managed Warfarin Dosing

PHARMACY POLICY AND PROCEDURE

Policy No._____

DEPARTMENT: Pharmacy
SECTION: Pharmacy Practice
SUBJECT: Pharmacist Managed Warfarin Dosing

PURPOSE: To provide guidelines to inpatient pharmacists for independently dosing warfarin when delegated that authority by physicians

POLICY/PROCEDURE:

I. Eligible patients:
   1. Patients will be eligible for this program if a physician has written an order for "Warfarin Dosing Per Pharmacy," "warfarin per pharmacy," "warfarin monitoring per pharmacy" or any other similar order.
   2. Patients will also be eligible for this program if a preprinted ordered is received indicating a checked/circled warfarin consultation (may be worded as warfarin dosing consult).
   3. If the pharmacist is unclear of the intent of the physician orders, they are to contact the physician for clarification.

II. Expectations of the pharmacist when an order for pharmacist managed warfarin order is received:
   1. Pharmacist will immediately assume the responsibility for assuring the patient's warfarin is dosed on a daily basis.
   2. Pharmacist will order baseline and daily INR levels under the authority of the Pharmacy and Therapeutics Committee if not already ordered.
   3. Pharmacist will utilize the Pharmacy and Therapeutics Committee approved "Anticoagulation Guidelines" for this service, but all final-dosing decisions will be based on the clinical judgment of the pharmacist. The pharmacist will seek physician input when needed.
   4. Pharmacist will always notify the original physician who consulted the pharmacy for warfarin management (or covering MD) when:
      - INR levels are >6
      - Any time clinically significant signs of thrombosis or bleeding are being reported
      - Any time they need further clarification of the clinical status of the patient
   5. Pharmacist will be expected to review all anticoagulation needs of their patients and discuss untreated needs with the physician and document in the chart using a modified SOAP note.
   6. Chart documentation will include an initial SOAP note and follow-up SOAP notes when a when significant issues occur. For the follow up notes, the pharmacist should communicate any major issues to the consulting physician verbally before leaving documentation. Examples if issues necessitating a follow-up SOAP notes are, but not limited to:
      - Significant warfarin adjustment is needed to manage a drug-drug interaction
      - Pharmacist intervention to avoid a drug-drug interaction
      - Documentation of how interruption of warfarin will be handled for an invasive procedure
      - Bleeding of thromboembolism events are reported
      - Recommendations for warfarin reversal are requested
   7. If a physician writes an order for warfarin on a pharmacist managed patient without writing an order to resume dosing responsibility, the pharmacist is expected to contact the physician to clarify who is managing the warfarin therapy.

Continued

Figure 5-3.

8. Pharmacist will fax a history of his or her inpatient warfarin dosing to the clinic responsible for the outpatient anticoagulation of the patient to assure continuity of care.
9. Pharmacist will be responsible for writing discharge order for the patient's warfarin therapy up to the first outpatient INR check set by the physician.
10. The pharmacist should assess if the follow-up INR date is appropriate. The recommendation for a follow-up INR for a new warfarin start is within 3 days. For chronic patients, a recheck should happen within 1 week. The pharmacist may exercise clinical judgment when follow-up plans outside of these times are desired.
11. Pharmacist will assist the provider in completing the anticoagulation discharge follow-up orders.

III. Expectations of the physician when delegating the authority to dose warfarin to the pharmacy.
1. Physician will maintain all ability to order warfarin if desired, however, they will be expected to write an order such as "Physician to manage/dose warfarin therapy" to indicate to the pharmacist that they are resuming dosing responsibility if previously delegated to the pharmacist.
2. Physician is still responsible for the overall anticoagulation needs of the patient, however, the pharmacist will assist the physician in this regard.
3. Physician should speak with the pharmacist anytime they are concerned with how the pharmacist is managing warfarin therapy for a patient.
4. Physician is expected to relate (verbal or progress note) to the pharmacist any pressing clinical concerns they have that could contribute to the pharmacist's clinical decision making.
5. Physician will be responsible for ordering the first outpatient INR, but the pharmacist will be responsible for dosing the warfarin up to that visit.
6. Physician is responsible for signing anticoagulation discharge orders.

Managing Anticoagulation Patients in the Hospital: The Inpatient Anticoagulation Service

Conservative Warfarin Initiation Algorithm[8]

Day	INR	Warfarin Dose, mg
1		5
2		5
3	<1.5	10
	1.5–1.9	5
	2–3	2.5
	>3	0
4	<1.5	10
	1.5–1.9	7.5
	2-3	5
	>3	0
5	<2	10
	2-3	5
	>3	0
6	<1.5	12.5
	1.5–1.9	10
	2–3	7.5
	>3	0

Figure 5-4.

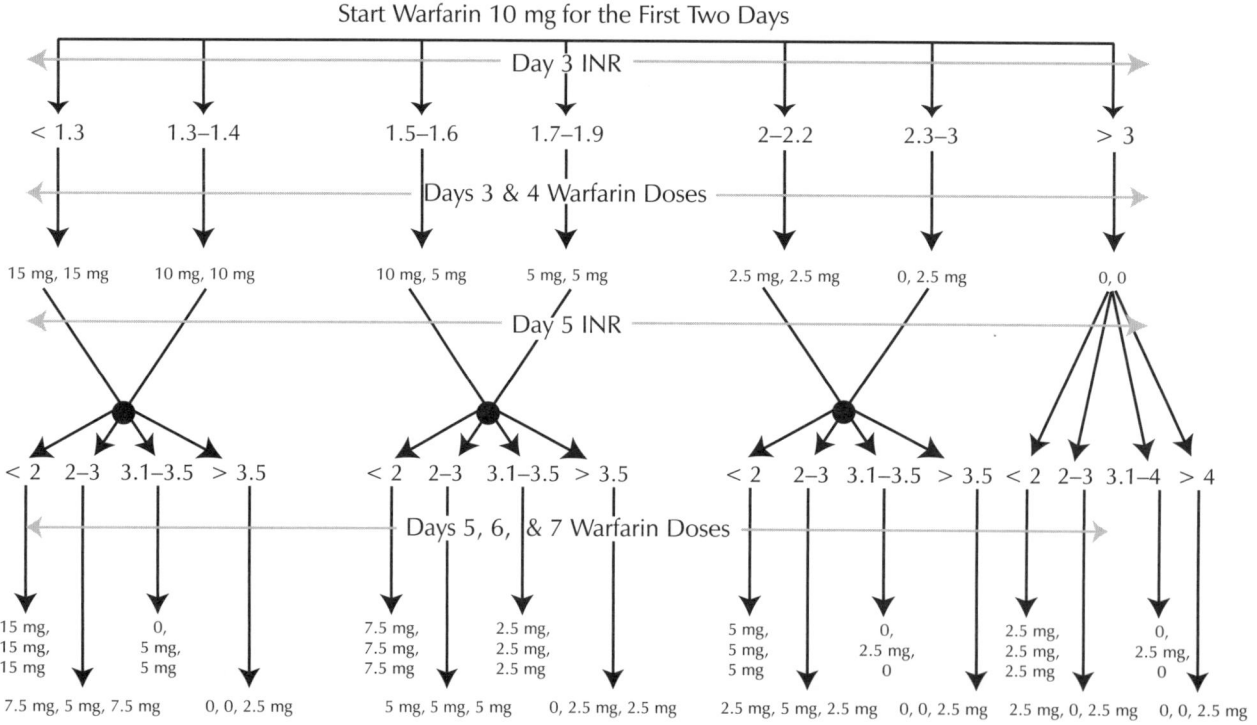

Figure 5-5. *It was studied in outpatient venous thromboembolism patients and is likely too aggressive for most hospitalized patients.[10]

Chapter 5 ■ Winning Support for the Inpatient Anticoagulation Service

Anticoagulation Discharge Follow-up Orders

ANTICOAGULATION FORM FOR ALL WARFARIN/COUMADIN PATIENTS

M.D./ PHARMACIST/NURSE TO COMPLETE:
Patient Discharge Diagnosis: _____

Diagnosis/Reason for Anticoagulation Therapy: _____

Length of Treatment for Warfarin: _____

Target INR Range: (if different from protocol): _____

Warfarin (Coumadin) Education Completed by Nurse/Pharmacist:
    Patient/family educated on medication
    Given warfarin (Coumadin) booklet
    Warfarin (Coumadin) prescription given to patient
    Patient given specific warfarin (coumadin) dose instructions until next INR
    Patient knows date and location of next protime/INR lab appointment
Nurse/Pharmacist Signature:_____

Low Molecular Weight Heparin (LMWH) Enoxaparin Education Completed by Nurse/Pharmacist:
    Patient/family viewed LMWH video
    Abdominal SQ injections reviewed with patient/family
    Patient/family verbalized/demonstrated ability to properly self-inject
    Low Molecular Weight Heparin discharge kit given to patient
    Low Molecular Weight Heparin prescription given to patient
    Patient given specific written/verbal dosage instructions
Nurse/Pharmacist Signature:_____

Physician/Anticoagulation Clinic to
Manage Warfarin/Coumadin on discharge:_____
_____

M.D. / Pharmacist / Nurse to complete:
Follow Up Protime Lab/INR Due Date:_____

Follow-Up Clinic/Lab Appointment Scheduled by HUC on Discharge:
Date/Time/Location:_____

DISCHARGE ANTICOAGULATION DOSAGE: To be completed by M.D./Pharmacist

Warfarin Tablet Size:_____

Dose_____Orally until next INR

Enoxaparin Dose:_____Sub Q until next INR

HUC TO FAX FOLLOWING INFORMATION TO ABOVE CLINIC/PHYSICIAN:
(see back of form for phone/fax numbers)
    1. **Completed Protime Flow Sheet**
    2. **Complete Discharge Medication List**
    3. **Interagency referral form (if applicable)**
    4. **Copy of this form**
HUC SIGNATURE:_____
Date/Time materials faxed:_____

Physician Signature:_____
Date:_____

Figure 5-6. Courtesy of St. Mary's Medical Center, Duluth, MN.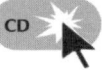

Managing Anticoagulation Patients in the Hospital: The Inpatient Anticoagulation Service

Warfarin Discharge Work Checklist

Patient Going Home
- ___ If patient has previously been on warfarin at home, verify tablet strength and amount of supply.
- ___ If the patient needs more tablets or has just started on warfarin for this admission, write a prescription on a prescription blank for warfarin if not already done. Write for approximately a 30-day supply and use the MD responsible for anticoagulation name and cosign the script.
- ___ Assure the "Anticoagulation Discharge Follow-Up Orders" are in the chart and fill out the pertinent sections.
- ___ Write the patient's home warfarin dose on the discharge instructions sheet.
- ___ Assure that a follow up INR has been arranged at a reasonable interval. (i.e., 2–3 days post discharge in a new patient or unstable patient, 1 week in a stable patient)
  - Avoid all outpatient INR draws on weekends and holidays. If it must be done in extraordinary circumstances, an outpatient provider MUST take responsibility for the patient.
- ___ Complete the patient's warfarin education by letting them know:
  - What strength tablet you have prescribed
  - How many tablets and milligrams they need to take each day
  - When their next INR is scheduled
  - When to start the warfarin at-home program
- ___ Include in the discharge summary what strength tablet the patient will be utilizing.
- ___ Print out an updated discharge summary profile for your patient including discharge dosing and follow up INR plan.
- ___ Fax our discharge summary sheet to the outpatient managing clinic/MD.

Patient Going to an Institutional Setting
- ___ Write an order for warfarin on the interagency transfer orders. BE SURE TO STATE WHEN THE NEXT DOSE OF WARFARIN IS DUE IN YOUR ORDER.
- ___ Assure an INR has been ordered at an appropriate interval. If not ordered or not an appropriate interval (i.e., 2–3 days post discharge in a new patient or unstable patient, 1 week in a stable patient) be sure to work with the warfarin attending MD to resolve the problem.
- ___ Write for today's warfarin dose in the physician orders.
  - Avoid all outpatient INR draws on weekends and holidays. If it must be done in extraordinary circumstances, an outpatient provider MUST take responsibility for the patient.
- ___ Assure the "Anticoagulation Discharge Follow-Up Orders" are in the chart and fill out the pertinent sections.
- ___ Print out an updated discharge summary profile for your patient including discharge dosing and follow up INR plan.
- ___ Fax our discharge summary sheet to the outpatient managing clinic/MD.

Figure 5-7.

Chapter 5 ■ Winning Support for the Inpatient Anticoagulation Service

Daily INR Policy

PHARMACY POLICY AND PROCEDURE MANUAL

Policy No._____

DEPARTMENT: Pharmacy
SECTION: Pharmacy Practice
SUBJECT: Warfarin Anticoagulation

PURPOSE: To assure the safety and timeliness of warfarin anticoagulation for the acute care areas

POLICY:
I. Warfarin administration in the acute care setting requires daily INR monitoring and dosing.

II. Warfarin is to be administered at 1700. A clinician (including pharmacists for patients for whom they are dosing warfarin) can overwrite the administration time according to clinical judgment.

PROCEDURE:
I. This policy applies to the acute care areas. Subacute areas are not covered by this policy.

II. Expectations of the pharmacist when they receive on order for warfarin in the acute care setting:
   1. Pharmacist will not accept warfarin orders of more than 24-hour duration. When the pharmacist receives a warfarin order for >24 hours duration, they will write an order in the chart stating SMDC policy requires warfarin to be dosed daily based on daily INRs.
   2. The pharmacist will order daily INRs if not already ordered.
   3. The pharmacist may elect to honor the first 24-hour dose of a warfarin order > 24 hours in duration if they feel it is appropriate given the patient's INR, clinical status, etc.
      - Example: An atrial fibrillation patient is admitted for pneumonia to the medical unit. They are not started on any significantly interacting medications. They are stable on warfarin 5 mg oral daily at home. Their admit INR is 2.5. The physician orders 5 mg of warfarin daily. In this case, the pharmacist may elect to honor the first 5 mg of this order since it is reasonable. However, further warfarin will need to be dosed daily based on a daily INR after this first day. In the case, the pharmacist should write an order for "Warfarin 5 mg oral today, further dosing will be dosed daily based on daily INRs by SMDC policy." They would also assure daily INRs have been ordered.
      - If a pharmacist does not think the first dose is appropriate, they shall contact the prescriber and recommend an alternative dose.
   4. A pharmacist shall personally contact the physician or on-call partner responsible for anticoagulation whenever an order for greater than 24 hours of warfarin is encountered. This contact should take place before 1700 the following day.
   5. Anytime a warfarin order is received or it appears a patient may need to restart warfarin at sometime in the future, the pharmacist will enter an order on the patient's MAR reminding the nurse to look for the day's warfarin dose.
   6. Whenever a pharmacist feels a patient needs anticoagulation and is not currently receiving therapy, this will be discussed with the responsible prescriber.

Figure 5-8. Courtesy of St. Mary's Medical Center, Duluth, MN.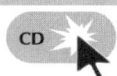

Managing Anticoagulation Patients in the Hospital: The Inpatient Anticoagulation Service

Vitamin K Use Policy

PHARMACY POLICY AND PROCEDURE MANUAL

Policy No._____

DEPARTMENT: Pharmacy
SECTION: Pharmacy Practice
SUBJECT: Vitamin K orders

PURPOSE: To assure the safest and most effective route of vitamin K is utilized

POLICY:
I. Oral vitamin K is the preferred route of administration whenever it is possible.

II. All orders for intramuscular (excluding use in neonates) and subcutaneous vitamin K will be automatically substituted by the pharmacy to oral vitamin K whenever possible.

III. All orders for intramuscular (excluding use in neonates) will be automatically substituted by the pharmacy to subcutaneous vitamin K if patients CANNOT take oral.

IV. All orders for intravenous vitamin K will be immediately dispensed and given via slow IV infusion.

PROCEDURE:
I. This policy applies to all hospital areas in the Saint Mary's/Duluth Clinic Health System serviced by the Department of Pharmacy.

II. Expectations of the pharmacist when they receive an order for intramuscular (excluding neonate use) and subcutaneous vitamin K.
   a. Pharmacist will review chart and/or consult with nursing personnel to determine if oral administration is possible. Factors to consider:
      - Patient is taking PO (clear liquids at minimum), or NG is usable, or feeding tube is usable
      - No abnormal GI absorption (low aspiration risk, no need for bowel rest, no obstruction, no vomiting, no continuous GI suction, no malabsorption syndrome)
   b. If oral administration is possible, the pharmacist will dispense oral vitamin K in the same milligram strength of the subcutaneous or IM order. The parenteral form of vitamin K will be used orally if needed for small doses of vitamin K (i.e., 1 mg).
      - Example: Pharmacist receives an order for vitamin K 5 mg subcutaneous. Vitamin K 5 mg orally will be substituted.
      - Example: Pharmacist receives an order for vitamin K 1 mg subcutaneous. Vitamin K 1 mg orally will be substituted. The parenteral product will be administered orally in this situation
   c. When this auto-substitution occurs, the pharmacist will write an order or call an order to the RN noting this substitution has occurred on behalf of the pharmacy and therapeutics committee.
   d. In the rare event the pharmacist receives an order for intramuscular and the oral route is not possible, the pharmacist will dispense subcutaneous vitamin K in the same milligram strength of the subcutaneous or IM order.
   e. When this auto-substitution occurs, the pharmacist will write an order or call an order to the RN noting this substitution has occurred on behalf of the pharmacy and therapeutics committee.
   f. Orders for subcutaneous vitamin K WILL BE DISPENSED when the patient CANNOT take oral.

III. There will be no auto-substitution of IV vitamin K. When IV vitamin K is ordered, it will be dispensed in a 50-mL piggyback to be given by slow IV infusion over 30 minutes.

IV. All pharmacists and physicians should refer to the "SMDC Vitamin K-Warfarin Reversal Guidelines" for detailed guidance on how to optimally dose and deliver vitamin K.

V. A physician can circumvent this policy at any time by writing "Dispense as written" or "DAW" in their vitamin K orders.

Figure 5-9. Courtesy of St. Mary's Medical Center, Duluth, MN.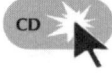

Chapter 5 ■ Winning Support for the Inpatient Anticoagulation Service
Warfarin Anticoagulation Reversal Guidelines

I. Caveats (see later sections for specific recommendations)

General
- Remember that patients receive anticoagulation to prevent **life-threatening thrombosis.**
- Consider the patient's **future anticoagulation needs when planning the reversal of warfarin anticoagulation.**

Vitamin K
- The effect of vitamin K on reversing warfarin anticoagulation is **delayed**, reaching its full effect at about **24 hours**.
- Excessively **large doses** of vitamin K **do not** reverse anticoagulation faster and may cause weeks of warfarin resistance. Any dose of vitamin K greater than **10 mg** should be considered excessive
- **Oral vitamin K** is the preferred preparation to be used in most situations.
- **Oral vitamin K** is **more** predictable in its bioavailability and has a **quicker onset** of action than subcutaneous vitamin K; it also offers additional **convenience** and **safety** in comparison to other dosage forms.
- **Intramuscular vitamin K** will not be used per SMDC policy to avoid hematoma risk.
- **Intravenous vitamin K** has a more predictable response and faster onset of action than other forms of vitamin K. However, IV vitamin K may cause **anaphylaxis** and slow infusion rates have never been proven to prevent anaphylaxis. It should be diluted in 50 mL and given via **piggyback infusion** over at least **30 minutes**. It is the **preferred route of administration** for **severe** bleeding situations.
- **Subcutaneous vitamin K** is not as effective on a mg-to-mg basis as IV vitamin K and does not work as quickly; but it does not carry the anaphylaxis risk of IV vitamin K. It is an alternative when a patient cannot take oral vitamin K and the situation is not emergent.

Fresh Frozen Plasma (FFP)
- FFP is a blood product containing a concentration of clotting factors. All of the risks of blood product transfusions apply to FFP.
- FFP replaces depleted clotting factors and is therefore the fastest way to reverse warfarin anticoagulation. It begins to work **immediately** with a full effect in **6 hours.**
- FFP is usually given in doses of **2 to 4 units** and is repeated every **6 to 12 hours** as needed. **4 units** should be used in a severe bleeding situation.

Continued

Figure 5-10. Courtesy of St. Mary's Medical Center, Duluth, MN.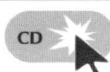

Managing Anticoagulation Patients in the Hospital: The Inpatient Anticoagulation Service

II. Management of overanticoagulation in patients without bleeding

	INR above target but less than 5	

Lower the dose or omit the dose, monitor more frequently, and resume therapy at a lower dose when the INR is at a therapeutic level.

	INR 5 to 9	
	Low Thrombotic Risk[2]	*High Thrombotic Risk[3]*
No risk factors for bleeding[1]	Omit the next 1 to 2 doses of warfarin.	Omit the next 1 to 2 doses of warfarin.
Risk factors for bleeding present[1]	Hold warfarin, give 1 to 2.5 mg oral vitamin K.	Omit the next 1 to 2 doses of warfarin and monitor closely for bleeding OR hold warfarin, give 1 to 2.5 mg oral vitamin K.

	INR greater than 9	
	Low Thrombotic Risk[2]	*High Thrombotic Risk[3]*
No risk factors for bleeding[1]	Hold warfarin, give 5 mg oral vitamin K	Hold warfarin, give 5 mg oral vitamin K
Risk factors for bleeding present[1]	Hold warfarin, give 10 mg oral vitamin K	Hold warfarin, give 5 to 10 mg oral vitamin K

In all above cases, monitor more frequently and resume therapy at a lower dose when the INR is at a therapeutic level if a reversible reason for the elevation cannot be identified

1. Risk factors for bleeding: History of GI bleed (not peptic ulcer disease WITHOUT bleeding), hypertension, cerebrovascular disease, ischemic stroke, congestive heart failure, renal insufficiency, concurrent aspirin, age greater than 75 years, and recent major surgery.

2. Low thrombotic risk:	Atrial fibrillation WITHOUT: <ul><li>history of severe left ventricular dysfunction (ejection fraction less than 25%)</li><li>clinically significant rheumatic heart disease</li><li>previous thromboembolic events within 6 months</li><li>cardioversion in the last month</li><li>bioprosthetic heart valve</li><li>severe left atrial enlargement</li></ul>
	More than 1 month since arterial thromboembolism
	Deep vein thrombosis prophylaxis
	More than 3 months since deep vein thrombosis or pulmonary embolism
3. High thrombotic risk:	Atrial fibrillation WITH: <ul><li>history of severe left ventricular dysfunction (ejection fraction less than 25%)</li><li>clinically significant rheumatic heart disease</li><li>previous thromboembolic events within 6 months</li><li>cardioversion in the last month</li><li>bioprosthetic heart valve</li><li>severe left atrial enlargement</li></ul> Less than 1 month since arterial thromboembolism Mechanical heart valves Less than 3 months since deep vein thrombosis or pulmonary embolism

Continued

Chapter 5 ■ Winning Support for the Inpatient Anticoagulation Service

III. Management of anticoagulated patients with bleeding

Minor bleeding:
- INR is low or in target range: make no changes and observe carefully
- INR above target but less than 5 (high): adjust warfarin appropriately, no vitamin K
- INR 5 to 9 (very high): hold warfarin, give 1 to 2.5 mg oral vitamin K
- INR greater than 9 (critical high): hold warfarin, give 5 to 10 mg oral vitamin K

Major bleeding:
- Any INR: clinical circumstances such as the severity of bleeding, risk of thrombosis, and the INR value will dictate the course of action. Generally in this situation the advice would be to hold warfarin, give 4 units FFP, and supplement FFP with 10 mg vitamin K by slow piggyback IV infusion over at least 30 minutes

In all above cases, monitor more frequently and resume therapy at a lower dose when the INR is at a therapeutic level if a reversible reason for the elevation cannot be identified.

<u>Minor bleeding example: bleeding gums</u>
<u>Major bleeding example: major GI bleed, CNS bleed, retroperitoneal bleed, etc.</u>

IV. Management of anticoagulated patients for emergent invasive procedures

Important facts to remember:
1. The peak effect of vitamin K on reversing warfarin anticoagulation takes 24 hours although you may start to see effects in 6 to 12 hours.
2. FFP replaces depleted clotting factors and is therefore the fastest way to reverse warfarin anticoagulation. It begins to work immediately with a full effect in 6 hours.

Low surgical risk of bleeding:
Goal is low therapeutic INR (INR—2 to 2.5)
- INR above target but less than 5: hold warfarin, consider giving 2.5 mg oral vitamin K, consider giving FFP
- INR 5 to 9 (very high): hold warfarin, give 2.5 mg oral vitamin K, consider giving FFP
- INR greater than 9 (critical high): hold warfarin, give 5 mg oral vitamin K, consider giving FFP

In all cases, recheck INR in 12 hours and re-administer vitamin K and/or FFP if needed.

Moderate surgical risk of bleeding:
Goal is subtherapeutic INR (INR ≤ 1.5)
- INR above 1.5 but less than upper target range: hold warfarin, give 2.5 mg oral vitamin K, consider giving FFP
- INR above target but less than 5: hold warfarin, give 2.5 mg oral vitamin K and FFP
- INR 5 to 9 (very high): hold warfarin, give 5 to 10 mg oral vitamin K and FFP
- INR greater than 9 (critical high): hold warfarin, give 10 mg oral vitamin K and FFP

In all cases, recheck INR in 12 hours and re-administer vitamin K and/or FFP if needed.

High surgical risk of bleeding:
Goal is complete reversal of anticoagulation (INR = 1)
- Hold warfarin, give FFP and 10 mg oral vitamin K

In all cases, recheck INR in 12 hours and re-administer vitamin K and/or FFP if needed.

Refer to the SMDC bridging guidelines for appropriate management of emergent invasive procedure patients post-op.

Low surgical risk of bleeding example: accessible laceration of the arm.
Moderate surgical risk of bleeding example: major abdominal surgery (bowel resection).
High surgical risk of bleeding example: brain surgery.

Continued

References

1. Ansell J, Hirsh J, Poller L, et al. The pharmacology and management of the vitamin K antagonists. *Chest.* 2004;126;204S-33S.
2. Crowther MA, Douketis JD, Schnurr T, et al. Oral vitamin K lowers the international normalized ratio more rapidly than subcutaneous vitamin K in the treatment of warfarin-associated coagulopathy. *Ann Intern Med.* 2002;137:251-4.
3. Whitling AM, Bussey HI, Lyons RM. Comparing different routes and doses of phytonadione for reversing excessive anticoagulation. *Arch Intern Med.* 1998;158:2136-40.

Direct Thrombin Inhibitor Orders Can Easily Be Adapted for Other Direct Thrombin Inhibitors

Direct Thrombin Inhibitor Orders

Please note that these orders are intended for treatment of patients who need immediate therapeutic anticoagulation and a heparin product is not appropriate (history and/or current heparin induced thrombocytopenia, anaphylaxis to heparin, etc.) THIS IS NOT INTENDED FOR USE IN THE CARDIAC CATHETERIZATION LABORATORY OR DURING BYPASS SURGERY; please consult hematology for guidance when a direct thrombin inhibitor is needed in these specialized situations.

INTRAVENOUS ARGATROBAN
1. Patient actual body weight _____ kg.
2. Draw baseline hematology profile, INR, bilirubin, albumin, and PTT.
3. Daily platelet and PTT
4. Hematology profile every 5 days while on argatroban
5. Start argatroban IV infusion at _____ mcg/kg/min (usual dose for HIT or therapeutic anticoagulation is 2 mcg/kg/min; if moderate to severe hepatic function [example: Child-Pugh class B or C], usual dose is 0.5 mcg/kg/min)
6. Notify pharmacy to dose and monitor the argatroban infusion. Pharmacy will order dose titrations and extra PTTs that may be needed.
7. Discontinue all heparin and low molecular weight heparin products **INCLUDING HEPARIN FLUSHES.**
8. If a pulmonary artery catheter (heparin coated) is being utilized, arrange removal.
9. PTT at 2 hours after start of infusion and daily. Review PTT results with a pharmacist for dose guidance.
10. Notify physician if bleeding or excessive bruising occurs.
11. Hematology consult? ____ yes ____ no   (if yes, please complete consult form)

_____
Physician/Credentialed Practitioner Signature

_____/_____/_____
      Date

Figure 5-11. Courtesy of St. Mary's Medical Center, Duluth, MN.

Managing Anticoagulation Patients in the Hospital: The Inpatient Anticoagulation Service

Policy and Procedure for Pharmacy to Dose Direct Thrombin Inhibitors

PHARMACY POLICY AND PROCEDURE MANUAL

Policy No._____

DEPARTMENT: Pharmacy
SECTION: Pharmacy Practice
SUBJECT: Pharmacist Managed Direct Thrombin Inhibitor Dosing

PURPOSE: To provide guidelines to SMMC inpatient pharmacists for independently dosing the direct thrombin inhibitors (DTI) argatroban when delegated that authority by physicians

POLICY/PROCEDURE:

I. Eligible patients:
   1. Patients will be eligible for this program if a physician has written an order for "argatroban per pharmacy," argatroban dosing per pharmacy," "direct thrombin inhibitor per pharmacy," or a similar order.
   2. Patients are also eligible anytime the direct thrombin inhibitor standing orders are utilized.
   3. If the pharmacist is unclear of the intent of the physician orders, he or she is to contact the physician for clarification.

II. Expectations of the pharmacist when an order for pharmacist managed direct thrombin inhibitor order is received:
   1. Pharmacist will immediately assume the responsibility for assuring the patient's direct thrombin inhibitor is correctly dosed.
   2. Pharmacist will assure the direct thrombin inhibitor standing orders have been utilized and order any necessary labs for the monitoring of the direct thrombin inhibitor under the authority of the Pharmacy and Therapeutics Committee.
   3. Pharmacist will utilize the Pharmacy and Therapeutics Committee approved "Direct Thrombin Inhibitor Guidelines" for this service, but all final dosing decisions will be based on the clinical judgment of the pharmacist. The pharmacist will seek physician input when needed.
   4. Pharmacist will always notify the original/responsible physician who consulted the pharmacy for DTI management (or covering MD) when:
      - clinically significant signs of thrombosis or bleeding are being reported.
      - he or she needs further clarification of the clinical status of the patient.
   5. Pharmacists will be expected to review all anticoagulation needs of their patients and discuss untreated needs with the physician. This specifically includes having knowledge of how to handle direct thrombin inhibitors in the setting of heparin-induced thrombocytopenia.
   6. Pharmacist will be expected to review all anticoagulation needs of his or her patients and discuss untreated needs with the physician and document in the chart using a modified SOAP note.
   7. Chart documentation will include an initial SOAP note and follow-up SOAP notes when significant issues occur. For the follow-up notes, the pharmacist should communicate any major issues to the consulting physician verbally before leaving documentation.
   8. If a physician writes an order for a new dose of a direct thrombin inhibitor on a pharmacist-managed patient without writing an order to resume dosing responsibility, the pharmacist is expected to contact the physician to clarify who is managing the direct thrombin inhibitor therapy.

III. Expectations of the physician when delegating the authority to dose DTI to the pharmacy:
   1. Physician will maintain all ability to order the direct thrombin inhibitor if desired, however, he or she will be expected to write an order such as "Physician to manage/dose argatroban therapy" to indicate to the pharmacist that he or she is resuming dosing responsibility if previously delegated to the pharmacist.

Continued

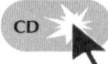

Figure 5-12. Courtesy of St. Mary's Medical Center, Duluth, MN.

2. Physician is still responsible for the overall anticoagulation needs of the patient, however, the pharmacist will assist the physician in this regard.
3. Physician should speak with the pharmacist anytime he or she is concerned with how the pharmacist is managing the direct thrombin inhibitor therapy for a patient.
4. Physician is expected to communicate (verbal or progress note) to the pharmacist any pressing clinical concerns he or she has that could contribute to the pharmacist's clinical decision making.
5. The physician shall have the sole authority to decide when to initiate and discontinue therapy, but the pharmacist will be available to advise the physician in this regard.

Managing Anticoagulation Patients in the Hospital: The Inpatient Anticoagulation Service

Dosing Guidelines and Monitoring Form for Argatroban Anticoagulation that Can Be Modified to Other Direct Thrombin Inhibitors

MD _____
Baseline PTT _____
aPTT Goal
(usual 1.5–3× baseline)
_____

HT _____
ABW _____

ARGATROBAN

DATE	TIME	PLT COUNT	aPTT	INFUSION RATE		RPH	WARFARIN DOSE	INR
				mcg/kg/min	ml/hr			

Continued

Figure 5-13. Courtesy of St. Mary's Medical Center, Duluth, MN.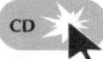

Indication—Prophylaxis or treatment of thrombosis in patients with immune-mediated heparin-induced thrombocytopenia (HIT). Also for patients with or at risk of HIT undergoing percutaneous coronary intervention (PCI).

Contraindications—Overt, major bleeding or previous hypersensitivity to argatroban

I. **BASELINE LABS NEEDED**—aPTT, INR, platelet count, bilirubin, albumin

II. **INITIAL DOSE** (If active thrombosis, <u>start ASAP</u> after heparin stopped. If no active thrombosis, may consider allowing 3–4 hours after heparin stopped to initiate or 10 hours after last therapeutic enoxaparin dose)

   A. Package insert recommends 2 mcg/kg/min continuous IV infusion (no bolus required); mean dose in trials was 1.6–1.7 mcg/kg/min
   B. **Hepatic dysfunction** (including but not limited to: cirrhosis, hepatitis, fatty liver)
      0.5 mcg/kg/min continuous IV infusion

III. **MONITORING**
   - The aPTT should be monitored 2 hours after infusion started, and 2–3 hours after a dose increase. Order aPTT every morning if stabilized.
   - Platelets should be checked daily (counts should improve within 3–4 days)

IV. **DOSAGE ADJUSTMENTS**
   - Titrate infusion to achieve an aPTT that is 1.5–3x the baseline level, not to exceed 100 seconds, titrate toward the lower range for those at risk of bleeding without a thrombus, and toward the higher range in those not at risk of bleeding with a thrombus
   - Dose increases in increments of 0.5 mcg/kg/min are typical, <u>unless</u> the initial dose is 0.5 mcg/kg/min in which increments of 0.25 mcg/kg/min are warranted.
   - **Doses of greater than 10 mcg/kg/min have not been formally studied (rarely should a dose exceeding 3.5 mcg/kg/min be required)**

V. **OVERDOSAGE / EXCESSIVE ANTICOAGULATION**
   - May be controlled by discontinuing the infusion or decreasing the infusion rate, depending on clinical situation and aPTT level. The aPTT should return to baseline within 2–4 hours after infusion stopped, but may take longer in patients with hepatic dysfunction.
   - No specific antidote is available, therefore if overdose occurs and emergent bleeding develops, blood transfusions may be required.

VI. **CONCOMITANT ADMINISTRATION WITH WARFARIN**
   Warfarin should not be started until the platelets are at least 100,000 and argatroban should not be discontinued before the platelets have reached a stable plateau. The combination of argatroban and warfarin results in an elevation of the INR, however this is a "false" elevation of the lab measurement and does not necessarily increase the risk of bleeding. Our warfarin dosing guidelines can still be used, but you will be trying to push the INRs higher than usual. Should only give vitamin K, FFP, or platelets if <u>life-threatening</u> bleeding occurs since these patients are at very high risk of developing both venous and arterial clots.

   A. With argatroban doses less than or equal to **2 mcg/kg/min**, argatroban can be discontinued when the INR is greater than 4, which generally corresponds to a "true" INR of 2–3. An INR should be drawn 4–6 hours after the argatroban infusion is stopped to make sure the INR is therapeutic. If the INR is subtherapeutic, the previous infusion rate should be restarted and the process repeated the following day.
   B. For argatroban doses greater than **2 mcg/kg/min**, the prolongation of the INR is less predictable, therefore it is recommended that when the INR exceeds 4, the infusion rate should be lowered to 2 mcg/kg/min for 4–6 hours at which time an INR should be drawn. If that INR is greater than 4, the above parameters (section A) should be followed; if less than 4, increase infusion as clinically needed.

Please remember these are only guidelines and you must use your clinical judgment when adjusting every rate depending on other clinical variables with each patient.

Managing Anticoagulation Patients in the Hospital: The Inpatient Anticoagulation Service

HEPARIN PROTOCOL
-- Clinical Pharmacist Guidelines --

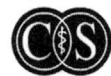

CEDARS·SINAI MEDICAL CENTER.
Department of Pharmacy Services

HEPARIN PROTOCOL
-- **Clinical Pharmacist Guidelines** --

I. PURPOSE: To establish guidelines for the management of heparin therapy by pharmacists. Heparin per Pharmacy is initiated by a physician's order for "heparin protocol", "heparin per pharmacy", or similar language.

> Note: Whenever the anticoagulation protocol order falls outside of the approved guidelines (e.g., unapproved indications, patients with severe hypercoagulable states), the pharmacist will communicate with the prescriber that the patient does not meet the P&T approved criteria for anticoagulation protocol and that the patient would be better managed by the attending physician. If the prescriber requests a PTT range that is outside the approved guidelines, the pharmacist may NOT accept the order. Rather, the physician should be contacted to change goal to *within* protocol range (78 to 115 seconds **OR** 70 to 101 seconds, based on the current thromboplastin batch - see section V.D.), as approved by the P&T Committee. (Incidentally, the thromboplastin reagent in the lab changes annually around June and we will communicate revised ranges when they become available annually.) The pharmacist can offer to attempt to achieve PTT values as close as possible to the requested goal. Likewise, if the requested range is < 20 seconds wide **AND** is outside the protocol range (see above and section V.D.), the pharmacist may NOT accept the order. The pharmacist should recommend increasing the range to ≥ 20 seconds (and within the protocol range), as approved by the P&T Committee.
> In either scenario, if the physician refuses to change the range, the pharmacist must decline the request to follow the patient per protocol

II. INITIAL ORDERS

  A. The following patient information should be obtained: patient's diagnoses and indication for anticoagulation; patient height, weight, age and gender. If unavailable in the chart, height and weight may be obtained by patient interview or by estimation. Note prescribing physician's name and phone # to facilitate communication when needed.

  B. For heparin therapy, ascertain whether a heparin drip, often started in the ER, is already infusing. Check for contraindications to heparin therapy.

  C. For heparin therapy ordered for treatment of CVA or TIA, a head CT result confirming absence of CNS bleed must be available

  D. Order baseline (pre-heparin loading dose) INR & PTT on a STAT basis, unless these have been obtained within the previous 24-48 hours.

  E. Order CBC (no diff) at least every other day, unless such an order already exists.
  For patients receiving heparin for acute coronary syndromes or immediately post-CABG, order CBC daily. In order to reduce the number of duplicate phlebotomy sticks, check before ordering the CBC to see if one has already been ordered.

Continued

Figure 5-14. Courtesy of Cedars-Sinai Medical Center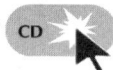

HEPARIN PROTOCOL
-- Clinical Pharmacist Guidelines --

F. Order: **NO** intramuscular injections. If the patient is receiving intramuscular medications, consult with the physician before initiating anticoagulation.

G. It is recommended that patients on continuous infusion heparin receive no concurrent aspirin at doses >162mg/day unless treated for a cardiac indication. For cardiac patients, any concurrent order for any dose of scheduled aspirin is OK.
For **non-cardiac** patients on aspirin doses exceeding 162mg/day, the pharmacist is to call the physician and inform him of the potential interaction. If the physician is not immediately available, a message should be left, but should not cause a delay in starting heparin. At the pharmacist's discretion, a supplemental Dear Doctor Note may be added as well.

H. If the patient is receiving an NSAID, contact the physician and determine if he/she would like it discontinued due to increased risk for bleeding. If the patient is ordered an NSAID during therapy, the pharmacist is to contact the physician and remind him/her that the patient is on IV heparin and that the NSAID poses an increased risk for bleeding.

I. If the patient is to be started on warfarin, order a daily INR.

III. INITIATING HEPARIN THERAPY

A. Loading Dose of Heparin [if one has not already been given and an infusion has not been started in the ER]:

NOTE:
- **No** loading dose for patients with CVA or TIA.
- **No** loading dose for patients who have been on warfarin prior to admission and have a baseline INR $\geq$ 1.4 (e.g. patients admitted for surgery). If no baseline INR is available, do not give loading dose if patient has taken warfarin within the last two days.

   1. For venous thromboembolism (DVT or PE): 80 units/kg IV push.
   2. For obese (i.e. >20% above ideal body weight) patients, use a corrected body weight (50% between IBW and TBW).
   3. Maximum loading dose for obese patients: 10,000 units
   4. Round off loading dose to nearest 1,000 units.

B. Initial Maintenance Infusion for Heparin:
   1. Heparin ordered as 25,000 units in 500 cc D5W or 0.45% NaCl (for diabetics with poorly controlled blood sugars).
   2. Initial infusion rate is dependent upon the patient's height, weight (use TBW), and sex (see attached Tables 1-A and 1-B).

Continued

HEPARIN PROTOCOL
-- Clinical Pharmacist Guidelines --

TABLE 1-A: INITIAL INFUSION RATES FOR HEPARIN (not ACS) - MALES (from AJHP 1985;42:1965)

Total Weight	Height in inches							
	5 ft.	5 ft 2 in.	5 ft. 4 in.	5 ft. 6 in.	5 ft. 8 in.	5 ft. 10 in.	6 ft.	6 ft. 2 in.
100lb = 45kg	850	850	900	950	1000	1050	1100	1150
110lb = 50kg	900	900	950	1000	1050	1050	1100	1150
120lb = 55kg	900	950	1000	1000	1050	1100	1150	1200
130lb = 59kg	950	1000	1000	1050	1100	1150	1200	1250
140lb = 64kg	1000	1000	1050	1100	1150	1200	1250	1250
150lb = 68kg	1000	1050	1100	1150	1150	1200	1250	1300
160lb = 73kg	1050	1100	1150	1150	1200	1250	1250	1300
170lb = 77kg	1100	1150	1150	1200	1250	1300	1350	1400
180lb = 82kg	1150	1150	1200	1250	1300	1300	1350	1400
190lb = 86kg	1150	1200	1250	1300	1300	1350	1400	1450
200lb = 91kg	1200	1250	1300	1300	1350	1400	1450	1500
210lb = 95kg	1250	1300	1300	1350	1400	1450	1500	1550
220lb = 100kg	1300	1300	1350	1400	1450	1450	1500	1550
230lb = 105kg	1300	1350	1400	1400	1450	1500	1550	1600
240lb = 109kg	1350	1400	1400	1450	1500	1550	1600	1650
250lb = 114kg	1400	1400	1450	1500	1550	1600	1650	1650
260lb = 118kg	1450	1450	1500	1550	1550	1600	1650	1700
270lb = 123kg	1450	1500	1550	1550	1600	1650	1700	1750
280lb = 127kg	1500	1550	1550	1600	1650	1700	1750	1800
290lb = 132kg	1550	1550	1600	1650	1700	1750	1750	1800
300lb =136kg	1550	1600	1650	1700	1700	1750	1800	1850
310lb =141kg	1600	1650	1700	1700	1750	1800	1850	1900

TABLE 1-B: INITIAL INFUSION RATES FOR HEPARIN (not ACS) - FEMALES (from AJHP 1985;42:1965)

Total Weight	Height in inches							
	5 ft.	5 ft 2 in.	5 ft. 4 in.	5 ft. 6 in.	5 ft. 8 in.	5 ft. 10 in.	6 ft.	6 ft. 2 in
80lb = 36kg	650	700	750	750	800	850	900	950
90lb = 41kg	700	750	750	800	850	900	950	950
100lb = 45kg	750	750	800	850	900	900	950	1000
110lb = 50kg	750	800	850	900	900	950	1000	1050
120lb = 55kg	800	850	900	900	950	1000	1050	1100
130lb = 59kg	850	900	900	950	1000	1050	1100	1100
140lb = 64kg	900	900	950	1000	1050	1050	1100	1150
150lb = 68kg	900	950	1000	1050	1050	1100	1150	1200
160lb = 73kg	950	1000	1050	1050	1100	1150	1200	1250
170lb = 77kg	1000	1050	1050	1100	1150	1200	1250	1300
180lb = 82kg	1050	1050	1100	1150	1200	1200	1250	1300
190lb = 86kg	1050	1100	1150	1200	1200	1250	1300	1350
200lb = 91kg	1100	1150	1200	1200	1250	1300	1350	1400
210lb = 95kg	1150	1200	1200	1250	1300	1350	1400	1450
220lb = 100kg	1200	1200	1250	1300	1350	1350	1400	1450
230lb = 105kg	1200	1250	1300	1350	1350	1400	1450	1500
240lb = 109kg	1250	1300	1350	1350	1400	1450	1500	1550
250lb = 114kg	1300	1350	1350	1400	1450	1500	1550	1600
260lb = 118kg	1350	1350	1400	1450	1500	1500	1550	1600
270lb = 123kg	1400	1400	1450	1500	1500	1550	1600	1650
280lb = 127kg	1400	1450	1500	1500	1550	1600	1650	1700
290lb = 132kg	1450	1500	1500	1550	1600	1650	1700	1750

3. Order rate in units/hr AND cc/hr. ALWAYS SPELL OUT "units."
4. Clearly specify infusion solution concentration if not the standard 50 units/mL concentration.

Continued

HEPARIN PROTOCOL
-- Clinical Pharmacist Guidelines --

     5.   If the initial infusion rate was written by the MD **AND**
- a. The initial infusion rate is within 15% of the infusion rate the protocol calls for (from Table 1-A or Table 1-B), wait and react to the PTT that was ordered If the resultant PTT is not within the desired range, use Table 2 or 3 listed in V.D. (depending on PTT goal) to adjust the infusion rate. If the PTT is far from desired range, the infusion rate may be adjusted to the infusion rate the protocol called for (from Table 1-A or 1-B)
- b. If the difference between the initial infusion rate ordered by the MD and the one per protocol table is ≥ 15%, cancel the PTT ordered and change the infusion rate to that called for by the protocol (from Table 1-A or 1-B)
- c. At any time, if there is no bolus (or re-bolus), order a PTT four (4) hours after infusion rate change

C. **FOR ACS** (unstable angina, ST elevation MI, non-ST elevation MI) ONLY
1. Loading dose
   - **a. 60 units/kg IV push**
   - b. Round off loading dose to nearest 1,000 units
   - c. Maximum loading dose: 5,000 units
2. Initial maintenance infusion
   - a. Heparin ordered in D5W or 0.45% NaCl as above
   - b. **12 units/kg/hour** based on adjusted body weight

D. For **acute** CVA, stroke in evolution, TIA or similar diagnoses (regardless of history/presence of atrial fibrillation/flutter) use the **Higher Bleeding Risk category** dosage adjustments

IV. **FOLLOW-UP**

A. Order a PTT 6 to 8 hours after initiation of heparin infusion if a bolus is given. If no bolus is administered, order a PTT 4 hours after the start of the infusion. If the infusion is begun late in the evening (e.g. after 8pm), consider ordering the PTT with morning labs.

B. If ordered by the physician, initiate warfarin therapy by protocol. Note: warfarin doses are administered at 1800 per Medical Center policy.
1. If patient is NPO, consult with physician.
2. If heparin is initiated after 1800, order the first dose of warfarin to be given within 6 hours of the start of heparin.
3. Follow warfarin protocol on subsequent hospital days.

C. Initiate an Anticoagulation Monitoring Form (see attachment).

D. Enter a complete note into the Progress Note section of the patient's medical record at initiation of therapy, on a daily basis, and for each action taken (e.g. PTT result and heparin infusion rate adjustment). Refer to the Pharmacy Policy and Procedure for Chart Notes for more information.

E. In addition, make an entry into the Interdisciplinary Plan of Care in the medical chart at initiation and discontinuation of heparin therapy and for significant events (e.g. bleeding complication) or patient education

Continued

Managing Anticoagulation Patients in the Hospital: The Inpatient Anticoagulation Service

HEPARIN PROTOCOL
-- Clinical Pharmacist Guidelines --

    F.   Continue to assess patient's bleeding risk and thrombosis risk daily. In addition, review patient's medication list daily for potentially interacting medications (e.g. NSAIDS, COX-2 inhibitors, etc.)

V.   LABORATORY RESULTS

    A.   Monitor PTT, platelet counts, hemoglobin, hematocrit as required by the protocol.
        1.   If the platelet count falls >30% from baseline (is usually diagnosed at > 50%) or falls below 100,000, contact the MD to discuss the possibility of heparin-induced thrombocytopenia (HIT). Alternative therapies (e.g. lepirudin, argatroban) may be discussed.
        2.   If the H/H drops significantly, review carefully for potential signs/symptoms consistent with bleeding complications; contact MD

    B.   Monitor PTT (and PT/INR if patient concurrently on Warfarin per Pharmacy) result as defined in these guidelines to titrate heparin infusion rate as per guidelines to achieve and maintain therapeutic PTTs within 24hrs (and therapeutic INR on day 4 for warfarin).

    C.   Use Table 2 or 3 to adjust the infusion rates and reorder PTTs. Round off infusion rates to the nearest 50 units/hr.

    D.   NOTE: Table 2 will be used the majority of the time. This table aims to achieve a PTT of 78 to 115 seconds.

        If the physician requests "conservative" dosing, or uses other language suggesting a desire to achieve lower levels of anticoagulation, Table 3 may be used. Additionally, for patients with ACS or any post-AMI patient who has received fibrinolytic therapy or for **acute** CVA, stroke in evolution, TIA or similar diagnoses (regardless of history/presence of atrial fibrillation/flutter), use the **Higher Bleeding Risk category** dosage adjustments in Table 3. This table aims to achieve a PTT of 70 to 101 seconds.
        If other ranges are provided by the physician as a goal, the pharmacist should contact the physician and suggest one or the other goal ranges from these two tables.

TABLE 2: DOSAGE CHANGES FOR HEPARIN PROTOCOL (Adapted from Arch Int Med 1992;152:1589)
Goal aPTT: 78 to 115 seconds

APTT (sec)	HOLD INFUSION	RATE ADJUSTMENT	NEXT APTT
< 60	= = = =	↑ 2.5 u/kg/hr	4 hr
61-77	= = = =	↑ 1 u/kg/hr	4 hr
78-115	= = = =	no change	next AM
116-132	60 min.	↓ 1 u/kg/hr	4 hr
> 132	60 min.	↓ 2.5 u/kg/hr	4 hr

Round off any infusion rate to nearest 50 unit/hr increment.

Continued

HEPARIN PROTOCOL
-- Clinical Pharmacist Guidelines --

TABLE 3: DOSAGE CHANGES FOR PATIENTS AT HIGHER BLEEDING RISK OR ACUTE CORONARY SYNDROME (Adapted from Chest 1998;114:561s-578s, Am J Med 2001;110:641-50)

Goal aPTT: 70 to 101 seconds

APTT (sec)	HOLD INFUSION	RATE ADJUSTMENT	NEXT APTT
< 57	= = = =	↑ 3 u/kg/hr	4 hr
57-69	= = = =	↑ 1.5 u/kg/hr	4 hr
70-101	= = = =	no change	next AM
102-114	60 min.	↓ 1.5 u/kg/hr	4 hr
> 114	60 min.	↓ 3 u/kg/hr	4 hr

Round off any infusion rate to nearest 50 unit/hr increment.

* Both tables adjusted for difference in CSMC aPTT

E. Pharmacist must investigate reasons for spuriously high or low aPTTs.
   1. Surprisingly low PTTs may occur due to:
      a. RN held heparin during IVPB administration.
      b. Heparin line clotted or disconnected from patient.
      c. Heparin held for procedure.
      d. Incorrect infusion given.
      e. PTT drawn at low end of circadian rhythm (about 1500) according to Hull et al (1992), where the mean PTT at 1500 was approximately 10 seconds lower than at the maximum PTT.
      f. Drug interaction (e.g. IV nitroglycerin).

   2. Surprisingly high PTTs may occur due to:
      a. Larger than expected effect from warfarin (expect 2-5 second increase).
      b. PTT drawn from heparin line with insufficient flush given.
      c. Incorrect infusion given
      d. PTT drawn at high end of circadian rhythm (about 0300, according to Hull et al (1992), the mean PTT at 0300 was approximately 10 seconds higher than at the minimum PTT.
      e. PTT drawn too early after bolus.

F. If a patient has two consecutive PTT readings of > 101 seconds (> 94 seconds for high risk patients), inform the physician. Note that nurses are instructed to contact the physician with reports of any active bleeding.

VI. **DISCONTINUING HEPARIN THERAPY**

   A. For venous thromboembolic indications, after a minimum of 5 days of heparin given concurrently with warfarin, if the INR has been within the desired range (INR 2.0-3.0 or 2.5-3.5, depending on indication) for at least 2 days, notify the physician to discontinue the heparin.

Continued

HEPARIN PROTOCOL
-- Clinical Pharmacist Guidelines --

    B.   If platelet count falls by ≥ 30% from baseline (even if the total count is >150,000) or falls below 100,000, contact the physician to suggest that this might be heparin-induced thrombocytopenia (HIT). Although rare, HIT is associated with a 25% risk of mortality and a 25% risk of amputation, due to coagulopathy. Although it usually occurs 6 to 12 days after starting heparin, it can occur earlier (e.g. day 1 or 2) if the patient has been exposed to heparin within the prior 3 months. . Additionally, rather than just discontinuing the heparin, the physician should be reminded that the patient should receive some other type of non-cross reacting anticoagulation (lepirudin or argatroban) as they are hypercoagulable. Also, warfarin therapy should not be initiated until the patient is adequately anticoagulated with the alternative anticoagulant; if the patient was receiving warfarin therapy at the time they presumptively developed HIT, the warfarin therapy should be suspended until the patient is adequately anticoagulated with the alternative anticoagulant, as they should be considered hypercoagulable until "therapeutically" anticoagulated

    C.   Document these actions in your chart note.

VII.   CANDIDATES FOR DISCHARGE FOR OUTPATIENT TREATMENT WITH LMWH

    A.   POPULATION: Adult patients requiring continued anticoagulation for treatment of DVT or uncomplicated PE meeting criteria for outpatient treatment with LMWH following 24 to 48 hours of treatment with IV Heparin (refer to Medical Center VTE Guideline).

    B.   GUIDELINES:

1. Admission to the Medical Center for initiation of IV (unfractionated) heparin as defined above. IV heparin should be continued for a minimum of 24-48 hours in the inpatient setting while the patient is being evaluated for outpatient therapy with LMWH

2. Oral anticoagulation therapy with warfarin should begin the evening of the first hospital day following diagnosis and initiation of heparin therapy, as described above.

3. The patient is assessed by the physician as a candidate for completion of the course of parenteral anticoagulation as an outpatient, based on the criteria in G4 of the VTE Guideline.

4. If the patient is determined to be a candidate for outpatient therapy after 24-48 hours of IV heparin therapy, LMWH shall be initiated in this manner
   - IV heparin is discontinued and the first dose of LMWH is administered between 30 and 60 minutes after the discontinuation.
   - LMWH dosage regimen: dalteparin 200 IU/kg SQ once daily
   - the patient is discharged after appropriate follow-up has been arranged: patient to be seen daily in MD office, clinic, procedure center or by home care nurses for the duration of LMWH therapy for clinical assessment, LMWH administration and labs, including INR

5. Therapy with LMWH is continued until the INR goal range (of 2.0 to 3.0 or 2.5 to 3.5) is attained with warfarin for 2 days AND the patient has received at least 5 days of parenteral (heparin plus LMWH) anticoagulation therapy.

Continued

Chapter 5 ■ Winning Support for the Inpatient Anticoagulation Service

HEPARIN PROTOCOL
-- Clinical Pharmacist Guidelines --

VIII. CLINICAL SUPPORT

The following individuals are available to provide assistance with this protocol and anticoagulation therapy management:

1. After-Hours Clinical Call: Pager #3092 (long-range: 310-790-0113) *(Alternating Manny or Hai)*
2. Hai Tran, Pharm.D. – Clinical Coordinator
    - pager #3092 (long-range: 310-790-0113); office phone ext: 31496
3. Frank Saya, Pharm.D. – Inpatient Manager
    - Office phone: ext: 35611
4. Manny Saltiel, Pharm.D. – Drug Information Pharmacist
    - Office phone: ext: 33784; pager #0948
5. Sylvia Martin-Stone, Pharm.D. – MUE Pharmacist – M-Th 0900-1500
    - Office phone: ext: 32890; pager# 1931
6. Wayne Schwartz, Pharm.D. – Clinical Pharmacist
7. Doug Douglas, Pharm.D. – Clinical Pharmacist

Appendix – Perioperative Management of Heparin Therapy[1]

- Pre-Op:
  Discontinue IV heparin 6 hours before surgery
  Discontinue SQ heparin 12 hours before surgery

- Post-Op:
  Restart IV heparin infusion (with no loading dose) or SQ heparin 12 hours post-operatively, longer if there is any evidence of bleeding from surgical site

Chapter 6

Justifying the Program to Hospital Administration: The Financial Perspective

Michael Gulseth

Chapter Outline

- Introduction
- Budget considerations for the pharmacy manager/director
- Conducting an economic assessment to justify starting an inpatient anticoagulation program
- Business plan development
  - Executive summary
  - Background and business description
- Market analysis
- Operational structure and processes
- Financial projections
- Implementation action plan
- Conclusion/references
- Making the pitch
- Conclusion
- Case study

Introduction

In Chapter 4 it was suggested that other options should be explored before pharmacy approaches hospital administration to add pharmacists to start an inpatient anticoagulation service. Other ideas included taking pharmacist duties away or reassigning them to technicians and hiring pharmacy students to help make pharmacists more efficient. However, many departments will have to hire more pharmacists to successfully launch a service. The purpose of this chapter is to provide the tools to help the program manager and pharmacy director to justify increased pharmacist staffing when other options have been exhausted.

Most business proposals that require a monetary investment also have the potential to generate revenue to cover the cost. This is how many other proposals for increased services in a health-system are justified as they will create more payment for services. Outpatient anticoagulation clinics have been justified, at least in part, in this fashion for years.[1]

The fundamental problem for pharmacists is that it is the difficulty in generating revenue in the inpatient setting for cognitive services because pharmacists are not universally considered providers (like nurse practitioners and physician assistants) by payers like Medicare Part B. Even the much-touted Medication Therapy Management Services that are supposed to be covered under Medicare Part D are only aimed at outpatients. Some hospital pharmacy departments have shown limited ways they have been able to generate revenue from cognitive services, but this is the exception, not the rule.[2]

Due to this current reality of pharmacy practice, this chapter will attempt to justify the addition of pharmacist resources in a different way than increasing revenue. Instead, justification will be based on improved patient outcomes (see Chapter 2 for literature review), the more efficient use of nurses and physicians, the decreased cost of managing bleeding and thromboembolic complications (see Chapter 2), and risk management. Unfortunately, many people with business acumen will call this a "soft dollar" argument because if dollars are spent in the proposed area, spending will need to be cut in another area to maintain the bottom line. Therefore, the argument needs to be made in as compelling a way as possible to overcome this huge hurdle.

Budget Considerations for the Pharmacy Manager/Director

A question that every program manager and pharmacy director will have to answer is how much time is needed by pharmacists to manage each patient. This is the only way to estimate how much additional staffing is needed. An answer to this question cannot be readily found in the literature and is further affected by the complexity of each individual patient and the scope of the service. Nonetheless, the time can be estimated based on other hospitals who have implemented the service or from pilot projects of such a service. On average, each warfarin patient managed and dosed by an inpatient pharmacist takes about 10–15 minutes each day depending on case mix and complexity at St. Mary's Medical Center in Duluth, MN. At the same hospital, evaluating the appropriate dosing of new low-molecular-weight heparin start takes 5 minutes on average. Each heparin aPTT evaluation and dosing took an estimated average time of 5–10 minutes at Fairview Southdale Hospital in Edina, MN. Again, all these values are estimates but can give a program manager and pharmacy director an idea of how much pharmacist time will need to be devoted to the service.

For most hospitals, other monetary investments into an inpatient anticoagulation program will be minimal. Considerations include more computers if an electronic system in tracking and monitoring patients is desired or funds to purchase personal data assistants (PDAs).[3] If the department wishes to have software written to organize the service, this may take additional resources. Patient education materials may also be needed, but many hospitals have separate budgets for patient education. Very few capital expenditures will likely be needed as an inpatient anticoagulation service provides care at the bedside and patient care units where most needed materials are readily available.

Conducting an Economic Assessment to Justify Starting an Inpatient Anticoagulation Program

Due to the difficulty with reimbursement of pharmacists for clinical services, providing a compelling financial argument based on cost savings is needed. The following steps for conducting this analysis are roughly adapted from the chapter "Evaluating and Justifying Clinical Pharmacy Services" in *Pharmacoeconomics and Outcomes*, published by American College of Clinical Pharmacy.[4] For a more in-depth discussion of justifying a clinical pharmacy service, this text is highly recommended. A case study accompanies each number demonstrating each point for an actual inpatient anticoagulation service.

1. *Decide how to structure the evaluation*
   Ideally, an evaluation of this type should compare the financial costs of the program to the potential benefits of the program. If one measures the benefits in terms of clinical outcomes (e.g., cost per pulmonary embolism prevented), it is a cost-effectiveness analysis. If one measures the benefits in terms of humanistic outcomes (e.g., cost per quality of life unit), it is a cost-utility analysis. For the purposes of justifying a clinical pharmacy program, some type of cost-benefit analysis is desirable.

   A cost-benefit analysis compares the costs of providing a service to the costs avoided by provision of this service. In other words, the clinical benefit is evaluated in a monetary fashion. Ideally, the service that is measured should be compared to a control (e.g., not having the service) to be considered a formal economic analysis. Just like any study involving pharmaceuticals, this is needed to establish causality. For example, the increased costs of a program could be compared to the input costs of not having a program (the input costs of not having a program will likely be $0). Then the difference in economic outcomes can be measured between the two groups based on things like Medicare charges.

   Performing rigorous cost-benefit economic analysis likely needs to be done in the confines of a research project, and this may be possible for some hospitals. Ideally, this is the best way to justify a new pharmacy service as the benefit in the institution seeking the program will be proven, but many will not have the substantial resources or expertise needed necessary to conduct this formal of an analysis. Other strategies are presented below to overcome this hurdle.

2. *Perspective of the analysis*
   Any pharmacoeconomic analysis must consider the perspective of the study. In other words, when estimating costs, whose costs are they? When estimating benefits, benefits to who? Common perspectives chosen in pharmacoeconomic analysis include society, insurance

companies, or hospitals. This chapter's Case Study will use the hospital's perspective when evaluating costs and benefits of the program as this will be the primary concern of any administrator over pharmacy.

3. *Measurement of resources*
Since this evaluation will be done from the hospital's perspective, the cost of the resources necessary to conduct the program must be estimated. Costs are typically broken into fixed and variable costs. Fixed costs are largely start-up costs and costs for equipment and overhead. These costs do not vary for each patient served. Variable costs are costs that occur with each patient served and include things like salary/benefits and patient education materials. Examples of the two types of cost that must be included in a financial analysis are shown in Table 6-1.[4,5]

4. *Measurement of outcomes*
Since a cost-benefit analysis framework will be utilized, the measurement of outcomes will be in the form of monetary resources saved. This is most applicable to patients who's hospitalization is being reimbursed in a capitated fashion like Medicare patients. Money saved with the implementation of an inpatient anticoagulation service would be any costs that occur in delivering care to a hospitalized patient outside of physician costs. Examples would include medication costs, nursing costs, and laboratory costs.

5. *Picking a study design*
Most institutions would have a very difficult time performing a full-blown randomized trial with a control group due to the expense and complexity of these studies. An excellent alternative to these studies are known as *quasiexperimental* trials. In a quasiexperimental trial, two non-randomized groups are compared at baseline to assure the groups are comparable. Then, the intervention is implemented in the experimental group and the differences in outcomes are noted. One way to do this would be to first identify two hospitalist teams that manage similar patient populations. Then take one team and let the physicians manage their patients in the usual care fashion. For the other team, have all of their anticoagulation patients managed by the pharmacists. Then, estimate the economic value of the program by comparing resource utilization. If an inpatient anticoagulation program has already been implemented or piloted in an area, a before service implementation and after service implementation design could also be used. In a before and after implementation design, the before group serves as the control group and the after group serves as the intervention group. Then the changes in costs and monetary resource utilization would be compared.

Even the above suggested study designs would take considerable time and effort to execute. What should be done to justify the program for hospitals that do not have the resources to conduct these types of analysis? While a rigorous evaluation is recommended whenever possible, if one is simply looking to conduct a quick analysis to support the program, literature generalization can be used (this is what is done in the Case Study accompanying this chapter). Literature generalization, in this case, involves taking data already published on the economic benefit of an inpatient anticoagulation program and generalizing it to one's practice site. It is important to assure the researched patients are similar to those encountered at the practice site. This data can be combined with known local site data when preparing the analysis.

When extrapolating literature to a practice site, it is important to be mindful of the analysis drawbacks. For example, many feel the quality of published economic analysis of clinical pharmacy services is mediocre.[4] It should be obvious that extrapolating poor quality data to a practice site is problematic. Another example

Table 6-1.
Fixed and Variable Costs to Consider in an Inpatient Anticoagulation Service[4,5]

Fixed Costs	Variable Costs
Computers/technology needed for start up	Wages for employees
Furniture/desk equipment	Benefits paid for employees
Overhead expenses assessed (would vary by institution)	Patient educational materials
Pharmacist education	

is that skill levels of pharmacists could lead to differences in care delivery at the institution trying to justify the program when compared to the program in the article. A third issue is that the financial numbers may be very old and will need to be adjusted for inflation. Finally, practice could have changed substantially since the analysis was conducted. Any financial analysis for an inpatient anticoagulation program based on literature extrapolation should address the preceding points to assure the reader understands the inherent assumptions.

6. *Sensitivity or statistical analysis*
All completed financial analysis should undergo statistical and sensitivity analysis when appropriate. For statistical analysis, care should be taken to select the appropriate test based on the data collected (i.e., nominal vs. continuous data, parametric vs. nonparametric data). Consultation with a biostatistician may be considered. Sensitivity analysis is necessary as much of the data used may be estimates only. For example, if economic data is to be projected into the future, the effects of inflation must be considered. Since the inflation rate in medical care has varied from 3%–5% over the last 10 years, it would be advisable to run the financial analysis for different inflation rates and see if benefits remain. This should be done for any economic measures that are open for uncertainty.[6]

7. *Analyze and include the financial analysis in a business plan*
When the analysis is complete, it should be carefully analyzed and reviewed by others. Were all possible costs and monetary outcomes considered? Was inflation accounted for? Were statistical tests used when needed? Were important data prone to uncertainty analyzed by sensitivity analysis? Were the critical assumptions of the analysis stated? Were study limitations included? After one is confident the financial analysis is appropriate, it should be included as the centerpiece of a business plan to be presented to hospital administration.

Business Plan Development

Many hospitals will require the pharmacy department to prepare a business plan to justify adding an inpatient anticoagulation service. This task will most likely fall on the program manager or director of pharmacy. Specific references are available to aid in writing business plans.[4,5] A sample business plan is provided in the Case Study.

The person writing the business plan should have a firm grasp of the issues currently confronting the health-system and show how the inpatient anticoagulation service will help solve those issues. The proposal should clearly link with the hospital's current goals. They should also review other successful business plans in the health-system to understand the desired style and substance. It is important to note that every hospital may have different elements that they desire covered in their business plans. What follows are some of the common elements many hospitals may want covered in their business plans.

Executive Summary

After a title page and table of contents, many business plans begin with an executive summary that is kept to one page. It should contain a summary of all the high points presented in the business plan. This page, like this rest of the proposal, should be written in lay language as many healthcare administrators do not have a health sciences background. This page is primary targeted at the administrator ultimately charged with making the final decision who may not have time to read the rest of the proposal. It should conclude with the best arguments from the business plan on why the program is needed.

Background and Business Description

So what exactly will the program do? What is the scope of the program? These are key elements to describe in the background section of the business plan. Flow diagrams showing the current process and contrasting that with the proposed process may be helpful. Visually showing how the program will improve care is a powerful tool to explain the service to those who are not familiar with clinical pharmacy services. Be sure to illustrate how the plan will likely save physician and nurse time as this is a powerful supporting argument for the service.

This section also needs to include a review of the published literature on similar programs. This data can provide a powerful augmentation to the financial arguments because it shows others have reaped the benefits of such as service. This section should also clearly show how the program helps the organization achieve its goals. An extremely important final issue is to show the level of internal and external support the program has. This is a place where the political homework can really pay off if the department can show the program is supported by crucial physicians, physician groups, the nursing department, and the pharmacy department.

Market Analysis

It is important to consider how many patients will qualify for the proposed service and will likely be enrolled in the service. This will be necessary for the financial projections. As most financial projections will want to look both at the short term and longer term financial implications, program expansion of services should be figured into this market analysis. Competition should also be considered in the market analysis. For example, will the program face competition for its services from other health professionals? Also, are other hospital pharmacy departments providing this service at competing hospitals? If so, the administration may not want to be perceived as delivering a different level of care.

Operational Structure and Processes

If the service has already been described in the background and business section, the critical element to cover here is how will the program be organized? In other words, who will manage the service for the pharmacy department? Who will deal with personnel issues related to the program? What are the specific duties of the pharmacists in regard to the program? From a clinical reporting perspective, organizationally, where will the program report (many programs would report directly to the pharmacy and therapeutics [P & T] committee or a subcommittee of P & T)? This section should also cover any space issues or equipment that will be needed for the service. The section should explain what and how many pharmacists will provide the service and how those pharmacists will be trained.

Financial Projections

The financial projection of the program is the single most important piece of the proposal. The argument, as mentioned above, likely needs to be based on costs savings which makes it a more difficult sell to an administrator. The steps outlined above should be utilized in making the financial projections. The more rigorous and scientific the analysis, the more compelling the projections will be to decision makers. Less rigorous analysis like that in the Case Study are possible in nearly any care setting, but may not be as convincing. Carefully consider how rigorous the analysis should be as this may make or break the proposal. Less rigorous analysis may succeed if the program enjoys broad political support prior to program implementation. A final piece that may help the less rigorous analysis to be successful is related to risk management.

Risk management, in regard to hospitals, means taking coordinated action to reduce the risk of a malpractice suit by maintaining a high quality of care delivered, taking steps to lessen the probably of a claim being filed when a potentially compensable event occurs, and protecting the hospital's assets once a lawsuit has been filed.[7] In a recent study analyzing medication errors reporting in a hospital, 7.2% were due to anticoagulants, and for those anticoagulation errors, 6.2% or these patients required medical intervention, and 1.5% needed a prolonged hospitalization.[8] Another recent report by Winterstein et al. showed that anticoagulant medications were responsible for 32.2% of preventable ADEs in a teaching hospital and this was double the amount caused by any other medication class.[9] A study by Forster et al. recently evaluated the risk of adverse drug events (ADEs) after hospital discharge.[10] In this study of 400 patient discharges to the ambulatory setting, it was found that 7% (4 of 56) of all warfarin prescriptions caused ADEs. All four ADEs due to warfarin were considered preventable by reviewers, one event was considered a serious severity, and the other three were considered life-threatening.[11] All four cases were deemed attributable to both poor dosing and follow up of warfarin.

Since it is clear that anticoagulants cause liability risk to a healthcare organization, a good question is how many malpractice claims are actually due to anticoagulants. A recent analysis of medication-related malpractice claims filed in the 1990s for a New England malpractice insurance company showed that anticoagulants were responsible for 8% of claims (10/129) and that six of these claims were considered preventable.[12] The same study found the mean cost of defending preventable ADEs to be $376,500. Clearly, a preventable ADE due to an anticoagulant that leads to a malpractice claim is a costly event, at least to the insurance company.

In the work *Managing Oral Anticoagulation Therapy*, 10 closed claims involving warfarin anticoagulation were analyzed.[7] Fifteen liability issues were identified in those cases (Table 6-2). Many of the issues, such as "no response to abnormal values" or issues with invasive procedures appear to be areas where an inpatient anticoagulation service can positively impact care.

Implementation Action Plan

This section should clearly show how all of the objectives to the program will be achieved. Further, an implementation timeline should be developed and responsibilities for implementation assigned. The action plan should ideally have measurable endpoints so achieving the goals of the program

Table 6-2.
Fifteen Liability Issues from Malpractice Claims Involving Warfarin[7]

1.	Inadequate response to out-of-range values
2.	Lack of warfarin reorder after invasive procedure
3.	Lack of warfarin being held before an invasive procedure
4.	Patient medication history was inadequate or missing
5.	No communication and coordination of care
6.	Poor or no patient teaching
7.	Poor documentation in the medical record
8.	Ordering and dispensing medication errors
9.	Noncompliant patient not identified
10.	Error in not giving vitamin K when indicated
11.	Lack of appropriate consultation
12.	Computer-generated protocol over reliance
13.	Poor physician attitude
14.	Lack of resident supervision and staffing issues
15.	Problems with telephone assessment

can be measured. The action plan can be aggressive or conservative in how long it will take to get the work done. The action plan is also an excellent area to discuss outside hiring if this is necessary to get the program off the ground. A key element to include in this section is how the quality of the service will be measured in the long term. It should also include a section on how the service will be promoted.

Conclusion/References

The conclusion should be a succinct section summarizing the key points of the business proposal. Repetition is an important tool to get the most important points across. The conclusion should not be as long as the executive summary, but should mention many of the same points. A busy executive may read only the executive summary and the conclusion of the proposal. References should also be added to the end of the business proposal.

Making the Pitch

If one only sends the written business proposal to decision makers and expects approval, they will likely fail. When submitting the proposal, try to get on the agenda of a committee that has the authority to make a decision on the program. Pick a talented speaker who knows the program well and is respected by administration. This will usually be the pharmacy director or anticoagulation program manager, but it would not need to be. Prepare roughly a 10–15 minute presentation with good visual aids and verbally make the pitch to the committee while they refer to the business plan for more specific questions. A powerful delivery may sway skeptical decision makers even if the business plan is not perfect. Never run over on the presentation time allotment, and be sure to repeat the key points like in the business proposal itself. Finally, the presenter should never be defensive during questioning. Instead, they should repeat the question both the make sure they understand the question, and give themselves time to think. Once this is completed, the question should be answered appropriately.

Conclusion

Creating a sound justification for an inpatient anticoagulation service is a difficult task, but it can be done. The justification should be based on improved patient outcomes, more efficiently utilization of physician and nurse time, decreasing the cost of managing bleeding and thromboembolic complications, and decreasing the liability risk of the organization. The financial justification should be well thought out. The availability of research time and resources will have a large bearing on how rigorous this evaluation will be. A business plan that captures the above elements should be prepared and shared both verbally and in writing with critical administrators. If all of these recommendations are followed, the chances for program approval will vastly be improved.

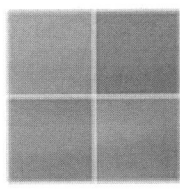

Case Study

The Director of Pharmacy from the case study in Chapter 4 directs his newly appointed anticoagulation program manager to perform an economic evaluation of the proposed anticoagulation program. The program will initially focus on the appropriate dosing and management of warfarin in orthopedic patients. This analysis is intended to justify the hiring of more pharmacists if the program pilot is successful and the program is to be rolled out in more areas. Utilizing the steps outlined in Chapter 6, he designs and conducts the analysis:

1. *Decide how to structure the evaluation*
   The program manager decides it is best to utilize a cost-benefit analysis. The hospital's administrators have been pushing this collaboration, but have been reluctant to invest more human resources in the department to support the collaboration. The pharmacy director and program manager both feel that they can free up some resources to conduct a pilot, but for the program to grow they will likely need to hire another pharmacist. Since a cost-benefit analysis could possibly show cost savings of the program even after adding resources, it seems to be the most appropriate analysis.

2. *Perspective of the analysis*
   The program manager decides to use the hospital's perspective for the analysis. The hospital's administration has been under severe pressure from the board of directors to hold down costs, so if the pharmacy department is to add resources, they must show hospital administration the possibility of avoiding future costs despite adding human resources.

3. *Measurement of resources*
   The resources required to expand the program beyond an orthopedic surgery patient pilot will be explored. The program will not incur fixed costs as the pharmacists are already stationed on the nursing units and do not require new computers or workstations to perform the service. The program will not cause overhead expenses carried by pharmacy to grow based on how the facility accounts for these expenses. Thus, the only expenses will be variable costs. Patient education materials are already available, so the only extra costs of the program will be from pharmacist salaries and benefits needed to be added to the payroll to run the service.

4. *Measurement of outcomes*
   The measurement in outcomes will be done in dollars as this is a cost-benefit analysis.

5. *Picking a study design*
   The program director does not have the time or resources to conduct a formal economic evaluation of the program. He decides to rely on the research of others. He will generalize what has been learned from other inpatient anticoagulation programs. He decides to rely heavily on the data from the Bond and Raehl analysis of inpatient anticoagulation programs.[1] Although the data does not describe the breadth of service provided at each hospital, it is from a broad array of hospitals and should help minimize differences in skill levels of pharmacists. It also deals with actual economic outcomes of not having a service. In his analysis, he will use not having a service as his control where the input costs are $0. This will be compared to the increased cost of having pharmacists staff the service. The analysis will also assume the increased Medicare charges realized for the patients at hospitals without the service persists today (the study was based on 1995 claims data). The hospital's 1995 Medicare cost/charge ratio will be used to covert the Medicare charges to costs. This number will then be increased by the medical consumer price index for each year until the current year.

6. *Sensitivity or statistical analysis*
   Since the analysis is only an estimate and relies on literature generalization, the program director determines that a statistical analysis is unnecessary. A sensitivity analysis will be conducted to consider different rates of inflation and the amount of time spent by pharmacists per patient.

7. *Analyze and include the financial analysis in a business plan*
   The program manager completes the financial analysis and includes this in a business plan to support the service. This business plan is provided below.

St. Joseph's Hospital Department of Pharmacy Business Plan for an Inpatient Anticoagulation Service

Executive Summary

The department of pharmacy was recently asked by the orthopedic surgeons to assist them in the dosing and management of warfarin, a powerful oral blood thinner. In response to this request, the department is requesting permission to launch an inpatient anticoagulation service to fulfill this request. This service would be piloted in the orthopedic arena and then be rolled out to all other areas of the hospital on a consult basis. One additional full time equivalent (FTE) of pharmacist will be necessary to launch the service.

Numerous studies of have shown both the clinical and economic benefit of pharmacist managing anticoagulation in hospitals. One prominent study evaluating these services in the Medicare patients estimated that, on average, these services save $370 of Medicare charges per patient in 1995 dollars.[1] After adjusting this value for inflation and converting it to costs, it is estimated this program could save the institution a minimum of $103,000 for Medicare patients alone and $210,000 if the Medicare savings are extrapolated to all patients. These saving are after the increased costs of hiring an additional pharmacist. These savings do not include possible avoidance of lawsuits due to the program (settlements estimated at $376,500 in the 1990s), or the amount of nursing and physician time saved.

The department already has engaged key physician groups and this program has broad political support. More importantly, the program will help the hospital meet its mission of "delivering world-class healthcare to the patients we serve."

Background and Business Description

Anticoagulant medications, which are powerful blood thinners, provide a particular challenge to caregivers when they are utilized inside of the hospital. These medications are known to have narrow therapeutic indexes meaning that too little of the medications could lead to devastating blood clots and too much of the medications could lead to serious bleeding complications. These facts, combined with high patient acuity in the modern day hospital, are a recipe for the occurrence of adverse drug events (ADEs). Due to this, anticoagulants such as warfarin, heparin, and low molecular weight heparins are all considered high-alert medications by the Institute for Safe Medication Practices (ISMP).[2] A recent report by Winterstein et al. showed that anticoagulant medications were responsible for 32.2% of preventable ADEs in a teaching hospital and this was double the amount caused by any other medication class.[3] This type of data is leading for more and more hospitals and accreditation bodies to call for pharmacists to become actively involved in the management of these medications for patients in the hospital.

The orthopedic surgeons recently approached the hospital pharmacy department requesting pharmacist help in the dosing of warfarin, an oral blood thinner, for the prevention of deep vein thrombosis (clots in the legs, a common problem after orthopedic surgery procedures). The department of pharmacy has also been aware of ADEs reported involving warfarin throughout the hospital including one sentinel event that underwent root cause analysis. The root cause analysis team had suggested that pharmacists become more actively involved in the dosing of warfarin. Therefore, the department of pharmacy is proposing piloting a service that doses and manages warfarin anticoagulation for the orthopedic surgery population. If this pilot is successful as expected, the department would like to expand the service throughout the hospital on a physician consult basis.

Pharmacists will monitor and dose warfarin anticoagulation for this program and will also monitor and address other anticoagulation needs of the patients they follow. To expand the service to other areas of the hospital, the department of pharmacy has determined that the pharmacist staffing in the department will need to be increased, thus the reason for this business proposal. The department will train and utilize the decentralized pharmacists to provide this service and increase their number on the floors.

The utility and benefit of pharmacists managing anticoagulation in hospitalized patients has been described in numerous studies. Two of the most interesting studies that likely apply to our setting will be briefly presented below.

Dager et al. evaluated the impact of inserting pharmacist consultation into the daily management of warfarin in a matched cohort of 120 patients. A significant reduction in the number of inpatient days on warfarin (9.5 days vs. 6.8 days; $p = 0.009$), days of INRs (the blood test utilized to monitor warfarin) over target (INR > 3.5) values (142 vs. 29; $p < 0.001$) or critical (INR > 6.0) values (50 vs. 6; $p < 0.001$) were observed. The INR was more likely in the therapeutic range at discharge in the pharmacist group ($p = 0.07$). Long-term outcomes on readmission for bleeding or recurrent thromboembolism measured out to 3 months postdischarge and showed a lower incidence of both in the cohort receiving pharmacist consultations. For every dollar spent on pharmacist

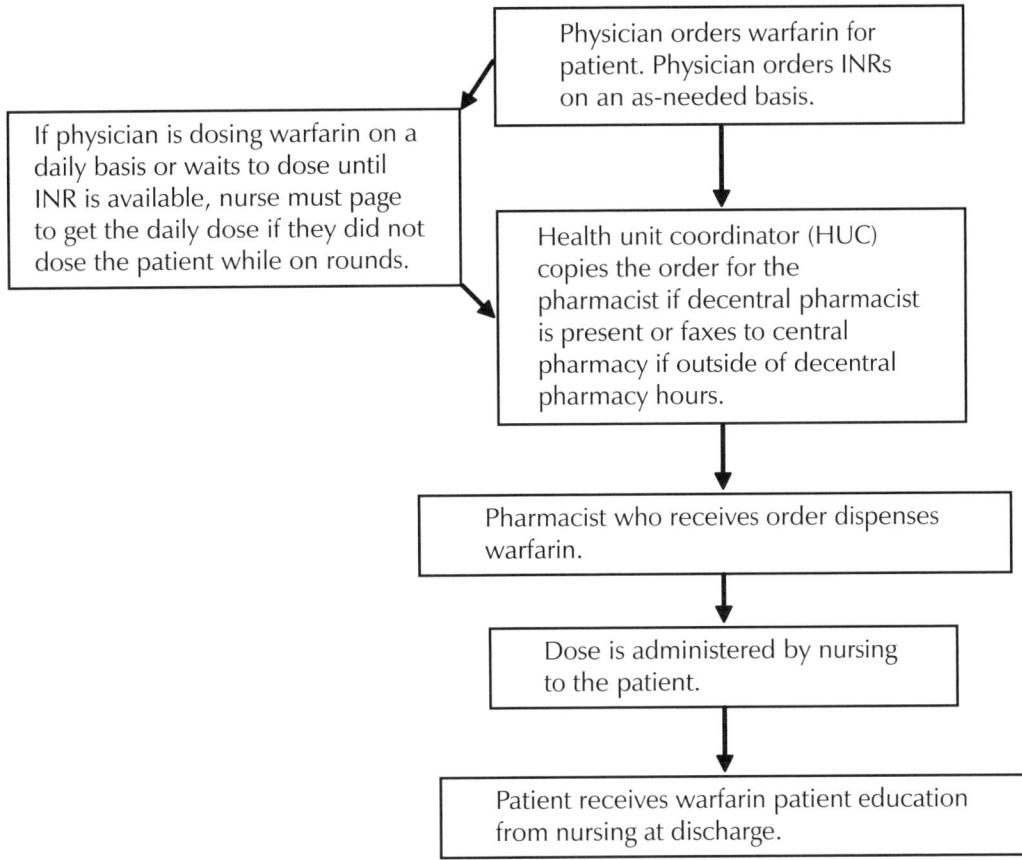

Figure 6-1. Current warfarin process.

staffing, $8 dollars in direct hospital cost savings were realized.[4]

Bond and Raehl investigated the potential impact of pharmacist involvement in managing anticoagulants by analyzing the 1995 Medicare and the National Clinical Pharmacy Services Databases. Hospitals with pharmacists providing management of either heparin or warfarin were observed to have significantly (all $p < 0.001$) lower anticoagulation-related mortality, length of hospital stay, bleeding complications, blood transfusion requirements, and cost of therapy. In hospitals with pharmacists monitoring heparin or warfarin, death rates were lower (11.4% and 6.2%, respectively), length of stay longer (10.5% and 5.7%, respectively) and Medicare charges higher (6.6% and 2.2%, respectively) compared to hospitals without pharmacist provided management. Each warfarin patient not managed by pharmacy, on average, resulted in $370 of excess Medicare charges. Noting that heparin and warfarin are commonly prescribed anticoagulants frequently associated with harmful prescribing errors, the authors concluded "pharmacy directors and clinical coordinators should develop pharmacist-provided anticoagulation management as an integral component of their core service mix."[1]

Due to the request of the orthopedic surgeons, the safety issues with warfarin anticoagulation, the positive data just presented, and the possibility that pharmacist warfarin dosing input may soon be mandated by the Joint Commission®,[5] the department of pharmacy convened a multidisciplinary panel. This group had representation from hospital medicine, cardiology, hematology/oncology, orthopedic surgery, nursing, and pharmacy. The group, and the medical sections represented, fully support this venture by the department of pharmacy.

Figures 6-1 and 6-2 demonstrate how an inpatient anticoagulation program focused on warfarin will change current care practices. Figure 6-1 shows the current process of managing a patient on warfarin anticoagulation. Figure 6-2 shows the new proposed process after implementation of the service. Please note that the revised process assures that INRs will be drawn for all patients on the service. The new system assures that nurses will not need to page physicians to get a current day's warfarin dose, a major inconvenience to both nurses

Managing Anticoagulation Patients in the Hospital: The Inpatient Anticoagulation Service

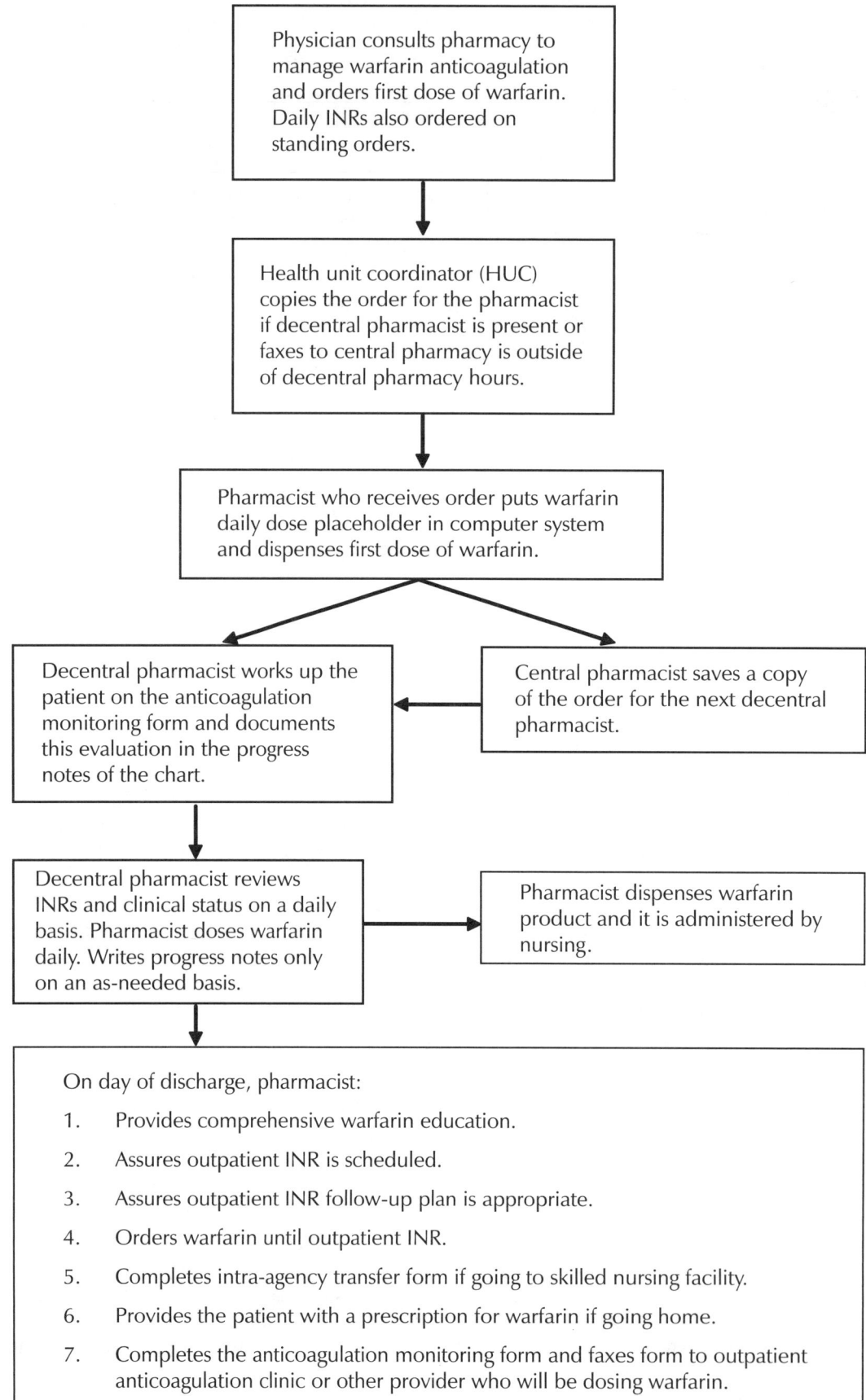

Figure 6-2. Proposed warfarin process.

and physicians. It assures all clinical issues that could affect warfarin dosing are being considered. Finally, it also assures thorough discharge planning has occurred ensuring smooth transitional care.

The department of pharmacy feels this fits well with the hospital's current goals. Table 6-3 shows how the anticoagulation program will help the hospital meet its current goals. The mission of this health-system is to "deliver world-class healthcare to the patients we serve." Considering the scientific articles showing the benefit of pharmacists managing anticoagulation and the unique skills pharmacists posses in managing medication therapy, the department feels this would truly be a way to "deliver world-class healthcare to the patients we serve."

Market Analysis

Currently, the hospital typically has 25–35 patients on warfarin at any one time. No significant increases in these numbers are expected in the next few years. No other providers in the health-system have expressed an interest in specifically managing warfarin anticoagulation in the hospital. Another local hospital pharmacy department is already providing this type of service and it currently enjoys strong support from patients, nurses, and physicians.

Operational Structure and Processes

If this program is approved, the department of pharmacy will appoint Bob Smith, Pharm.D., BCPS to be the anticoagulation program manager. Dr. Smith is a clinical manager for the department. He will coordinate all training and implementation of systems needed to support the program. Dr. Smith also has extensive experience dosing and managing anticoagulants from a previous job. He will be the pharmacist in charge of doing the dosing initially and he will train others to perform the service after he has smoothed the processes. As the program expands, Dr. Smith will also deal with personnel performance issues as they arise. The planning committee also wants the pharmacy department to form an expert subcommittee to chronically monitor anticoagulation issues. They want the committee to evaluate new anticoagulants as they enter the market, analyze data regarding old anticoagulants that may affect practice, evaluate adverse drug events involving anticoagulants that are reported, and continuously monitor the quality of the inpatient anticoagulation service. This committee will be co-chaired by Dr. Smith and Dr. Dwight Jones, a physician and hematologist. This new subcommittee will report directly to the Pharmacy and Therapeutics Committee. Dr. Jones will also serve as a physician champion for the inpatient anticoagulation program and will help promote use of the program to his peers. He will also serve as a clinical resource for the pharmacists when needed.

Financial Projections

Based on the Bond and Raehl data presented above, we conducted a cost-benefit analysis of the proposed inpatient anticoagulation program.[1] Key assumptions of this analysis are:

1. Since the hospital does not currently have an inpatient anticoagulation service, our patients are incurring increased costs of care like the article.
2. Increased reimbursement will not be generated by program implementation.
3. Our pharmacists will have similar ability in managing warfarin as those in the study. This is likely since the study was from a broad array of hospitals.

Table 6-3.
How the Inpatient Anticoagulation Program Will Help the Hospital Achieve Its Goals

Hospital Goal	Benefit of the Anticoagulation Program
Assure the financial viability of the hospital	Program will likely lower the overall costs of therapy for patients (see financial analysis)
Assure patient safety is a top priority	Program will standardize how these patients are managed likely improving patient safety
Streamline current workflows to reduce workload on nurses	Nurses will not have to call physicians to get doses for warfarin saving them time; physicians will not have to track down INRs on a daily basis, saving them time
Promote interdisciplinary collaboration	Pharmacists will work very closely with physicians when managing their patients; will likely lead to closer physician/pharmacist relationships

4. Care has not changed enough to affect results of this analysis which was based on 1995 data.
5. The costs of providing care have escalated since 1995.
6. Utilizing our 1995 cost-charge ratio for Medicare will realize a good estimate of increased costs (article is based on increased Medicare charges).
7. The only difference in cost before program implementation and after program implementation is the variable costs of having more pharmacist staffing to provide the service. All education will be provided with already budgeted resources.

Estimation of How Much Additional Pharmacist Time will Be Needed To Provide The Service

The staffing of the pharmacy department is already very tight. The department has already tried to make the pharmacists more efficient by delegating many duties to others in the department. The only option to try to get this service off the ground is to add pharmacist personnel. When the program is fully implemented house wide, the department expects to actively manage 20–30 patients daily (about 80% utilization) as some physicians will not utilize the service (usually 25–35 total patients on warfarin). Other departments estimate the time spent per patient at 10–15 minutes on average. This equated to an additional 23 hours (10 minutes/patient × 20 patients × 7 days) – 52 hours (15 minutes/patient × 30 patients × 7 days) of pharmacist time needed per week. The department is requesting adding one FTE pharmacist to launch this service. The cost of one FTE pharmacist with benefits is about $125,000.

Estimation of the Current Increased Cost Per Patient in the Current System

The Bond and Raehl article estimated increased 1995 Medicare charges of $370 per patient. St. Joseph's Hospital's 1995 Medicare cost/charge ratio (includes both operating and capital cost/charge ratios) was 0.516. Thus, estimated increased cost of care to each warfarin patient <u>not</u> managed by an inpatient anticoagulation service is about $191 in 1995 dollars. Table 6-4 shows how the 1995 costs likely have risen until the current day. Adjusted by the medical care services consumer price index (CPI) yearly, the estimated costs to the hospital of not having a service is currently $287 per patient.[6]

Estimation of How Much Money Could Be Saved by the Hospital

In 2005, the hospital dispensed warfarin to 1631 different warfarin patients and 1108 of those patients were Medicare patients like those in the Bond and Raehl article. Assuming 80% utilization rate of the service, 1305 patients could be managed each year with 886 of those being Medicare patients. If the cost savings apply to all patients, not just Medicare, spending $125,000 on another pharmacist could realize a cost savings of about $375,000 (net cost savings of $250,000). Applying the cost savings to Medicare patients only, the hospital would save about $254,000 (net cost sav-

Table 6-4.

Estimating 2006 Increased Costs of Care

Year	Medical Service Consumer Price Index (CPI) for this Year[6]	Estimated Increased Costs of Care Adjusted by CPI	Estimated Increased Costs of Care Adjusted by 3% Inflation Rate	Estimated Increased Costs of Care Adjusted by 5% Inflation Rate
1995	Baseline year	$191	$191	$191
1996	3.7%	$198	$197	$201
1997	2.9%	$204	$203	$211
1998	3.2%	$210	$209	$221
1999	3.4%	$217	$215	$232
2000	4.3%	$227	$221	$244
2001	4.8%	$238	$228	$256
2002	5.1%	$250	$235	$269
2003	4.5%	$261	$242	$282
2004	5%	$274	$249	$296
2005	4.8%	$287	$257	$311

ings of $129,000). If instead of $287 saved for each patient, 3% inflation rate per year is used ($257 per patient), the savings would be about $335,000 (net $210,000) for all patients and $228,000 (net $103,000) for Medicare patients. See Table 6-5 for a visual of this most conservative estimation of cost savings.

Risk Management

A recent analysis of medication-related malpractice claims filed in the 1990s for a New England malpractice insurance company showed that anticoagulants were responsible for 8% of claims (10/129) and that six of these claims were considered preventable. The same study found the mean cost of defending preventable ADEs to be $376,500.[7] While the hospital carries malpractice insurance to cover these events, it is important to note this significant financial risk to the organization.

Implementation Action Plan

Table 6-6 summarizes the implementation timeline for this project, if approved. Dr. Bob Smith is assigning responsibilities to assure all of these steps are executed. An experienced, residency trained pharmacist will be recruited to add to the current pharmacist staffing of the floors. The hire will coincide with launching the pilot so this pharmacist is fully trained at the time the service is ready to expand beyond the pilot stage. The program will also collect and analyze data similar to that of Dager et al. to see if it can match their measures of quality.[4]

Conclusion

Anticoagulants pose significant risk to the organization, but pharmacists have proven their ability to safely manage these agents in the inpatient setting. The department of pharmacy feels an inpatient anticoagulation program focused on warfarin management will not only improve patient safety, but decrease the total costs of care even after pharmacist resources are added. It will also save physician and nurse time. Approving the inpatient anticoagulation program will help the hospital "deliver world-class healthcare to the patients we serve."

Case Study References

1. Bond CA, Raehl CL. Pharmacist-provided anticoagulation management in United States hospitals: death rates, length of stay, Medicare charges, bleeding complications, and transfusions. *Pharmacotherapy*. 2004;24(8):953-63.
2. Unknown. ISMP's List of High-Alert Medications. *Institute for Safe Medication Practices* [Web page]. Available at: http://www.ismp.org/Tools/highalert-medications.pdf. Accessed May 26, 2006.
3. Winterstein AG, Hatton RC, Gonzalez-Rothi R, Johns TE, Segal R. Identifying clinically significant preventable adverse drug events through a hospital's database of adverse drug reaction reports. *Am J Health-Syst Pharm*. 2002;59(18):1742-9.
4. Dager WE, Branch JM, King JH, et al. Optimization of inpatient warfarin therapy: impact of daily consultation by a pharmacist-managed anticoagulation service. *Ann Pharmacother*. 2000;34(5):567-72.
5. Unknown. Draft Candidate 2007 National Patient Safety Goals, Requirements and Implementation

Table 6-5.

Most Conservative Projection of Cost Saving of an Inpatient Anticoagulation Service for Medicare Patients Only

Potential Cost Savings of Anticoagulation Program	Rounded to Nearest Thousand
1108 Medicare patients × 80% managed by pharmacy × $257/patient (3% inflation rate since 1995)	$228,000
Increased cost of anticoagulation program	
Fixed costs	
Computers/technology needed for start-up (already available)	$0
Furniture/desk equipment (already available)	$0
Overhead expenses	$0
Education expenses (will be provided with current resources)	$0
Variable costs	
One FTE pharmacist salary	$100,000
One FTE pharmacist benefits	$25,000
Patient education materials (budgeted elsewhere)	$0
Total costs	$125,000
Total net savings of program	**$103,000**

Table 6-6.
Warfarin Action Plan

Measurable Endpoint	Due Date for Completion
Gain approval of pharmacy warfarin dosing policy/procedure and guideline	July 31, 2006
Finalize warfarin monitoring form	July 31, 2006
Present warfarin didactic lectures to pharmacy staff	August 15, 2006
Modify orthopedic orders to facilitate pharmacist dosing	September 1, 2006
Present information item on the program at orthopedics committee	September 1, 2003
Meet with outpatient anticoagulation providers to plan smooth patient transitions	September 1, 2006
Meet with health unit coordinators to inform them of what is happening with warfarin	September 1, 2006
Hire an additional full-time pharmacist	September 1, 2006
Launch pilot service on orthopedics	September 8, 2006
Promote the service to physicians outside of orthopedics	November 15, 2006
Launch house-wide service	December 1, 2006
Train all pharmacists (hands-on) and assure test on didactic lectures completed	Ongoing
Formulate an electronic anticoagulation data tracking system	December 31, 2006
Develop a system to monitor program quality	December 31, 2006
Form new anticoagulation sub-committee of P & T	December 31, 2006

Expectations. *Joint Commission on Accreditation of Healthcare Organizations*. Available at: http://www.jointcommission.org/NR/rdonlyres/4901A094-80A7-4AD6-86CD-4754B896A986/0/07_npsg_hap_cah.pdf. Accessed May 31, 2006.

6. Unknown. Consumer Price Index - All Urban Consumer. *United States Department of Labor Bureau of Labor Statistics* [Web page]. Available at: http://data.bls.gov/PDQ/servlet/SurveyOutputServlet. Accessed September 1, 2006.

7. Rothschild JM, Federico FA, Gandhi TK, Kaushal R, Williams DH, Bates DW. Analysis of medication-related malpractice claims: causes, preventability, and costs. *Arch Intern Med.* 2002;162(21):2414-20.

References

1. Hughes RA, Wilson Norton JL. Reimbursement for anticoagulation management services. In: Ansell JE, Oertel LB, Wittkowsky AK, eds. *Managing Oral Anticoagulation Therapy*. Gaithersburg, MD: Aspen Publishers; 2000.
2. Michalets EL, Williams E. Reimbursement for pharmacists' cognitive services in the inpatient setting. *Am J Health-Syst Pharm.* 2001;58(2):164-6.
3. Paradiso-Hardy F, Seto A, Ong S, Bucci C, Madorin P. Use of a personal digital assistant in a pharmacy-directed warfarin dosing program. *Am J Health-Syst Pharm.* 2003;60(19):1943-6.
4. Schumock G, Butler M. Evaluating and justifying clinical pharmacy services. In: Grauer D, Lee J, Odom T, Osterhaus J, Sanchez L, Touchette D, eds. *Pharmacoeconomics & Outcomes*. Kansas City, MO: American College of Clinical Pharmacy; 2003.
5. Wilson Norton JL. Business plan. In: Ansell JE, Oertel LB, Wittkowsky AK, eds. *Managing Oral Anticoagulation Therapy*. Gaithersburg, MD: Aspen Publishers; 2000.
6. Unknown. Consumer Price Index - All Urban Consumer. *United States Department of Labor Bureau of Labor Statistics* [Web page]. Available at: http://data.bls.gov/PDQ/servlet/SurveyOutputServlet. Accessed September 1, 2006.
7. Ryan EM. Risk management and anticoagulation therapy. In: Ansell JE, Oertel LB, Wittkowsky AK, eds. *Managing Oral Anticoagulation Therapy*. Gaithersburg, MD: Aspen Publishers; 2000.
8. Fanikos J, Stapinski C, Koo S, Kucher N, Tsilimingras K, Goldhaber SZ. Medication errors associated with anticoagulant therapy in the hospital. *Am J Cardiol.* 2004;94(4):532-5.
9. Winterstein AG, Hatton RC, Gonzalez-Rothi R, Johns TE, Segal R. Identifying clinically significant preventable adverse drug events through a hospital's database of adverse drug reaction reports. *Am J Health-Syst Pharm.* 2002;59(18):1742-9.
10. Forster AJ, Murff HJ, Peterson JF, Gandhi TK, Bates DW. Adverse drug events occurring following hospital discharge. *J Gen Intern Med.* 2005;20(4):317-23.
11. Forster AJ, Murff HJ, Peterson JF, Gandhi TK, Bates DW. Appendix: Adverse Drug Events. *Journal of General Internal Medicine* [Web Page]. Available at: http://www.blackwellpublishing.com/products/

journals/suppmat/jgi/jgi30390/jgi30390.doc. Accessed September 8, 2006.

12. Rothschild JM, Federico FA, Gandhi TK, Kaushal R, Williams DH, Bates DW. Analysis of medication-related malpractice claims: causes, preventability, and costs. *Arch Intern Med.* 2002;162(21):2414-20.

Chapter 7

Pharmacist Education and Training

Michael Gulseth

Chapter Outline

- Introduction
- Design of the education program
  - Educational techniques
  - Precepting
- How to assess the competency of pharmacists dosing anticoagulants
- Strategies to train pharmacists and assure competence
- Conclusion
- References

Introduction

A long-standing debate in pharmacy is whose responsibility is it to further develop the skills, attitudes, knowledge, and abilities of individual pharmacists in providing direct patient care? Namely, is this the job of the health system or of the individual? While most pharmacists would argue that a professional has an obligation to maintain proficiency in their area, it is a lot to ask of pharmacists to begin to manage inpatients on anticoagulants without providing educational support to do so. In other words, when launching an inpatient anticoagulation service, the pharmacists in the department have a professional obligation to further their skills in the area, but the department should also provide training to ensure safe patient care will be provided. This will also help win the support of less enthusiastic members of the department.[1]

Design of the Education Program

When designing any type of education program, a good rule of thumb is to start with the end in mind. In other words, what are the skills and abilities that will be needed by the pharmacists when providing this service? By critically answering this question, it will make it much easier to write educational objectives for the program.

So how does one write good educational objectives? First, the educational objective must be focused on the learner. In other words, what will the learner be able to do when the program is complete? Second, the objective must be measurable. When writing objectives, avoid using verbs like *understand, appreciate, learn,* and *comprehend,* as they are not measurable. Instead use verbs that are clearly measurable, such as *define, describe, list, state, explain, give examples of, predict, compute, demonstrate, solve, use, differentiate, discriminate, point out, select, design, formulate, modify, write, appraise, compare, explain,* and *justify*. Third, the objective should say under what conditions the objective should be demonstrated. For example, an educational objective for an inpatient anticoagulation program involving warfarin could be, "Given a patient's chart and access to departmental resources and the patient, the pharmacist shall be able to justify the dose of warfarin picked each day." Finally, a good educational objective should describe under what criteria the objective should be demonstrated. A simple revision to the previous statement would accomplish this: "Given a patient's chart and access to departmental resources and the patient, the pharmacist shall be able to justify the dose of warfarin picked each day 100% of the time."[2]

It should be quite obvious from the verbs mentioned above that some of them imply a higher level of learning than others. For example, "appraising" the current literature to determine where a new anticoagulant would fit in therapy is much more difficult than "describing" how the same new anticoagulant exerts its mechanism of action. These different levels of learning are described by Bloom's taxonomy of learning for the cognitive domain. This taxonomy is shown Figure 7-1 along with examples of how different levels of learning could be demonstrated by a pharmacist working in an inpatient anticoagulation service. The goal of any education program for pharmacists practicing in an inpatient anticoagulation service should be to elevate them to the "evaluation" level of learning.[2]

Educational Techniques

Another important consideration when designing the educational program is to correctly match the educational technique for the level of learning needed to be attained. Table 7-1 shows appropriate educational techniques to teach different levels of learning. After reviewing Table 7-1, it should

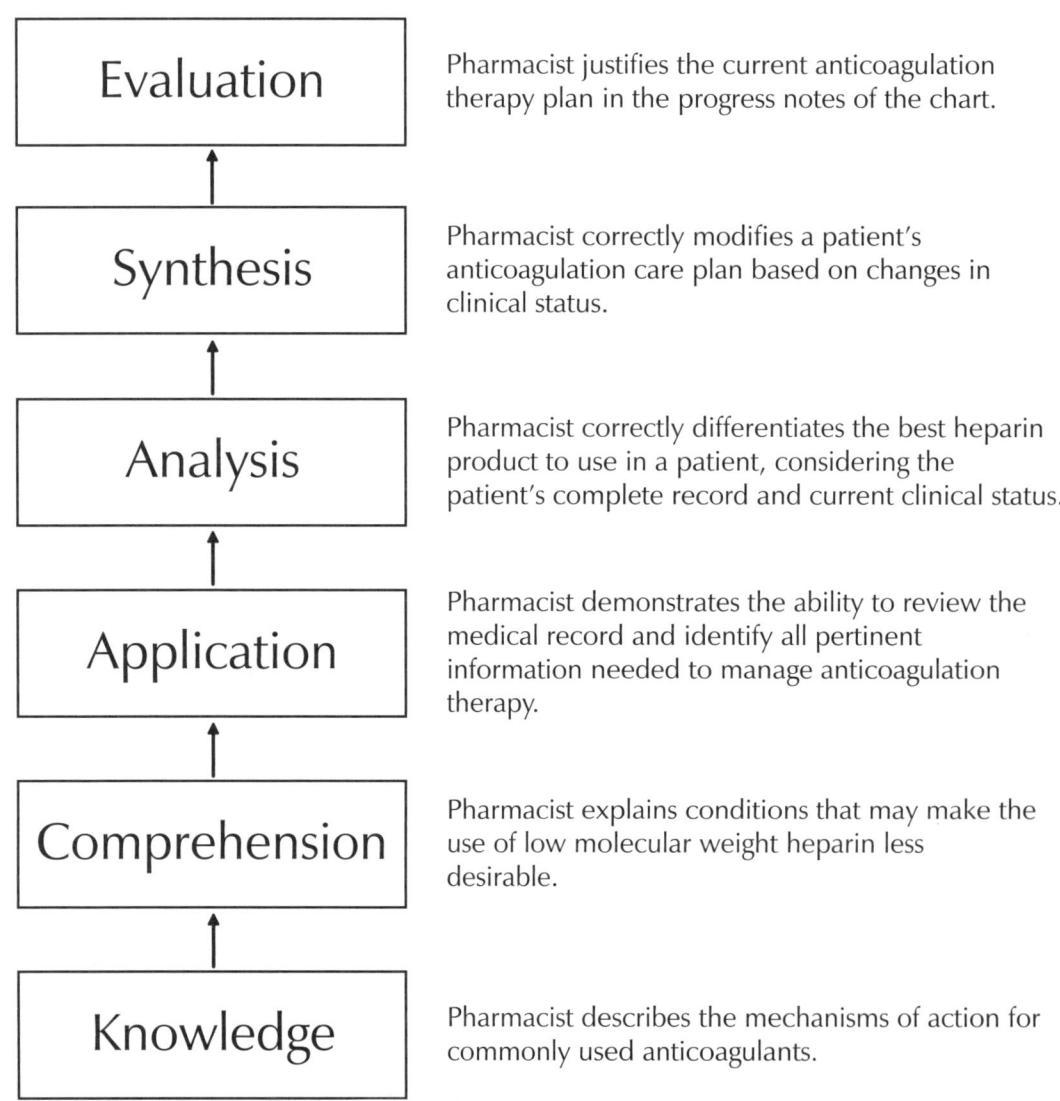

Figure 7-1. Bloom's taxonomy of learning for the cognitive domain and examples of how this may apply to pharmacists practicing in an inpatient anticoagulation service. *Source*: Ref. 2

become clear that to achieve the highest level of learning needed to run an inpatient anticoagulation service that the pharmacists will likely need more education than just a lecture and test. So what are different educational techniques that can be utilized?[3]

To obtain the "knowledge" level of learning, reading and lecture can be useful techniques. Developing or assigning readings (as in Part 2 of this book) and lectures to start an inpatient anticoagulation program are a relatively easy way to get started with training, but they must be kept up to date and certainly should not be the only training provided as they do not facilitate higher levels of learning. Guided discussion and interactive lectures are good techniques to build comprehension. Guided discussion and interactive lectures involves the instructor asking carefully framed questions to stimulate thinking and understanding of content. The receivers of the education should be encouraged to express thoughts in their own words while attempting to understand the material. A key to both is two-way communication between both learning and teacher. All of the rest of the techniques teach skills at a level beyond comprehension.[3]

Case presentations involve a skilled clinician going through a case and presenting how they approached the problems and came to the solutions they implemented. The learners should have the chance to ask questions about points they do not understand. Case-based teaching also involves presenting a carefully crafted case, but the learner is challenged to make decisions at critical junctures. The decisions are challenged by a highly skilled instructor forcing the student further their understanding of the material. Simulation and role playing attempt to emulate real situations and the pace of actual practice. Unfortunately, they require a high level of instructor skill and time to pull off correctly. Finally, practice-based teaching is perhaps the best learning technique to educate pharmacists in providing care in inpatient anticoagulation patients. The reason it is an excellent option is the easy availability of patients to work with under the direct supervision of a knowledgeable preceptor. The key for this technique to work is to assure one on one preceptorship is assigned and that the best preceptors are utilized.[3]

Precepting

What pharmacists make the best preceptors? First, let's review the role of the preceptor in pharmacist development. Figure 7-2 is a schema similar to Bloom's taxonomy of learning for the cognitive domain. Foundation skills and knowledge is similar to the knowledge and comprehension levels in Bloom's. Practical application is similar to application, analysis, and synthesis levels of Bloom's. Finally, culminating integration is like the evaluation level of Bloom's. Notice that Figure 7-2 shows that the best preceptor techniques vary based on the skill level of the learner. Thus, excellent preceptors are pharmacists who will vary their teaching techniques to the level of the learner. In the context of an inpatient anticoagulation program, that means the preceptor does not throw someone to the wolves, expecting them to dose and manage all the patients when they have no experience doing it. Instead, they would model behavior first and only ask them to start trying the manage the patients when the learner seems ready. Even then, they would directly supervise the pharmacist as they are working through cases coaching them along. Finally, as they become more proficient, they would take a step back and only facilitate the learners activities, perhaps letting the learner do all the work without supervision, but then signing off on their decisions after they are reviewed.[3]

Table 7-1.
Matching the Instructional Method to the Level of Learning Desired

Bloom's Levels of Cognitive Learning	Appropriate Instructional Methods
Knowledge	Reading Lecture
Comprehension	Guided discussions Interactive lecture
Application Analysis Synthesis	Case presentation Case-based teaching Simulation/role-play Practice-based teaching
Evaluation	

Source: Adapted from ref. 3.

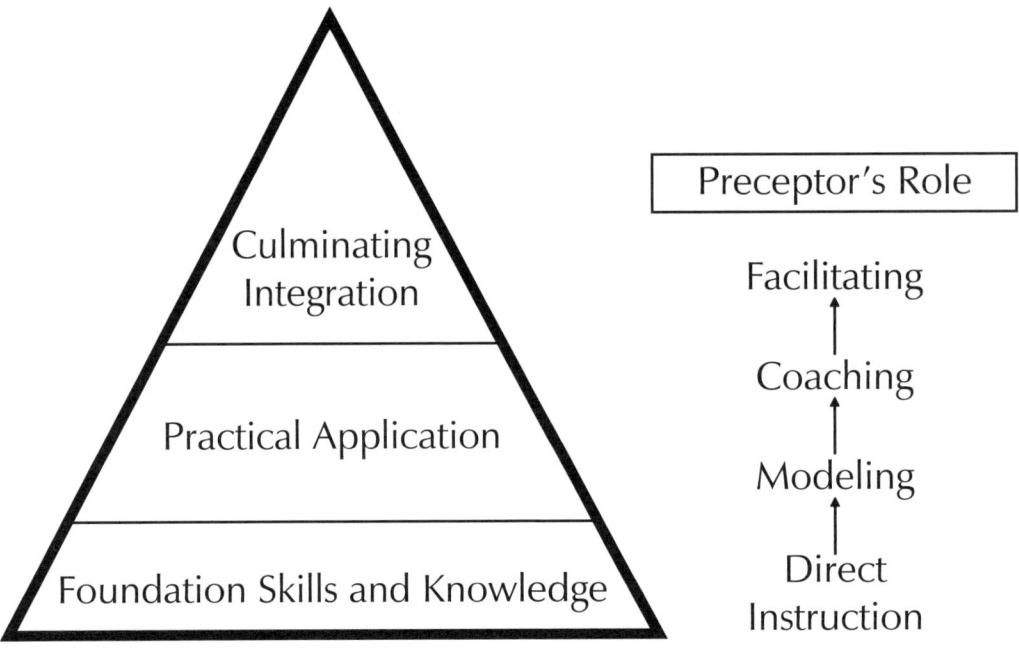

Figure 7-2. The learning pyramid. *Source:* Ref. 2.

Another quality to look for in anticoagulation care preceptors are to choose pharmacists with high moral reasoning skills. Who are these pharmacists? They are those pharmacists who consider delivering inadequate care as morally unacceptable. Further, they work at being competent and consider it a standard of professional behavior.[4] These are typically some of the most respected pharmacists in a department as they function at the highest clinical levels.

Preceptors chosen for the training program will also have good written and oral communication skills.[5] When performing chart documentation, they will demonstrate the skills discussed in Chapter 4. They also will know how to communicate with nurses and physicians in a respectful yet assertive manner. They must also be able to teach that the clinical world is not black and white, and often difficult judgments must be made. When making these difficult judgments in the presence of the learner, they further must be able to explain their reasoning. Finally, they must be able to give insightful, yet fair feedback to the learner. Suggested steps in giving excellent feedback is given in Table 7-2.[6]

In conclusion, the educational program needed to launch an inpatient anticoagulation service should be carefully planned. Educational objectives should be developed for the program with the end product in mind. The educational techniques chosen should facilitate the highest levels of learning. Pairing up inexperienced pharmacists with a mentor-preceptor to learn how to care for anticoagulation patients is a necessity. The pharmacists chosen to precept need to be thoughtfully picked.

How to Assess the Competency of Pharmacists Dosing Anticoagulants

After the educational program and teaching techniques are chosen, the anticoagulation program manager will need to decide how they will assess the competence of the pharmacists who will provide the service. Not only is this necessary to assure the training program has met its educational objectives and the right thing to do, it is required by the Joint Commission®. The Joint Commission® requires that "Competence to perform job responsibilities is assessed, demonstrated, and maintained."[7] It is important not to confuse competency with proficiency. Competency is the ability to do a job correctly. Proficiency is the ability to perform the function effectively and efficiently. Are excellent pharmacists practicing in an inpatient anticoagulation service also proficient? Yes, but this is much more difficult to assess and cannot be expected immediately after someone is found competent to provide the service. Thus, the following will focus on how to assure competence of pharmacists providing an inpatient anticoagulation service.[8]

Professional competence can be thought of as having three components. First, the practitioner must have the skill to perform the service. For an

Table 7-2.
Suggested Steps for Preceptors to Give Feedback to Learners

1. Prepare the learner to receive feedback.
2. Convince learners that you are trying to help them improve.
3. Base any feedback on first-hand data.
4. Deliver feedback when the timing is right and it is expected.
5. Be as specific as possible when providing feedback. Use specific examples whenever possible.
6. Provide feedback in a descriptive, nonjudgmental manner.
7. Limit how much feedback is given at any one time. The learner can only absorb so much.
8. If the preceptor shares opinions based on performance rather than on objective data, this should be clearly stated.
9. Encourage learners to participate in the feedback process by asking them how they felt they did first.

Source: Adapted from ref. 6.

inpatient anticoagulation service, this will mostly be cognitive and communication skills. Second, the practitioner must have the attitude and values of a professional. They need to put the patient first and accept responsibility for their actions. Finally, they must be able to execute judgment. Commonly, this is the ability to see the gray area of issues and the ability to pick the best alternative of management options for a particular situation.[7]

So, how does one assess the competence of pharmacists who will practice in an inpatient anticoagulation program? The literature suggests three possible options for assessing professional competence:

1. Cognitive tests. The strength of cognitive tests is the objectivity of the assessment and generalization to related tasks if the test is complete. They are also easy to design and implement in practice. The drawbacks of tests is they do not do a good job testing the higher levels of learning which are the skills that must be used when providing the service.
2. Simulations (please note this is a different context than the teaching technique mentioned above). Most current simulations would involve a pharmacist working up a hypothetical patient case. This technique may provide good insight into what a pharmacist would do in similar situations and it has the benefit that mistakes can be made since no real patients are involved. The biggest drawback is the difficulty in assessment because more than one answer is often possible. Further, the cases usually do not have the depth and complexity of cases in actual practices.
3. Direct observations. An excellent way to assess competence through direct observation is to first have the trainee evaluate and manage patients in actual practice under the supervision of the trainer/preceptor. Then, the performance of the trainee is then evaluated against a set of objective criteria of skills that should be demonstrated in practice to be competent. The strength of this method is that it is real-world and gives a good indication of how the pharmacist will practice when independent. It also assesses a higher level of cognitive function than nearly all tests. The drawback is that the answer to how to approach each situation may not be clear cut and it requires one-on-one precepting.[7]

Strategies to Train Pharmacists and Assure Competence

A strategy that has worked well for many institutions that combines many of the above methods is as follows:

1. Provide lectures and reading to the pharmacists who will provide the service. These teaching techniques are appropriate to build baseline knowledge. Appropriate readings would include those found in Part 2 of this book. The CD resource also contains sample lectures that could be presented.
2. Provide a second educational session that is interactive in nature. This program should focus on working through hypothetical cases and force the attendees to try to make decisions on how to manage these patients. These patients should be as realistic as possible, but it may be wise to start with easier patients and end with more complex patients. This technique will help raise the cognitive level of pharmacists beyond the "knowledge" level.

3. Design a test that assesses both baseline knowledge and includes cases for pharmacists to work through. The test should be graded. The tester should meet with the pharmacist to clear up confusion on any areas where they struggled. This combines the testing and simulation methods of assessing competence.
4. Pair up the trainee pharmacists with pharmacists who are excellent at providing the service and have strong morale reasoning. The preceptor pharmacist should closely observe the trainee's work. When the both trainer and trainee think the trainee is ready, the preceptor should document that the trainee has demonstrated competence in practice by referring to a standard set of objectives. An example of a set of objective criteria to assure competence of an inpatient anticoagulation pharmacist is provided in Figure 7-3. This approach assures the new pharmacist can safely take care of real world patients and is practicing at the highest cognitive level. During the initial roll out, this may require the program manager to "train the trainers" until they have demonstrated the competence and proficiency to train others.

Conclusion

Pharmacist education and competence assessment is one of the most important steps in launching a new inpatient anticoagulation service. It should be an area that consumes a considerable amount of the program manager's time. It is important not only to assure safe care if being given to patients,

Skills for Inpatient Anticoagulation Pharmacists	Yes	No
Pharmacist correctly identifies all anticoagulation patients that must be managed by the pharmacy department.		
Pharmacist correctly applies all pharmacy policies involving anticoagulants by correctly using them in practice.		
Pharmacist correctly identifies the indication for anticoagulation therapy.		
Pharmacist correctly lists the patients pertinent past medical history.		
For patients previously on warfarin, the pharmacist accurately documents the most recent dose utilized.		
Pharmacist correctly identifies all risk factors for bleeding and thrombosis in individual patients.		
Pharmacist correctly identifies all medications that may interact with warfarin and intervenes when necessary.		
Pharmacist can differentiate the appropriate anticoagulant to utilize based on an individual patient situation.		
Pharmacist correctly identifies the correct evidence based INR range based on a patient's medical history.		
Pharmacist can formulate appropriate dosing and monitoring regimens for all anticoagulants managed.		
Pharmacist correctly identifies changes in patient status that may alter the current therapeutic plan.		
Pharmacist correctly modifies the therapeutic plan based on changes in patient status.		
Pharmacist is able to justify therapeutic decisions both verbally and in writing.		
Pharmacist correctly educates patients regarding anticoagulation therapy.		
Pharmacist appropriately communicates anticoagulation therapeutic plan to outpatient anticoagulation provider.		
Pharmacist appropriately and succinctly writes progress notes in the chart that are both informative and comply with departmental policy.		

Figure 7-3. Objective criteria to assure an inpatient anticoagulation pharmacist is competent in practice; pharmacists must be able demonstrate all skills in practice before independent practice.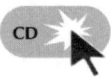

but also to ensure internal support for the program. The education program must strive to both teach and assess the highest levels of cognitive function and will likely require more than just lectures and reading. For competence assessment, only providing a test to measure competence in strongly discouraged; instead, it is recommended to combine testing, simulation, and practice observation to assure competence of the pharmacists providing the service.

References

1. Nimmo CM, Guerrero RM, Taylor JT. Planning departmental and individual training programs. In: Nimmo CM, ed. *Staff Development for Pharmacy Practice*. Bethesda, MD: American Society of Health-System Pharmacists; 2000:101-7.
2. Nimmo CM. Developing training materials and programs: creating educational objectives and assessing their attainment. In: Nimmo CM, ed. *Staff Development for Pharmacy Practice*. Bethesda, MD: American Society of Health-System Pharmacists; 2000:109-18.
3. Nimmo CM. Developing training materials and programs: facilitating learning in staff development. In: Nimmo CM, ed. *Staff Development for Pharmacy Practice*. Bethesda, MD: American Society of Health-System Pharmacists; 2000:119-31.
4. Galt K. *Developing Clinical Practice Skills for Pharmacists*. Bethesda, MD: American Society of Health-System Pharmacists; 2006.
5. Ginsberg DB, Vermeulen LC. Necessary skills to be an effective preceptor. In: Cuellar LM, Ginsberg DB, eds. *Preceptor's Handbook for Pharmacists*. Bethesda, MD: American Society of Health-System Pharmacists; 2005.
6. Nimmo CM. Developing training materials and programs: practice-based teaching. In: Nimmo CM, ed. *Staff Development for Pharmacy Practice*. Bethesda, MD: American Society of Health-System Pharmacists; 2000:143-8.
7. Murdaugh LB. *Competence Assessment Tools for Health-System Pharmacies*. 3rd ed. Bethesda, MD: American Society of Health-System Pharmacists; 2005.
8. Nimmo CM. Assessing the need for training. In: Nimmo CM, ed. *Staff Development for Pharmacy Practice*. Bethesda, MD: American Society of Health-System Pharmacists; 2000:95-100.

Chapter 8

Patient Education Needs

Michael Gulseth

Chapter Outline

- Introduction
- Health literacy evaluation
- Cultural considerations
- General patient education tips
- Patient education materials for the patient and pharmacist
- Internet patient education resources
- Conclusion
- References
- Appendix 8-1: Patient education materials: warfarin
- Appendix 8-2: Patient education materials: injectable anticoagulants such as enoxaparin and dalteparin

Introduction

Many pharmacy-run inpatient anticoagulation programs will charge the pharmacist with providing patient education before the patient is discharged. This a great way to get pharmacists in front of patients and it supports Objective 1.4 of the 2015 Initiative from the American Society of Health-System Pharmacists.[1] Even if pharmacy does not personally provide patient education, the key is that someone in the hospital must be designated to perform discharge education of anticoagulation patients. The education should have both a face-to-face and written component, and the patient's background should be considered when providing the education. An in-depth discussion on how to provide excellent patient education/counseling is beyond the scope of this book, but this chapter will provide a discussion of two timely patient education topics, health literacy and cultural considerations, and provide some general patient education tips. The chapter concludes with useful patient education resources that can be found on the internet.

Health Literacy Evaluation

The Institute of Medicine endorses the following definition of health literacy: "the degree to which individuals have the capacity to obtain, process, and understand basic health information and services needed to make appropriate health decisions."[2] It is estimated that 90 million American adults have difficulty understanding and acting on health information. This lack of health literacy is a huge financial burden to the healthcare system as these patients likely use many more resources than those who are health literate.[2]

Health literacy of individual patients is influenced by many factors. Examples are level of education, culture, language, knowledge, listening, speaking, arithmetical ability, writing, and reading skills. It is also known that the following groups are more prone to health literacy problems[2]:

- Older patients
- Patients with limited education
- Patients with limited English proficiency

- Poor patients
- Minority patients

Considering how often patients in the above categories are encountered by many practitioners, it should become clear that health literacy should be considered by every healthcare professional when educating patients.

Has low health literacy been linked to problems with anticoagulants? Machtinger et al. evaluated the understanding of warfarin therapy among an ethnically diverse population of a public hospital. All patients were taking warfarin therapy to prevent stroke from atrial fibrillation or valvular heart disease. They found that 22% of patients did not fully understand why they were taking warfarin and 41% did not know what a stroke was.[3] Lasater et al. evaluated low-income anticoagulation clinic patients and found that low literacy level was correlated with a lack of anticoagulation control.[4] Estrada et al. evaluated the effect of low literacy and numeracy (math) skills on INR control in English speaking warfarin patients greater than 50 years old. They found that lower literacy rates led to greater INR variability. Patients with lower numeracy skills also had more INR variability and excess time above the therapeutic range. Neither group had a statistically significant difference for time in the therapeutic range, however, the low numeracy group trended toward that negative finding ($p = 0.1$).[5] Fang et al. assessed the effect of limited or adequate health literacy on warfarin knowledge, adherence, and warfarin control in English and Spanish speaking patients. While adherence and warfarin control did not appear to differ between groups, warfarin knowledge was lower in the limited health literacy group.[6]

So what is the implication of these findings? When designing a patient education program for anticoagulants, the written materials should be written at a low education level (the patient education sheets provided below are written at a 6th-grade level). Pharmacists and other health professionals engaged in patient education of any kind need to be aware of health literacy issues. For example, a knowledgeable pharmacist in this area would likely know a patient with limited English proficiency is at risk of poor health literacy. This pharmacist would strive to provide the educational materials in the patient's native tongue and would arrange a professional translator to be present when the face to face education is to occur. This issue was important enough for the Institute of Medicine (IOM) to recommend:

> Professional schools and professional continuing education programs in health and related fields, including medicine, dentistry, *pharmacy*, social work, anthropology, nursing, public health, and journalism, should incorporate health literacy into their curricula and areas of competence.[2]

Cultural Considerations

Another important consideration when educating patients on anticoagulants is the patient's cultural background. For example, some Vietnamese have profound respect for authority and will not question healthcare providers. Some Latinos believe illness is caused by supernatural or spiritual agents. If the pharmacist providing the education does not attempt to understand these beliefs, the effectiveness of the education could suffer.[7]

Ann Zweber recently recommended the following steps in the *American Journal of Pharmaceutical Education* for pharmacists to ensure their own cultural competence[8]:

1. Examine your own cultural background.
2. Learn about the cultures you serve.
3. Demonstrate sincere interest in your client's culture. Ask open-ended questions.
4. Recognize cultural differences.
5. Don't generalize or stereotype. Determine individual perceptions, beliefs, preferences, and needs.
6. Make the pharmacy environment welcoming and attractive based on clients' cultural backgrounds.
7. Negotiate and educate to develop therapeutic plans which are compatible with cultural beliefs.
8. Use culturally sensitive educational approaches and materials.
9. Learn some phrases of the predominant non-English speaking population in your community.
10. Be aware of culturally based resources in your community. Have materials available for referral if needed.
11. For language barriers, use a trained interpreter if possible. If not, a family member may be helpful.
12. Pictograms may help convey some messages.

By increasing cultural competence, pharmacists will be able to connect the education to what is important to the patient.

General Patient Education Tips

Here are some final tips to provide high quality patient education[7]:

- Understand the patient's values. Link the value of the anticoagulant medication to their values when possible.
- Make sure the setting where the education is being provided is as private as possible. If the patient shares a room, consider closing the curtain to increase the sense of privacy or provide the education when the other patient is absent.
- Promote that patients must become an active participant in their treatment. This may be very challenging yet important with some cultural backgrounds.
- Use open-ended questions whenever questioning is needed. This makes the patient verbalize what they are thinking rather than providing "yes" and "no" answers. For example, when educating on enoxaparin, instead of asking, "Do you understand how to inject the medication?" ask instead "Would you now explain to me how you plan to inject the medication?" A good tip to ensure a question is open-ended is to use the five "W" questions (who, what, where, when, why) and the "H" question (how).[9]
- Consider having the patient explain back to you the most important points you have imparted to assure he or she understands. This both helps reinforce the major points in the patient's mind while giving the pharmacist a chance to "fill in the gaps."
- Provide written supplemental resources to all patients. Assure it is on an appropriate reading level as described above.
- Utilize other teaching techniques that may be helpful such as videos, DVDs, on-line demonstrations, etc., that may assist in teaching difficult concepts. This may be particularly useful with injectable training.

Patient Education Materials for the Patient and Pharmacist

When the conversation is complete, it is important to provide patients with supplementary materials to take with them to refer to and keep for their own records. Medication information handouts such as those found at www.safemedication.com and in *The Medication Teaching Manual*, published by ASHP, are good for this purpose. Also, giving patients a dosing calendar in addition to the handouts can assure that they know exactly how to take their medication. Examples of these types of materials are included in Appendixes 8-1 and 8-2 on warfarin and injectable anticoagulants such as enoxaparin and dalteparin. Other excellent resources for warfarin education materials and templates can be found in *Managing Oral Anticoagulation Therapy: Clinical and Operational Guidelines* available from Facts and Comparisons.

For the pharmacist, using checklists such as the ones provided in Appendixes 8-1 and 8-2 can help to ensure that all of the important issues are covered when talking to a patient. The checklist can be kept with patients' files as part of their medication record.

Internet Patient Education Resources

Many other resources to aid in anticoagulation patient education can be readily found on the internet from respectable sources. A sample of useful sights and comments on the sites can be found in Table 8-1. Many of these sites have downloadable patient materials or materials that can be ordered for use at a hospital. These sites also provide useful ideas on what to include in the hospital anticoagulation education program.

Finally, sites that are deemed excellent could also be given to patients as recommended home reading provided they or a family member has internet access.

Conclusion

Excellent patient education is a key to providing anticoagulation services in any setting. The programs must be able to train patients with low health literacy and from all cultures. Pharmacists should be given a refresher on how to provide excellent patient education and supplement their verbal training of patients with written material. The internet contains many excellent patient education resources for anticoagulants that come from reputable sources and can be an excellent aid for an inpatient anticoagulation program.

References

1. Unknown. ASHP 2015 Initiative. *American Society of Health-System Pharmacists*. Available at: http://www.ashp.org/2015/Obj1.cfm?cfid=18711029&CFToken=13024978. Accessed November 4, 2006.
2. Unknown. Health Literacy: A Prescription to End Confusion. *Institute of Medicine*. Available at: http://www.nap.edu/catalog/10883.html#toc. Accessed November 4, 2006.
3. Win K, Schillinger D. Understanding of warfarin therapy and stroke among ethnically diverse anticoagulation patients at a public hospital. *Abstr J Gen Intern Med*. 2003;18(suppl 1):278 (abstract).
4. Lasater L. Patient literacy, adherence, and anticoagulation therapy outcomes: A preliminary report. *J Gen Intern Med*. 2003;18(suppl 1):179 (abstract).
5. Estrada CA, Martin-Hryniewicz M, Peek BT, Collins

Table 8-1.
Useful Anticoagulation Patient Education Websites

Website	Sponsor	Comment
www.afadvisor.org	AF (atrial fibrillation) Advisor, a group of expert physicians	Excellent patient information on atrial fibrillation and it covers why anticoagulation is necessary to prevent stroke. The site also has downloadable patient education materials and pamphlets that can be ordered.
www.ecu.edu/anticoagulation	Brody School of Medicine at East Carolina University	Site contains low health literacy friendly patient brochures on anticoagulation topics.
www.clotcare.com	ClotCare	Site contains some answers to frequently asked questions by patients.
www.nattinfo.org	The National Alliance for Thrombosis and Thrombophilia	Site contains stories from patients living with thrombophilia and other support materials for thrombophilia patients.
www.tigc.org	Thrombosis Interest Group of Canada	Site contains education for patients on oral anticoagulation and about the risk of developing deep vein thrombosis due to traveling.
www.med.umich.edu/cvc/prof/anticoag	University of Michigan Anticoagulation Service	Site contains downloadable patient handouts on living with anticoagulation and patient information on the amount of vitamin K in different foods.
www.arixtra.com and www.arixtra.com/docs/LLC_PatEdBlkt.pdf	GlaxoSmithKline	Site has patient education materials on knee replacement, ordering form for a fondaparinux patient starter kit, and a patient education brochure.
www.coumadin.com	Bristol-Myers Squibb	Traditionally an excellent site for warfarin patient education materials, however, the site was under reconstruction at the time of writing this text.
www.jantoven.com/patient/index.html	Upsher-Smith Laboratories	Site contains both a patient education guide and a patient education brochure on warfarin including vitamin K content of common foods.
www.dvt.net	Sanofi Aventis	Site contains numerous patient resources regarding deep vein thrombosis including handouts and animations.
www.fragmin.com and http://www.fragmin.com/documents/How_to_inject_FRAGMIN.pdf	Pfizer	Site contains illustrations of deep vein thrombosis, materials to aid patients in administering dalteparin, and order forms for a dalteparin training kit.
www.innohepusa.com/corporateweb/innohepus/home.nsf/Content/Home	Pharmion	Site contains limited patient education materials on deep vein thrombosis.
www.lovenox.com	Sanofi Aventis	Site contains patient education materials on deep vein thrombosis and different kinds of anticoagulants.
www.americanheart.org	American Heart Association	Site contains extensive materials for patients with different thrombotic diseases and for anticoagulants.

Website	Sponsor	Comment
heartcenteronline.com	HeartCenterOnline	Site contains many patient education materials on heart disease and on anticoagulants.
www.nhlbi.nih.gov/health/dci/Diseases/Dvt/DVT_WhatIs.html and www.nhlbi.nih.gov/health/dci/Diseases/pe/pe_what.html	National Institutes of Health	Site contains government sponsored patient education on DVT and PE.
ods.od.nih.gov/factsheets/cc/coumadin1.pdf	National Institutes of Health	Site contains a patient handout on warfarin and vitamin K.
www.stroke.org	National Stroke Association	Site contains patient education materials on how to prevent stroke and on antithrombotics used to prevent future strokes.
pfrc.med.nyu.edu/handouts/alpha.html#w	NYU Medical Center	Site contains numerous patient education handouts on disease states and one specifically on warfarin.
www.mybloodthinner.org/	Project SOS Rx	Site is a patient education website completely dedicated to promoting the safe use of warfarin.
www.warfarinfo.com/	Warfarin Institute of America	Site is dedicated to providing information to patients on warfarin. It contains extensive educational materials.

C, Byrd JC. Literacy and numeracy skills and anticoagulation control. *Am J Med Sci*. 2004;328(2):88-93.

6. Fang MC, Machtinger EL, Wang F, Schillinger D. Health literacy and anticoagulation-related outcomes among patients taking warfarin. *J Gen Intern Med*. 2006;21(8):841-6.
7. Galt K. *Developing Clinical Practice Skills for Pharmacists*. Bethesda, MD: American Society of Health-System Pharmacists; 2006.
8. Zweber A. Cultural competence in pharmacy practice. *Am J Pharm Ed*. 2002;66:172-6.
9. Ginsberg DB, Vermeulen LC. Necessary skills to be an effective preceptor. In: Cuellar LM, Ginsberg DB, eds. *Preceptor's Handbook for Pharmacists*. Bethesda, MD: American Society of Health-System Pharmacists; 2005.
10. Unknown. *Medication Teaching Manual*. 8th ed. Bethesda, MD: American Society of Health-System Pharmacists; 2004.
11. Unknown. Medication Guide Coumadin Tablets. *Bristol-Myers Squibb Company*. April, 2006. Available at: www.fda.gov/Cder/Offices/ODS/MG/warfarinMG.pdf Accessed November 4, 2006.
12. Grant P. Warfarin and cranberry juice: an interaction? *J Heart Valve Dis*. 2004;13(1):25-6.
13. Rindone JP, Murphy TW. Warfarin-cranberry juice interaction resulting in profound hypoprothrombinemia and bleeding. *Am J Ther*. 2006;13(3):283-4.
14. Suvarna R, Pirmohamed M, Henderson L. Possible interaction between warfarin and cranberry juice. *Br J Med*. 2003;327(7429):1454.
15. Unknown. Dalteparin Sodium Injection. *American Society of Health-System Pharmacists*. Available at: http://www.safemedication.com/displaydrug.cfm?id=696006. Accessed November 4, 2006.

Appendix 8-1: Patient Education Materials: Warfarin

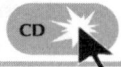

Contents

1. A warfarin education handout from the Medication Teaching Manual published by ASHP.[10] All patient education materials from this manual are written at a 6th-grade level in lay language.
2. The FDA-approved medication guide intended to be given to patients taking branded Coumadin® tablets.[11] References 1 and 2 above can serve as an excellent starting point for designing a new warfarin patient education tool at a hospital.
3. Patient education check-off sheet for a pharmacist to use when educating to assure all pertinent issues with warfarin have been shared in person with the patient. A record of this education should be placed in the permanent medical record.
4. A warfarin calendar that can be filled in by hand or on the computer and given to patients to assure they clearly know how they are to take warfarin each day.

Reference 1: Patient Education Handout from *The Medication Teaching Manual*

Warfarin

(war′ far in)

Other Names: Coumadin

Why is this medication prescribed?

Warfarin is used to prevent blood clots from forming or growing larger. It is often prescribed for patients with certain types of irregular heartbeat and after a heart attack or heart valve replacement surgery. It works by stopping the formation of substances that cause clots.

This medication is sometimes prescribed for other uses; ask your doctor or pharmacist for more information.

How should this medicine be used?

Warfarin comes as a tablet to take by mouth. It usually is taken once a day. Follow the directions on your prescription label carefully, and ask your doctor or pharmacist to explain any part you do not understand. Take warfarin exactly as directed. Do not take more or less of it or take it more often than prescribed by your doctor.

Continue to take warfarin even if you feel well. Do not stop taking warfarin without talking to your doctor.

What special precautions should I follow?

Before taking warfarin,

- tell your doctor and pharmacist if you are allergic to warfarin, aspirin, tartrazine (a yellow dye in some medications and processed foods), or any other drugs.
- tell your doctor and pharmacist what prescription and nonprescription medications you are taking, especially other heart medications; antibiotics; aspirin and other non-steroidal anti-inflammatory drugs such as ibuprofen (Advil, Motrin) and naproxen (Aleve, Naprosyn); cimetidine (Tagamet); medications for cancer, depression, diabetes, digestive problems, epilepsy, gout, high cholesterol, and thyroid problems; and vitamins. Many medications interfere with the effectiveness of warfarin. It is important that you tell your doctor every medication that you take, including nonprescription medications. Do not take any new medications without talking to your doctor.
- tell your doctor and pharmacist what herbal products you are taking, especially bromelains, coenzyme Q10, danshen, dong quai, garlic, Ginkgo biloba, and St. John's wort. Do not start taking any herbal products without talking to your doctor.

- tell your doctor if you have had your prostate removed, have or have ever had a stroke, kidney or liver disease, high blood pressure, a thyroid condition, diabetes, tuberculosis, a bleeding disorder, ulcers, leukemia, vitamin C deficiency, colostomy bag, or intestinal disease.
- tell your doctor if you are pregnant, plan to become pregnant, or are breast-feeding. If you become pregnant while taking warfarin, call your doctor.
- if you are having surgery, including dental surgery, tell the doctor or dentist that you are taking warfarin. Your doctor may tell you to stop taking warfarin 3 days before your procedure. Follow these directions.
- ask your doctor about the safe use of alcohol while you are taking warfarin.

What special dietary instructions should I follow?

Do not increase your consumption of foods containing vitamin K, such as liver, green leafy vegetables, broccoli, and cauliflower, without discussing your diet with your doctor.

What should I do if I forget a dose?

Take the missed dose as soon as you remember it. However, if it is almost time for the next dose, skip the missed dose and continue your regular dosing schedule. Do not take a double dose to make up for a missed one. Record the date of the missed dose and tell your doctor at your next visit, since missing a dose of warfarin may alter your blood clotting tests. If you miss doses for two or more days, call your doctor immediately.

What side effects can this medication cause?

Although side effects from warfarin are not common, they can occur. Warfarin may turn your urine red-orange; this effect is harmless. If you think your urine contains blood, call your doctor immediately. Tell your doctor if any of these symptoms are severe or do not go away:

- headache
- upset stomach
- diarrhea
- fever
- skin rash

If you experience any of the following symptoms, call your doctor immediately:

- unusual bleeding or bruising
- black or bloody stools
- blood in the urine
- tiredness
- unexplained fever
- chills
- sore throat
- stomach pain

What storage conditions are needed for this medication?

Keep this medication in the container it came in, tightly closed, and out of reach of children. Store it at room temperature and away from excess heat and moisture (not in the bathroom). Throw away any medication that is outdated or no longer needed. Talk to your pharmacist about the proper disposal of your medication.

What other information should I know?

Keep all appointments with your doctor and the laboratory. Your doctor will order certain lab tests to check your response to warfarin.

Warfarin prevents blood from clotting so it may take longer than usual for you to stop bleeding if you are cut or injured. Avoid activities that have a high risk of causing injury. Call your doctor if bleeding is unusual.

Carry an identification card or wear a bracelet that indicates that you take warfarin. Ask your pharmacist or doctor how to obtain this card or bracelet. List your name, medical problems, drugs and dosages, and doctor's name and telephone number on the card. Tell any doctor or dentist that you visit that you are taking warfarin.

If you have an illness that causes vomiting, diarrhea, or fever for more than a few days, call your doctor. These problems can change the effectiveness of warfarin.

Do not let anyone else take your medication. Ask your pharmacist any questions you have about refilling your prescription.

(Selected Revisions April 2003.)

Chapter 8 ■ Patient Education Needs

Reference 2: FDA Coumadin® Medication Guide

Author note: The handout mentions avoiding cranberry products. This is a controversial recommendation and is based on very limited patient data.[12-14]

Bristol-Myers Squibb Company

Distributed by:
Bristol-Myers Squibb Company
Princeton, New Jersey 08543 USA

COUMADIN® and the color and configuration of COUMADIN tablets are trademarks of Bristol-Myers Squibb Pharma Company.

Copyright © Bristol-Myers Squibb Company 2006

Printed in USA
1205733
1205735   Revised April 2006

MEDICATION GUIDE
COUMADIN® (COU-ma-din) Tablets
(Warfarin Sodium Tablets, USP) Crystalline

Read this Medication Guide before you start taking COUMADIN (Warfarin Sodium) and each time you get a refill. There may be new information. This Medication Guide does not take the place of talking to your healthcare provider about your medical condition or treatment. You and your healthcare provider should talk about COUMADIN when you start taking it and at regular checkups.

What is the most important information I should know about COUMADIN?

- **Take your COUMADIN exactly as prescribed to lower the chance of blood clots forming in your body.** (See "**What is COUMADIN?**").
- **COUMADIN is very important for your health, but it can cause serious and life-threatening bleeding problems.** To benefit from COUMADIN and also lower your chance for bleeding problems, you must:
  - **Get your regular blood test to check for your response to COUMADIN.** This blood test is called a PT/INR test. The PT/INR test checks to see how fast your blood clots. Your healthcare provider will decide what PT/INR numbers are best for you. Your dose of COUMADIN will be adjusted to keep your PT/INR in a target range for you.
  - **Call your healthcare provider right away if you get any of the following signs or symptoms of bleeding problems:**
    - pain, swelling or discomfort
    - headaches, dizziness, or weakness
    - unusual bruising (bruises that develop without known cause or grow in size)

31

Approved 2.0   Item 2 proposed.pdf

- nose bleeds
- bleeding gums
- bleeding from cuts takes a long time to stop
- menstrual bleeding or vaginal bleeding that is heavier than normal
- pink or brown urine
- red or black stools
- coughing up blood
- vomiting blood or material that looks like coffee grounds

- **Many other medicines, including prescription and non-prescription medicines, vitamins and herbal supplements can interact with COUMADIN and:**
  - **affect the dose you need, or**
  - **increase COUMADIN side effects.**

  Tell your healthcare provider about all the medicines you take. Do not stop medicines or take anything new unless you have talked to your healthcare provider. Keep a list of your medicines with you at all times to show your healthcare provider and pharmacist.

- Do not take other medicines that contain warfarin. **Warfarin is the active ingredient in COUMADIN.**
- **Some foods can interact with COUMADIN and affect your treatment and dose.**
  - **Eat a normal, balanced diet.** Talk to your doctor before you make any diet changes. **Do not eat large amounts of leafy green vegetables.** Leafy green vegetables contain Vitamin K. Certain vegetable oils also contain large amounts of Vitamin K. Too much Vitamin K can lower the effect of COUMADIN.
  - **Avoid drinking cranberry juice or eating cranberry products.**
  - **Avoid drinking alcohol.**
- **Always tell all of your healthcare providers that you take COUMADIN.**
- **Wear or carry information that you take COUMADIN.**

What is COUMADIN?

COUMADIN is an anticoagulant medicine. It is used to lower the chance of blood clots forming in your body. Blood clots can cause a stroke, heart attack, or other serious conditions such as blood clots in the legs or lungs.

Who should not take COUMADIN?

Do not take COUMADIN if:

- **your chance of having bleeding problems is higher than the possible benefit of treatment.** Your healthcare provider will decide if COUMADIN is right for you. Talk to your healthcare provider about all of your health conditions.
- **you are pregnant or plan to become pregnant.** COUMADIN can cause death or birth defects to an unborn baby. Use effective birth control if you can get pregnant.
- **you are allergic to warfarin or to anything else in COUMADIN.**

What should I tell my healthcare provider before starting COUMADIN?

Tell your healthcare provider about all of your health conditions, including if you:

- **have bleeding problems**
- **fall often**
- **have liver or kidney problems**
- **have high blood pressure**
- **have a heart problem called congestive heart failure**
- **have diabetes**
- **drink alcohol or have problems with alcohol abuse.** Alcohol can affect your COUMADIN dose and should be avoided.
- **are pregnant or planning to become pregnant.** See "Who should not take COUMADIN?"
- **are breastfeeding.** COUMADIN may increase bleeding in your baby. Talk to your doctor about the best way to feed your baby. If you choose to breastfeed while taking COUMADIN, both you and your baby should be carefully monitored for bleeding problems.

Tell your healthcare provider about all the medicines you take including prescription and non-prescription medicines, vitamins, and herbal supplements. See "What is the most important information I should know about COUMADIN?"

How should I take COUMADIN?

- **Take COUMADIN exactly as prescribed.** Your healthcare provider will adjust your dose from time to time depending on your response to COUMADIN.
- **You must have regular blood tests and visits with your healthcare provider to monitor your condition.**
- **Take COUMADIN at the same time every day.** You can take COUMADIN either with food or on an empty stomach.

- **If you miss a dose of COUMADIN, call your healthcare provider.** Take the dose as soon as possible on the same day. Do not take a double dose of COUMADIN the next day to make up for a missed dose.
- **Call your healthcare provider right away if you take too much COUMADIN.**
- **Call your healthcare provider if you are sick with diarrhea, an infection, or have a fever.**
- **Tell your healthcare provider about any planned surgeries, medical or dental procedures.** Your COUMADIN may have to be stopped for a short time or you may need your dose adjusted.
- **Call your healthcare provider right away if you fall or injure yourself, especially if you hit your head.** Your healthcare provider may need to check you.

What should I avoid while taking COUMADIN?

- Do not start, stop, or change any medicine without talking with your healthcare provider.
- Do not make changes in your diet, such as eating large amounts of green, leafy vegetables.
- Do not change your weight by dieting, without first checking with your healthcare provider.
- Avoid drinking alcohol.
- Do not do any activity or sport that may cause a serious injury.

What are the possible side effects of COUMADIN?

- COUMADIN is very important for your health, but it can cause serious and life-threatening bleeding problems. See "**What is the most important information I should know about COUMADIN?**"
- **Serious side effects of COUMADIN also include:**
  - **death of skin tissue (skin necrosis or gangrene).** This can happen soon after starting COUMADIN. It happens because blood clots form and block blood flow to an area of your body. Call your healthcare provider right away if you have pain, color, or temperature change to any area of your body. You may need medical care right away to prevent death or loss (amputation) of your affected body part.
  - **"purple toes syndrome."** Call your healthcare provider right away if you have pain in your toes and they look purple in color or dark in color.

Other side effects with COUMADIN include allergic reactions, liver problems, low blood pressure, swelling, low red blood cells, paleness, fever, and rash. Call your healthcare provider if you have any side effect that bothers you.

Bristol-Myers Squibb Company

These are not all of the side effects of COUMADIN. For more information, ask your healthcare provider or pharmacist.

How should I store COUMADIN?

- Store COUMADIN at room temperature between 59° and 86° F. Protect from light.
- **Keep COUMADIN and all medicines out of the reach of children.**

General Information about COUMADIN

Medicines are sometimes prescribed for purposes not mentioned in a Medication Guide. Do not use COUMADIN for a condition for which it was not prescribed. Do not give COUMADIN to other people, even if they have the same condition. It may harm them.

This Medication Guide summarizes the most important information about COUMADIN. If you would like more information, talk with your healthcare provider. You can ask your healthcare provider or pharmacist for information about COUMADIN that was written for healthcare professionals.

If you would like more information, call 1-800-321-1335.

Rx only

COUMADIN is distributed by:
Bristol-Myers Squibb Company
Princeton, New Jersey 08543 USA

COUMADIN® is a registered trademark of Bristol-Myers Squibb Pharma Company. COUMADIN (Warfarin Sodium), the COUMADIN color logo, COLORS OF COUMADIN, and the color and configuration of COUMADIN tablets are trademarks of Bristol-Myers Squibb Pharma Company.

**The brands listed (other than COUMADIN®) are registered trademarks of their respective owners and are not trademarks of Bristol-Myers Squibb Company.

This Medication Guide has been approved by the U.S. Food and Drug Administration.

1205733
1205735

April 2006

Reference 3: Patient Training Check-off List: Warfarin

Patient Education Point	Yes	No
1. Patient has been educated that warfarin is a blood thinner.		
2. Patient has been educated on why he or she has been prescribed warfarin.		
3. Patient has been educated that warfarin can cause bleeding.		
4. Patient has been educated on the necessity of regular INR monitoring.		
5. Patient has been educated to take the exact amount of warfarin prescribed each day and that the dosing regimen could possibly vary from day to day.		
6. Patient has been educated that medication aids such as pill boxes, calendars, etc., are a good idea to aid with warfarin therapy.		
7. Patient has been educated on his or her target INR range.		
8. Patient has been educated on the signs of bleeding problems.		
9. Patient has been educated to seek immediate medical attention for severe bleeding issues.		
10. Patient has been educated that warfarin has many drug interactions.		
11. Patient has been educated to notify their provider managing warfarin prior to taking any new medications including over the counter products and herbal products.		
12. Patient has been educated to always keep a current medication list.		
13. Patient has been educated on the effect of vitamin K on warfarin.		
14. Patient has been educated on what foods contain high amounts of vitamin K.		
15. Patient has been encouraged to eat a diet with a stable amount of vitamin K intake.		
16. Patient has been educated on the effects of alcohol (ethanol) on warfarin.		
17. Patient has been educated that warfarin is not intended for pregnant patients or those who plan to become pregnant.		
18. Patient has been educated to take warfarin at the same time every day, preferably in the evening.		
19. Patient has been educated on what to do if he or she misses a dose of warfarin.		
20. Patient has been educated to call the healthcare provider managing warfarin if he or she gets diarrhea, has an infection, or has a fever, as this can affect warfarin responsiveness.		
21. Patient has been educated to contact the healthcare provider managing warfarin if he or she will have any planned surgeries or other medical and dental procedures.		
22. Patient has been educated to seek medical attention for serious falls, particularly if the fall injures his or her head.		
23. Patient has been educated to avoid contact sports and activities that may cause serious injury.		
24. Patient has been educated that he or she should either carry an ID badge or bracelet saying he or she is on warfarin.		
25. Patient has been instructed that special arrangements may need to be made for monitoring during extended travel and that all extended travel plans should be shared early with his or her anticoagulation provider.		
26. Patient has been given written warfarin education materials to supplement verbal education.		

Reference 4: Patient Warfarin Calendar

Your current tablet strength is _____ mg. The pharmacist has filled out this calendar for you. Please take your warfarin as indicated until your next INR check. Following this check, ask your healthcare provider to help you fill out a new calendar for use until your next blood test. It is important to tell your healthcare provider if you missed any doses of warfarin or accidentally took too much warfarin.

Date							
Dose	mg	mg	mg	mg	mg	mg	mg
Number of Tablets	_____ tablet(s)	_____ tablet(s)	_____ tablet(s)	_____ tablet(s)	_____ tablet(s)	_____ tablet(s)	_____ tablet(s)
Dose taken? (place X to indicate)							

Your next blood test (INR) will be drawn at _____ on _____ (date) at _____ (time).

Appendix 8-2: Patient Education Materials: Injectable Anticoagulants such as Enoxaparin and Dalteparin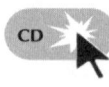

Contents

1. An enoxaparin handout taken from the *Medication Teaching Manual* published by ASHP.[10]
2. A dalteparin handout taken from MedMaster also published by ASHP.[15]
   References 1 and 2 could be used as a template for making handouts on fondaparinux or subcutaneous heparin. The manufacturers for enoxaparin, dalteparin, and fondaparinux also offer patient starter kits with demonstration videos and sharps containers. These can be very helpful for patient training.
3. A patient training check-off list much like the warfarin sheet. A record of this education should be placed in the permanent medical record.
4. A patient calendar dosing aid that is intended for injectable anticoagulants.

Reference 1: Patient Education Handout

Enoxaparin Injection

(ee nox a pa′ rin)

Other Names: Lovenox

Important Warning

> If you have epidural or spinal anesthesia or a spinal puncture while taking a "blood thinner" such as enoxaparin, you are at risk for collection of blood in the spinal column that could cause you to become paralyzed. Tell your doctor if you are taking other anticoagulants ("blood thinners") such as warfarin (Coumadin), abciximab (ReoPro), anagrelide (Agrylin), aspirin or nonsteroidal anti-inflammatory drugs (ibuprofen, naproxen), cilostazol (Pletal), clopidogrel (Plavix), dipyridamole (Persantine), eptifibatide (Integrilin), sulfinpyrazone (Anturane), ticlopidine (Ticlid), and tirofiban (Aggrastat).
>
> If you experience any of the following symptoms, call your doctor immediately: numbness, tingling, leg weakness or paralysis, and loss of control over your bladder or bowels.
>
> Talk to your doctor about the risk of taking enoxaparin. Keep all appointments with your doctor.

Why is this medication prescribed?

Enoxaparin is used to prevent blood clots in the leg in patients who are on bedrest or who are having hip replacement, knee replacement, or stomach surgery. It is used in combination with aspirin to prevent complications from angina (chest pain) and heart attacks. It is also used in combination with warfarin to treat blood clots in the leg. Enoxaparin is in a class of medications called low molecular weight heparins. It works by stopping the formation of substances that cause clots.

How should this medicine be used?

Enoxaparin comes as an injection in a syringe to be injected just under the skin (subcutaneously) but not into your muscle. It is usually given twice a day. You will probably begin using the drug while you are in the hospital and then use it for a total of 10–14 days. Follow the directions on your prescription label carefully, and ask your doctor or pharmacist to explain any part you do not understand. Use enoxaparin exactly as directed. Do not inject more or less of it or inject it more often than prescribed by your doctor.

Continue to use enoxaparin even if you feel well. Do not stop taking enoxaparin without talking to your doctor.

Your healthcare provider will teach you how to give yourself the shot or arrangements will be made for someone else to give you the shot. Enoxaparin is usually injected in the stomach area. You must use a different area of the stomach each time you give the shot. If you have questions about where to give the shot, ask your healthcare provider. Each syringe has enough drug in it for one shot. Do not use the syringe and needle more than one time. Your doctor, pharmacist, or healthcare provider will tell you how to throw away used needles and syringes to avoid accidental injury. Keep syringes and needles out of reach of children.

To inject enoxaparin, follow these instructions:

1. Wash your hands and the area of skin where you will give the shot.
2. Look at the syringe to be sure the drug is clear and colorless or pale yellow.
3. Take the cap off the needle. Do not push any air or drug out of the syringe before giving the shot unless your healthcare provider tells you to.
4. Lie down and pinch a fold of skin between your finger and thumb. Push the entire needle into the skin and then press down on the syringe plunger to inject the drug. Hold onto the skin the entire time you give the shot. Do not rub the site after you give the shot.

What special precautions should I follow?

Before taking enoxaparin,

- tell your doctor and pharmacist if you are allergic to enoxaparin, heparin, any other drugs, or pork products.
- tell your doctor and pharmacist what prescription and nonprescription medications you are taking, especially those listed in the IMPORTANT WARNING section and vitamins.
- tell your doctor if you have an artificial heart valve and if you have or have ever had kidney disease, an infection in your heart, a stroke, a bleeding disorder, ulcers, or a low platelet count.
- tell your doctor if you are pregnant, plan to become pregnant, or are breast-feeding. If you become pregnant while taking enoxaparin, call your doctor.
- if you are having surgery, including dental surgery, tell the doctor or dentist that you are taking enoxaparin.

What should I do if I forget a dose?

Inject the missed dose as soon as you remember it. However, if it is almost time for the next dose, skip the missed dose and continue your regular dosing schedule. Do not inject a double dose to make up for a missed one.

What side effects can this medication cause?

Although side effects from enoxaparin are not common, they can occur. Tell your doctor if any of these symptoms are severe or do not go away:

- upset stomach
- fever
- irritation or burning at site of injection

If you experience any of the following symptoms or those listed in the IMPORTANT WARNING section, call your doctor immediately:

- unusual bleeding or bruising
- black or bloody stools
- blood in urine
- swollen ankles and/or feet

What storage conditions are needed for this medication?

Keep this medication out of reach of children. Store the syringes at room temperature and away from excess heat and moisture (not in the bathroom). Do not use the syringe if it leaks or if the fluid is dark or contains particles. Throw away any medication that is outdated or no longer needed. Talk to your pharmacist about the proper disposal of your medication.

What other information should I know?

Keep all appointments with your doctor and the laboratory. Your doctor will order certain lab tests to monitor your enoxaparin therapy.

Enoxaparin prevents blood from clotting so it may take longer than usual for you to stop bleeding if you are cut or injured. Avoid activities that have a high risk of causing injury. Call your doctor if bleeding is unusual.

Do not let anyone else use your medication. Your prescription is probably not refillable.

(Selected Revisions April 2003.)

Chapter 8 ■ Patient Education Needs

Reference 2: Patient Education Handout

Dalteparin Sodium Injection

(dal te pa' rin)

Other Names: Fragmin

Important Warning

> If you have epidural or spinal anesthesia or a spinal puncture while taking a 'blood thinner' such as dalteparin, you are at risk for internal bleeding that could cause you to become paralyzed.
>
> Tell your doctor if you are taking abciximab (ReoPro); anagrelide (Agrylin); other anticoagulants ('blood thinners') such as warfarin (Coumadin); aspirin, ibuprofen (Advil, Motrin, or Nuprin), indomethacin (Indocin), ketoprofen (Actron, Orudis), naproxen (Aleve, Anaprox, Naprosyn), or other nonsteroidal anti-inflammatory drugs (NSAIDs); cilostazol (Pletal); clopidogrel (Plavix); dipyridamole (Persantine); eptifibatide (Integrilin); sulfinpyrazone (Anturane); ticlopidine (Ticlid); and tirofiban (Aggrastat).
>
> If you experience any of the following symptoms, call your doctor immediately: numbness, tingling, leg weakness or paralysis, and loss of control over your bladder or bowels. Talk to your doctor about the risk of taking dalteparin.

About your treatment

Your doctor has ordered dalteparin sodium, an anticoagulant ('blood thinner'), to prevent harmful blood clots from forming. The drug will be injected under the skin (subcutaneously) once a day. This medication is sometimes prescribed for other uses; ask your doctor or pharmacist for more information.

Your health care provider (doctor, nurse, or pharmacist) may measure the effectiveness and side effects of your treatment using laboratory tests and physical examinations. It is important to keep all appointments with your doctor and the laboratory. The length of treatment depends on how you respond to the medication.

Precautions

Before administering dalteparin,

- tell your doctor and pharmacist if you are allergic to dalteparin, heparin, enoxaparin (Lovenox), any other drugs, or pork products.
- tell your doctor and pharmacist what prescription and nonprescription medications you are taking, especially those listed in the IMPORTANT WARNING section and vitamins.
- tell your doctor if you have or have ever had liver or kidney disease or diabetes.
- tell your doctor if you are pregnant, plan to become pregnant, or are breast-feeding. If you become pregnant while taking dalteparin, call your doctor.

Administering your medication

Before you administer dalteparin, look at the solution closely. It should be clear and free of floating material. Observe the solution container to make sure there are no leaks. Do not use the solution if it is discolored, if it contains particles, or if the container leaks. Use a new solution, but show the damaged one to your health care provider.

Managing Anticoagulation Patients in the Hospital: The Inpatient Anticoagulation Service

It is important that you use your medication exactly as directed. Do not change your dosing schedule without talking to your health care provider.

Side effects

Although side effects from dalteparin are not common, they can occur. Tell your health care provider if the following symptom is severe or does not go away:

- upset stomach

If you experience any of the following symptoms or those listed in the IMPORTANT WARNING section, call your doctor or health care provider immediately:

- unusual bleeding
- vomiting or spitting up blood or brown material that resembles coffee grounds
- bloody or black, tarry stools
- blood in urine
- red or dark-brown urine
- easy bruising
- excessive menstrual bleeding
- fever
- dizziness or lightheadedness

Storing your medication

- Your health care provider will probably give you several days supply of dalteparin at a time. You will be told to store it at room temperature.

Store your medication only as directed. Make sure you understand what you need to store your medication properly.

Keep your supplies in a clean, dry place when you are not using them, and keep all medications and supplies out of reach of children. Your health care provider will tell you how to throw away used needles, syringes, tubing, and containers to avoid accidental injury.

Signs of infection

If you are receiving dalteparin under your skin, you need to know the symptoms of a catheter-related infection (an infection where the needle enters your skin). If you experience any of these effects near the infusion site, tell your health care provider as soon as possible:

- tenderness
- warmth
- irritation
- drainage
- redness
- swelling
- pain

Reference 3: Patient Training Check-off List for Injectable Anticoagulants

Patient Education Point	Yes	No
1. Patient has been educated that _____ (medication) is a blood thinner.		
2. Patient has been educated on why he or she has been prescribed _____ (medication).		
3. Patient has been educated that _____ (medication) can cause bleeding.		
4. Patient has been educated to inject the dose of _____ (medication) at the prescribed times each day.		
5. Patient has been educated that a dosing calendar may be useful to help not forget injections.		
6. Patient has been educated on the signs of bleeding problems.		
7. Patient has been educated to seek immediate medical attention for severe bleeding issues.		
8. For patients also on warfarin, the patient has been educated that it is okay to use _____ (medication) together with warfarin until the INR is in range and stable.		
9. Patient has been educated on what to do if he or she misses a dose of _____ (medication).		
10. Patient has been educated to contact the healthcare provider managing _____ (medication) if he or she will have any planned surgeries or other medical and dental procedures.		
11. Patient has been educated to seek medical attention for serious falls, particularly if the fall involves damage to his or her head.		
12. Patient has been educated to avoid contact sports and activities that may cause serious injury.		
13. Patient has been given written _____ (medication) education materials to supplement education.		
14. Patient has viewed instructional video on self-injecting the medication.		
15. Patient has been educated to wash and dry hands thoroughly prior to giving an injection.		
16. Patient has been educated to sit or lay in a comfortable position to prepare for the injection.		
17. Patient has been educated to look closely at the medication solution prior to injection for discoloration or particulate matter and to avoid injection if present.		
18. Patient has been educated to inject the medication into the abdomen and least 2 inches from navel.		
19. Patient has been educated to rotate injection sites.		
20. Patient has been educated to clean the planned injection site with an alcohol swab.		
21. Patient has been educated on how to remove the needle cap		
22. Patient has been educated on how the pinch the skin and actually give the injection.		
23. Patient has been educated not to rub the injection site.		
24. Patient has been educated on how to engage the needle safety system.		
25. Patient has been educated to place the used needle in a sharps container.		
26. When the treatment course is complete, patient has been educated on how to dispose of the sharps container with used syringes.		
27. Patient demonstrates the ability to give themselves the injection prior to discharge.		
28. Patient has been educated to continue therapy until instructed to stop by their anticoagulation therapy management provider.		

Managing Anticoagulation Patients in the Hospital: The Inpatient Anticoagulation Service

Patient Injectable Anticoagulant Calendar

You have been prescribed _____. You should inject ____ mg of _____ _____ times per day. The pharmacist has filled out this calendar for you. Please inject _____ as instructed at the same times each day until you are told to stop by your healthcare provider.

Date														
Dose	mg		mg		mg		mg		mg		mg		mg	
Time														
	AM	PM	AM	PM	AM	PM	AM	PM	AM	PM	AM	PM	AM	PM
Dose taken? (place X to indicate)														

Chapter 9

Monitoring and Maintaining Program Quality

Michael Gulseth

Chapter Outline

- Introduction
- Continuous quality improvement overview
- Planning the changes (plan)
- Implementing the changes (do)
- Study the effects of the changes (study)
- Act on the study results and repeat the cycle (act)
- Conclusion
- Case study
  - Plan
  - Do
  - Study
  - Act
- References

Introduction

Implementation of an inpatient anticoagulation program is the culmination of a lot of hard work by a lot of people. As stated previously, it is a critical step to improve the safe use of anticoagulants in the hospital. Like many programs launched in the healthcare setting, the anticoagulation program will need to be tweaked and improved over time. But how does one tweak and improve a program? How does one even know the program has issues that need to be improved? How do further refinements to the program get made? How are new opportunities for care improvement realized? How can the department continuously justify the resources being dedicated to the program with likely little reimbursement for cognitive services? This is the role of continuous quality improvement (CQI). CQI should be practiced by the anticoagulation program to realize future opportunities and justify its existence.

Continuous Quality Improvement Overview

A department of pharmacy engaging in CQI acknowledges that all services can be improved and collects data both to decide what needs to be improved and determine if changes made have improved care. These pharmacy departments design their services to meet the needs of their primary customers, patients, and secondary customers, physicians and nurses.[1] Departments practicing this philosophy are constantly generating data to assess the quality of the care provided, and then acting on the finding to improve care. This cycle is constantly repeated to make further and further improvements in care.[2,3]

An in depth discussion of CQI is beyond the scope of this book. Instead, this chapter will jump right into a helpful continuous quality improvement process known as the "Plan, Do, Study, Act" (PDSA) methodology. This is not the only methodology available (for example, another well-known methodology is Six Sigma®), however, PDSA is an easy methodology to adopt that is simple to learn and understand. Further, it is a recommended strategy of the Institute for Healthcare Improvement, a national leader in promoting healthcare quality.[2]

Planning the Changes (Plan)

Planning the inpatient anticoagulation service has already been discussed in detail in Chapter 4. What has not been discussed is that the anticoagulation planning team must think about quality and define what they think quality will look like. The PDSA Case Study at the end of this chapter walks through a team utilizing PDSA methodology and gives examples of how quality could be defined.

Here are some tips in picking the quality measures. First, the team should clearly identify what they are trying to accomplish. For an inpatient anticoagulation service, the aim of the team likely involves improving the appropriate use of these high-risk medications in patients. Second, the team should ask themselves how will they know improvement has been made? For an inpatient anticoagulation service, it may be a decrease in adverse drug events like bleeding due to anticoagulants or prevention of recurrent thrombosis from baseline. Or, it could be decreases in surrogate markers that may indicate risk of those hard endpoints such as percentages severely elevated INRs. The key is that the improvement must be measurable and time specific so it can be trended over time. Further, a goal should be set for performance. Reviewing the literature in Chapter 2 may be helpful for determining these goals. Finally, the action taken, in this case implementing an inpatient anticoagulation service, should be designed in a way that is felt will likely improve the quality of care. Implementing the program is the "do" step.[2]

Implementing the Changes (Do)

The "do" step in improving the safety on anticoagulants, as it relates to this book, would be to pilot the inpatient anticoagulation program in the way planned in Chapter 4. To improve medication systems, the Institute for Healthcare Improvement (IHI) recommends[2]:

- Developing a culture of safety
- Reducing harm from high-hazard medications
- Improving medication core processes
- Improving medication reconciliation

As one can easily see, an inpatient anticoagulation program is a "do" step that, when correctly implemented, addresses all four of these areas. An inpatient anticoagulation program creates a culture of safety by showing the organization is serious about avoiding problems with high-risk medications. It is a fundamental change to the traditional medication process and an excellent program will address transitional care issues on both admission and discharge.

Before a department implements an inpatient anticoagulation program, it is helpful if they have collected the same quality data for the time period prior to implementation. This data could also be collected retrospectively once the program is implemented. This way, the program can demonstrate any improvements to care that are made compared to a baseline. This concept is shown in the Case Study.

Study the Effects of the Changes (Study)

When deciding what to measure for monitoring quality, IHI recommends that three types of measures be implemented. First, if possible, measure the outcomes of the service. As mentioned previously, the services impact on bleeding rates or re-thrombosis rates from baseline would be great examples of this type of measure. The second measures are process measures. These measures assure the process is being run in the planned fashion. For example, the program manager could do perform random chart audits of 10 charts per month to assure progress notes are being written as planned or if other policies of the program are being followed. See Table 9-1 for an example data collection form for the type of analysis. The third measures are balancing measures. These measures assure that the changes implemented have not affected other core services in an adverse fashion. For example, the pharmacy department may want to monitor the quality of the clinical pharmacokinetics program if the same pharmacist performs both functions. Examples of outcome and process measures can be found in the Case Study.

Another problem that might be encountered by the program manager when testing changes is deciding where the resources will come from to collect the quality data. Some hospitals have implemented an Access databases to automate this data collection along with aiding program organization.[4] Even if this is not possible, random sampling of 10 patients a month may provide good data. Instead of using pharmacists to collect this data, investigate if the organization may have nurses in the quality department to do these audits. Another idea is to utilize pharmacy students on rotation as not only will it provide resources to conduct the study, it will be a great experience for them to

Chapter 9 ■ Monitoring and Maintaining Program Quality

Table 9-1.
Process Measure Data Collection Form

Process Quality Audit for Warfarin

Measure	1	2	3	4	5	6	7	8	9	10
Date of birth is recorded										
Patient height is recorded										
Patient weight is recorded										
Reason for admission is recorded										
Target INR range has been indicated										
Past medical history is recorded										
When appropriate, warfarin dose prior to admission is recorded (place check mark if a new warfarin start)										
Indication for anticoagulation is recorded										
Concurrent medications are listed										
Box is checked indicating a progress note has been written in the chart after the initial consultation										
All INRs are recorded daily										
The discharge dosing is clearly noted										
The planned INR follow-up day is noted										
Box has been checked indicating that discharge form has been faxed to anticoagulation or other appropriate clinic										
Box has been checked indication the patient has been educated on warfarin										

A pharmacy student audits 10 patients a month in the computer program to assure all of the key processes are completed. A check mark indicates the function was performed. The goal is 100% compliance. All instances of non-compliance are referred to the program manager to determine the reason for lack of adherence to the system.

125

learn the importance of collecting data to support practice changes. A final idea is that for some of the measures, it may even be possible to train an administrative aide or technician to collect the data.

So how often should quality data regarding the program be reported? First, this text would recommend collecting quality data on a monthly basis. The results of quality analysis should be reported up through the organization every 3–6 months. Reporting the quality data is not only important for planning further improvements and refinements of the system. Reporting the measures makes the pharmacy department look good as it shows how serious the department is regarding assuring safe and effective care is being delivered. This data is even more effective in supporting further practice advancement if it can be compared to a baseline performance as shown in the Case Study.

Act on the Study Results and Repeat the Cycle (Act)

Reporting the success of changes as described above is an important step to create the institutional buy in of the positive effects of an inpatient anticoagulation program. However, the anticoagulation program manager must also realize that "bumps in the road" will be encountered and that these may get reflected in the quality data. It is important for the program manager to carefully consider the quality data of the program on a monthly basis, and be prepared to plan new changes when needed and repeat the PDSA study cycle. To know what changes are needed, the program manager needs some knowledge on how to interpret the quality data.

First, the program manager needs to understand that the anticoagulant program is a system of processes. Figures 6-1 and 6-2 in the Chapter 6 Case Study illustrate how these systems might be graphically described. To consistently improve the performance of a system (thus consistently improving quality data), redesign the system to make it less prone to failure (i.e., in this case, abandoning the traditional way of managing anticoagulants in the hospital and establishing an inpatient anticoagulation service). Graphically, an anticoagulation program focused on managing warfarin that improves care would generate data that might look something like Figures 9-1 and 9-2 in the Case Study. Notice the clear and consistent change in performance (with the exception of November) from when the program was implemented compared to before implementation. If a program does not create clear and consistent improvement in the measures picked and the team agrees on the soundness of the measures, the system may need to be fundamentally redesigned to create the improvement desired.[1]

The second important concept the program manager must realize that sometimes the system will not function as designed. When this happens, "blips" of slips in quality will be evident when tracking data. This is depicted visually in Figures 9-1 and 9-2 of the Case Study for November. When these blips in data occur, the program manager should analyze the raw data for that time period to find out how the system broke down. Examples of situations that could lead to the system not performing as designed could include:

- Inadequate staffing leading to a pharmacist performing the function rushing through work.
- A new staff member managing anticoagulation without proper training.
- The wrong INR was reported for a patient causing an error in dosing.

To ensure the continued success of the program, the program manager must directly address the breakdowns in the system to assure they do not happen again. If system processes can be tweaked to ensure the same mistake <u>cannot</u> happen again, this is the option that should be chosen.[1]

It is also important to act on data that looks good. In the Case Study, Figures 9-1 and 9-2 show what look to be an improvement in care after the service was implemented. This data should be promoted through the organization as suggested above and the data also suggests that this pilot should be implemented in other areas. When spreading the change, be sure to address any problems encountered during the pilot so they do not happen again. Also, spreading the change is an example of how the PDSA cycle repeats itself as one would "plan" to spread the anticoagulation program to new areas, actually implement the program ("do"), "study" the effects of the program in the new areas, and "act" on the results of those evaluations.

The PDSA methodology is intended to run multiple times to continuously improve quality. So, if after expanding a pilot anticoagulation service focused on managing warfarin to all areas based on PDSA data, why not see if some of the changes could be adapted to other anticoagulants? New quality measures could be designed to measure the impact of the service on things like managing patients on unfractionated heparin, direct thrombin inhibitors, or other anticoagulants. This is a way anticoagulation programs can help justify their expansion into new areas.

Conclusion

The principles of CQI should be applied to launching an inpatient anticoagulation service. Without this being practiced, the service will have no way to know if it has improved quality or if problems in quality are being encountered on a long-term basis. The PDSA methodology is an easy way to help measure the effects of these changes and justify future actions. Maintaining a high quality anticoagulation service backed by strong quality data helps:

- demonstrate the excellent work of pharmacists caring for patients.
- protect pharmacist patient-care services from budget cuts.
- serve as a means to further expand an inpatient anticoagulation service.

Case Study

The St. Joseph's Hospital Department of Pharmacy has completed all planning outlined in Chapter 4 and has received approval for increasing pharmacist staffing to support of an inpatient anticoagulation program focused on managing warfarin. The hospital has a strong culture of practicing CQI and the department is expected to generate data demonstrating improvement in quality. The team decides to utilize the PDSA methodology to demonstrate these improvements in care.

Plan

As mentioned above, much of the planning for the program has already occurred, but the team had not yet identified how they will measure quality. They decide that the most important measures would be hard outcomes like re-thrombosis and bleeding rates when compared to baseline, but realize they do not have the resources to conduct chart audits to perform this type of study. Instead, they decide to benchmark themselves against some of the data generated by Dager et al.[5] The hospital and orthopedic surgeons have been particularly concerned by some serious bleeding events caused by warfarin and want to prevent excessively prolonged INRs. Despite the different populations from the Dager article, they set a goal of exceeding the performance of traditional care for percentage of INRs greater than 3.5 and 6 in the study. They also wish to at least equal the performance of the pharmacist group for those same measures. These measures will be reported up through the organization. Internally, the pharmacy department will develop process measures to assure core processes designed for patient care are being followed. The department also will continue to track the quality measures they follow for other services (kinetics and nutrition monitoring) to help assure the new program is not degrading services from older programs (i.e., these are balancing measures).

The team has to plan how the data will be obtained in such a way to minimize the use of human resources for data collection. They decide to contact the laboratory and obtain a list of all INRs drawn for orthopedic patients during the 6 months prior to program implementation. This will be compared with data generated during the 6 months after program implementation. The quality department has agreed to lend the department a nurse to conduct this data collection. To automate prospective data collection, organization, and storage after program implementation, the pharmacy department will have an information technology pharmacist design a secure Access based database program based on the work of Schneider et al.[4] For the process measures, pharmacy students on rotation will audit the database program for 10 patients a month to assure all critical patient care issues have been addressed (checklist to be used by student is Table 9-1). The clinical manager of the pharmacy department will continue to monitor the quality measures from other services as a balancing measure.

Do

The program is implemented by the St. Joseph's Hospital Department of Pharmacy on the orthopedic unit and utilizes the new computer database to manage patients. Small glitches in the system are quickly addressed when they arise. The quality nurse collects the data prior to program implementation. The inpatient anticoagulation program is very popular with the orthopedic nursing and medical staff.

Study

The outcome measures of the program are closely analyzed at 6 months. Figures 9-1 and 9-2 depict the percentage of INRs greater than 3.5 and 6 on a monthly basis before and after program implementation. It also shows the quality goals set by the program. The program manager makes the following observations from these figures:

- The manager is pleased that the department is exceeding the performance of physicians and pharmacists in the Dager study, but realizes that may not have been the correct quality goal.[5] He believes this is likely due to differences in the type of patients the pharmacy is managing compared to those in the Dager study. He considers setting lower targets for performance.

- The percentage of INRs that were greater than 3.5 or 6 appear to clearly and consistently drop after the pharmacy department began managing patients. The program manager knows this is how data appears when a new system improves the quality of a service.
- The performance of the pharmacists managing warfarin was not very good in November. In November, the process measures also showed lack of 100% compliance (data not shown) with standard procedures. The program manager quickly realizes what led to this data. During November, he received concerned comments from the outpatient anticoagulation clinic regarding how the patients were managed. He quickly realized, at the time, that a pharmacist who had not been trained had been managing the patients that month due to a scheduling misunderstanding with the clinical manager. The pharmacist was reassigned after performing the function poorly for 2 weeks, a mistake which the program manager regrets. He has taken steps with the clinical manager to assure this never happens again. The program manager also realizes this is what quality data looks like when systems do not function as designed.

% INRs >3.5 By Month

Figure 9-1. Percentage of INRs greater than 3.5. Benchmarks derived from Dager et al.[5]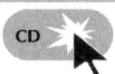

Chapter 9 ■ Monitoring and Maintaining Program Quality

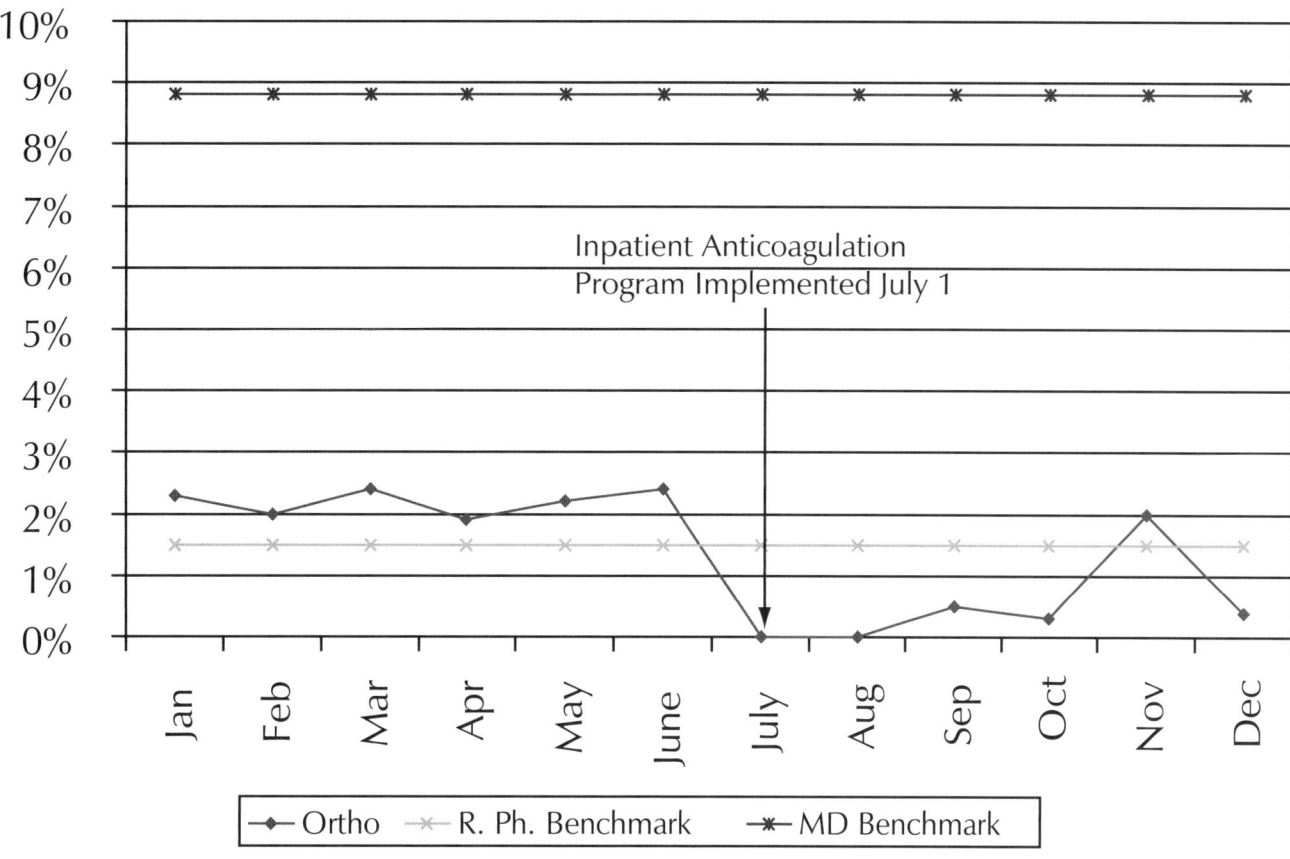

Figure 9-2. Percentage of INRs greater than 6. Benchmarks derived from Dager et al.[5]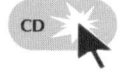

Act

The program manager decides on the following course of action based on his analysis of the data:

- He will recommend house-wide implementation of the program to the pharmacy and therapeutics committee based on what appears to be an improvement in quality.
- He will report this up through the organization to demonstrate the excellent work pharmacists do in providing patient care.
- He will reconvene his planning team to decide on better quality goals for orthopedics, but feels the current goals may be appropriate for non-orthopedic patients.
- He has already met with the clinical manager to assure no untrained pharmacists manage warfarin again.
- He will repeat the PDSA process with the house-wide implementation.

References

1. Kritchevsky SB, Simmons BP. Continuous quality improvement. Concepts and applications for physician care. *JAMA*. 1991;266(13):1817-23.
2. Unknown. How to improve. *Institute for Healthcare Improvement*. Available at: http://www.ihi.org/IHI/Topics/Improvement/ImprovementMethods/HowToImprove/. Accessed November 15, 2006.
3. Zimmerman CR, Smolarek RT, Stevenson JG. Peer review and continuous quality improvement of pharmacists' clinical interventions. *Am J Health-Syst Pharm*. 1997;54(15):1722-7.
4. Schneider BL, Gulseth MP, Cusick MA, Sisson DC, Tomsche JJ. Computer program to assist pharmacy management of an inpatient warfarin dosing service. *Am J Health-Syst Pharm*. 2005;62(22):2393-6.
5. Dager WE, Branch JM, King JH, et al. Optimization of inpatient warfarin therapy: impact of daily consultation by a pharmacist-managed anticoagulation service. *Ann Pharmacother*. 2000;34(5):567-72.

Part 2

Anticoagulant Knowledge 101

Chapter 10: Essential Warfarin Knowledge
Scott Neel

Chapter 11: Heparin, Low Molecular Weight Heparin, and Fondaparinux
Edith Nutescu, William Dager

Chapter 12: Essential Direct Thrombin Inhibitor Knowledge
William Dager

Chapter 13: Helpful References and Preparing for the Future
Michael Gulseth

Chapter 10

Essential Warfarin Knowledge

Scott Neel

Chapter Outline

- Objectives
- Pharmacology
- Pharmacokinetics/pharmacodynamics
  - Drug interactions
  - Warfarin-disease interactions
  - Genetic issues affecting warfarin dosing
  - Diet and vitamin K
- Indications
  - Stroke prevention in atrial defibrillation
  - DVT prophylaxis
  - DVT treatment
  - Valvular heart disease and prosthetic heart valves
  - Ischemic stroke
  - Antiphospholipid antibody syndrome (APS)
- Dose management
- Laboratory monitoring
- Management of non-therapeutic INRs
- Management of warfarin for invasive procedures
- Warfarin and hemorrhage risk
- Warfarin adverse effects
- Precautions and contraindications
  - Warfarin and pregnancy
- Generic versus brand warfarin
- Conclusion
- Patient cases
- References

Objectives

1. Understand the clotting cascade and important properties of vitamin K dependent clotting factors.
2. Identify indications and contraindications for warfarin therapy.
3. Recognize specific disease, herbal, and drug interactions associated with warfarin therapy.
4. Given a patient case, develop an appropriate treatment plan for patients outside goal INR.
5. Develop a patient specific pre- and post-treatment plan for patients requiring interruption of warfarin therapy.

Despite the vast amount of clinician experience with warfarin, developed at the University of Wisconsin in 1948, safe management of warfarin remains a challenge for usual care environments and practitioners.[1] Given the tremendous number of medications available in the U.S., warfarin remains among thirteen other medications the Institute for Safe Medication Practices considers a high alert medication for 2005.[2] Warfarin is also a frequently prescribed medication in the United States with approximately 21.2 million prescriptions in 2003.[3] Although there have been hopes and near successes for an oral replacement to warfarin, warfarin remains the predominant oral anticoagulant used in North America.[4,5]

Pharmacology

Warfarin reduces clot formation by disrupting the liver's production of functional vitamin K dependent clotting factors II, VII, IX, and X (Figure 10-1). A simplified explanation is that warfarin binds the enzyme vitamin K epoxide reductase (VKOR) in the liver interfering with the regeneration of natural vitamin K[1] from its inactive form, (oxidized) vitamin K 2-3 epoxide.[6] The clotting factors II, VII, IX, and X require gamma-carboxylation of their precursors in order to produce their procoagulant effect. This gamma-carboxylation step, gives the protein the calcium mediated ability to bind negative charged phospholipid surfaces, this being a requirement for the clotting factor's procoagulant activity.[6] Warfarin therefore causes production of partially carboxylated and decarboxylated proteins having reduced pro-

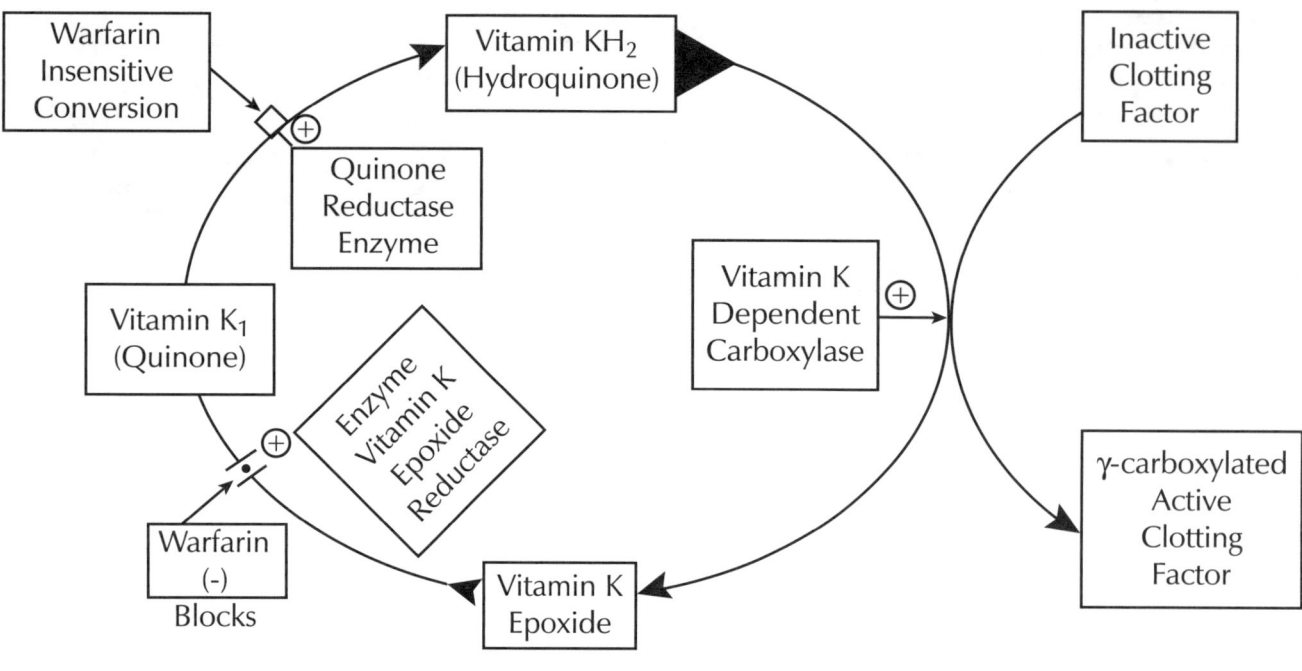

Figure 10-1. Vitamin K cycle. Warfarin blocks the conversion of vitamin K epoxide to vitamin C.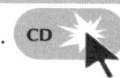

coagulant activity.[7-10] Warfarin also interferes with the synthesis of other vitamin K dependent proteins like endogenous anticoagulant proteins C and S as well as other proteins located in bone, cartilage, and other tissues unrelated to coagulation.[11,12]

Important concepts to understand in anticoagulation are intrinsic versus extrinsic clotting factors, clotting factor half-lives, warfarin's inhibition of anticoagulant proteins C and S, and warfarin's delayed onset (Figure 10-2). Warfarin does not inhibit activity of existing clotting factors. Depletion of these factors through normal catabolism and replacement with newly synthesized dysfunctional clotting factors must occur before therapeutic response to warfarin is established. Vitamin K dependent clotting factors differ in degradation half-lives; factor II (prothrombin) 48–120 hours (~60), factor VII 2 to 6 hours (~6), factor IX 18-40 (~25) hours, and factor X 30–70 hours (~35.6) (see Figure 10-2). In theory, response therefore requires approximately 5 days of warfarin and depletion of functional factors II and X to achieve effective anticoagulation.[6] Factor VII is in the extrinsic pathway and inhibition does not provide effective anticoagulation despite causing early INR elevation (Figure 10-2). The half-lives of anticoagulant proteins C and S are approximately 8 and 30 hours. Since warfarin reduces activity of anticoagulant proteins C and S having shorter half-lifes than factors II and X, in theory, a hypercoagulable state may be induced early in therapy.[1] Due to delayed depletion of factors X and II, and earlier reduction of anticoagulant proteins C and S, injectable anticoagulant overlap is often required when immediate anticoagulation is needed. Opinions regarding duration of overlap vary; although many authorities recommend a minimum of 5 days overlap and that the INR be in range and stable before heparin discontinuation.

Pharmacokinetics/ Pharmacodynamics

Warfarin is an equal mixture of two optically active isomers, R- and S-warfarin. The warfarin S isomer is more potent and each isomer is metabolized through different pathways.[13] Warfarin is available in an oral or injectable formulation. The IV formulation is used less frequently; however, this route prevents disruption of stabilized warfarin in hospitalized patients who have lost all enteral routes. Following oral administration with a functional GI tract, maximum plasma concentration occurs in approximately 90 minutes.[13,14] Warfarin's half-life ranges from 36 to 42 hours.[6] Warfarin is extensively bound to plasma proteins 97%–99%, predominantly albumin, and then accumulates in microsomes of the liver.[15] Warfarin dose response among patients is highly variable secondary to inter-patient differences in: metabolism, vitamin K diet, receptor affinity, quantity of vitamin K dependent clotting factors, genetic factors, disease states, binding proteins, laboratory testing, drug interactions, and compliance.[6,16,17]

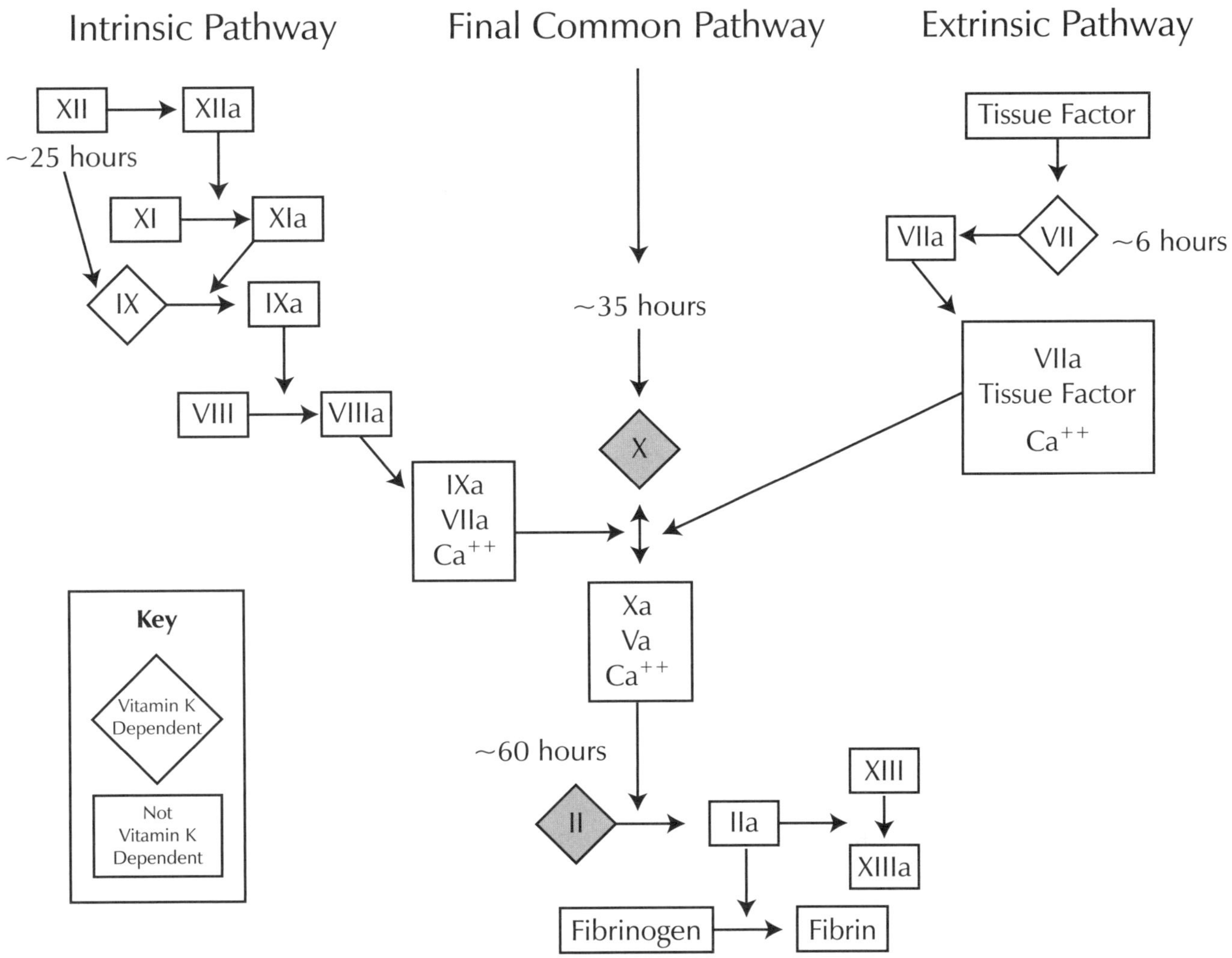

Intrinsic Pathway

Final Common Pathway

Extrinsic Pathway

Figure 10-2. Coagulation cascade and vitamin K–dependent clotting factor half-lives. Shaded clotting factors are critical warfarin targets.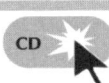

Clinical Pearls

Hospital pharmacists managing warfarin will encounter patients who cannot take warfarin enterally. If the INR is in range or close to in range, and the pharmacist and physician agree warfarin is still safe, using IV warfarin can prevent disruption of stabilized patients. This avoids use of other injectable anticoagulants and re-titration of warfarin. These patients often require lower IV doses from baseline despite equal bioavailability of oral warfarin secondary to acute illnesses, medication used to treat the illness, and/or decreased nutritional intake of vitamin K.

Due to the long half-life of warfarin, every dose taken within the last 7 days must be considered when making dosing decisions. However, the inpatient pharmacist will discover the doses taken 2–3 days ago will have the most prominent effect on current day INR and these require careful consideration when making dose adjustments.

> ### Clinical Pearls
>
> Patient and medical staff education on warfarin interactions reduce hospital admissions by improving warfarin management and preventing warfarin misadventures. Hospital admissions secondary to warfarin drug interactions provide an opportunity to educate the prescriber, patient's outpatient pharmacy, and patient on interaction screening. These admissions also require completion of an adverse drug reaction form. These interventions on preventable warfarin adverse drug events help prevent future occurrences.
>
> Interactions involving inhibition of S-warfarin metabolism are more severe and often require pre-emptive warfarin dose adjustments or interchange to safer alternatives.
>
> Interactions involving the five times less potent R-isomer can often be managed by daily INR monitoring and often don't cause as dramatic INR elevations.
>
> Clearly determining if a medication, even those known to interact, caused an INR elevation in hospitalized patients is difficult because acute illnesses may also elevate the INR. A good example is a patient receiving metronidazole for *Clostridium difficile* colitis. When an INR bump occurs, is it from the metronidazole, the severe diarrhea, poor vitamin K intake, or all of the above? Often, it is a combination of factors and the presumed "drug interaction" may become less pronounced as the patient recovers from illness.

Drug Interactions

Medication interactions can affect warfarin response in the following ways:

- binding warfarin and reducing GI absorption (cholestyramine).[17,18]
- decrease clotting factor production by inhibiting vitamin K recycling (2nd and 3rd generation cephalosporins).[19-22]
- change metabolism of clotting factors by the liver (thyroxin,[23] methimazole[24]).
- directly increasing or decreasing warfarin metabolism in the liver.

Inhibitors of 2C9 and S-isomer[25] warfarin metabolism include metronidazole,[26] ritonavir,[27] sulfinpyrazone,[28] amiodarone, fluconazole, and trimethoprim-sulfamethoxazole.[29] Inhibitors of 1A2 and 3A4 metabolizers of R-isomer warfarin[27,30] include quinolones,[31-33] omeprazole,[6,26,34] cimetidine,[6,26,34] and macrolides.[35-37] A comprehensive list of warfarin interactions by probability of occurrence are provided in Tables 10-1 and 10-2.[30] R-isomer interactions can also be clinically relevant and require increased monitoring but tend to be less dramatic than S-isomer interactions.[34,38] The *Chest* guidelines suggest increased INR monitoring following virtually any medication/herbal addition or withdrawal.[39,40] Following addition of interacting medications, hospitalized patients should have daily INRs. Some interactions like amiodarone are delayed and take longer before stabilization occurs.

Information regarding interactions between herbals and warfarin is scant. Published reports are often from case reports and experience from clinicians managing anticoagulation clinics. Clinically relevant herbal interactions are listed in Table 10-2.[30] Herbal supplements are not standardized with regard to purity, content, or potency, it is therefore difficult to estimate the degree of interaction with an herbal product. Therefore, it is best to discourage warfarin patients from taking herbal supplements. While medications and herbals may not have metabolism interactions with warfarin, agents altering platelet function increase risk of bleeding. Agents include aspirin, clopidogrel, dipyridamole, nonsteroidal anti-inflammatories (NSAIDs), high-dose penicillin, garlic, ginger, gingko biloba, ginseng, fish oils, vitamin E, and others.[40] Aspirin's effects on bleeding with warfarin has been studied more than others. The extent of increased bleeding correlates with aspirin dose and warfarin intensity; however, aspirin in combination with warfarin always increases bleeding over warfarin alone.[39,40] Aspirin and NSAIDs also increase bleeding by causing gastric erosions. There is little published data regarding the safety of combining warfarin with Plavix® nor do the Chest guidelines discuss this combination, as they do the combination of aspirin 81 mg and warfarin. Most experienced anticoagulation specialists generally feel the combination of Plavix® and warfarin is rarely justified and carries a higher risk of bleeding than combining warfarin and 81 mg aspirin. There are, perhaps, rare circumstances in which the benefits outweigh the risks of increased bleeding. This might include early status post drug eluding stent placement in a patient requiring warfarin for another justified indication. In these circumstances, patients require

Table 10-1.
Clinically Significant Interactions with Warfarin by Level of Causation and Drug Group

Level of Causation	Anti-infectives	Cardiovascular Drugs	Analgesics, Anti-inflammatories, and Immunologics	CNS Drugs
Potentiation				
I Highly Probable	Ciprofloxacin Cotrimoxazole Erythromycin Fluconazole Isoniazid (600 mg/d) Metronidazole Miconazole oral gel Miconazole vaginal suppositories Voriconazole	Amiodarone Clofibrate Diltiazem Fenofibrate Propafenone Propranolol Sulfinpyrazone (biphasic with later inhibition)	Phenylbutazone Piroxicam	Alcohol (if concomitant liver disease) Citalopram Entacapone Sertraline
II Probable	Amoxicillin/clavulanate Azithromycin Clarithromycin Itraconazole Levofloxacin Ritonavir Tetracycline	Fluvastatin Quinidine Ropinirole Simvastatin	Acetaminophen Acetylsalicylic acid Celecoxib Dextropropoxyphene Interferon Tramadol	Disulfiram Choral hydrate Fluvoxamine Phenytoin (biphasic with later inhibition)
III Possible	Amoxicillin Amoxicillin/tranexamic rinse Chloramphenicol Gatifloxacin Miconazole topical gel193 Nalidixic acid Norfloxacin Ofloxacin Saquinavir Terbinafine	Amiodarone-induced toxicosis Disopyramide Gemfibrozil Metolazone	Celecoxib Indomethacin Leflunomide Propoxyphene Rofecoxib Sulindac Tolmetin Topical salicylates	Felbamate
IV Highly Improbable	Cefamandole Cefazolin Sulfisoxazole	Bezafibrate Heparin	Levamisole Methylprednisolone Nabumetone	Fluoxetine/diazepam Quetiapine
Inhibition				
I Highly Probable	Griseofulvin Nafcillin Ribavirin Rifampin	Cholestyramine	Mesalamine	Barbiturates Carbamazepine
II Probable	Dicloxacillin Ritonavir	Bosentan	Azathioprine	Chlordiazepoxide
III Possible	Terbinafine	Telmisartan	Sulfasalazine	
IV Highly Improbable	Cloxacillin Nafcillin/dicloxacillin Teicoplanin	Furosemide		Propofol

Source: Adapted with permission from reference 30.

Table 10-2.
Clinically Significant Interactions with Warfarin by Level of Causation and Drug Group (Continued)

Level of Causation	Potentiation		
	GI Drugs and Food	Herbal Supplements	Other Drugs
I Highly Probable	Cimetidine Fish oil Mango Omeprazole	Boldo-fenugreek Quilinggao	Anabolic steroids Zileuton
II Probable	Grapefruit juice	Danshen Dong quai Lycium barbarum L PC-SPES	Fluorouracil Gemcitabine Levamisole/fluorouracil Paclitaxel Tamoxifen Tolterodine
III Possible	Cranberry juice Orlistat	Danshen/methyl salicylate	Acarbose CMF (cyclophosphamide/ methotrexate/fluorouracil) Curbicin Danazol Ifosphamide Trastuzumab
IV Highly Improbable			Etoposide/carboplatin Levonorgestrel
	Inhibition		
I Highly Probable	High vitamin K content foods/enteral feeds Avocado (large amounts)		Mercaptopurine
II Probable	Soy milk Sucralfate	Ginseng	Chelation therapy Influenza vaccine Multivitamin supplement Raloxifene hydrochloride
III Possible	Sushi containing seaweed		Cyclosporine Etretinate Ubidicarenone
IV Highly Improbable		Green tea	

Abbreviations: CNS, central nervous system; GI, gastrointestinal.
Source: Adapted with permission from reference 30.

> **Clinical Pearl**
>
> Patients who experience acute liver dysfunction (hypotensive episodes, liver metastasis, etc.) while in the hospital will be extremely sensitive to warfarin. Vigilance is necessary when managing warfarin in these patients (daily INRs and warfarin adjustments) and sometimes holding warfarin until liver function recovers is required. Close consultation with the attending physician is advised in these situations.

very close monitoring and additional education with regard to medication interactions.

When deciding whether to combine warfarin with anti-platelet agents, the pharmacist must carefully weigh risks versus benefits for a specific patient.

Warfarin-Disease Interactions

Since the liver is responsible for production and metabolism of clotting factors and metabolism of warfarin, altered warfarin response with hepatic disease is not surprising.[40-45] Liver dysfunction is associated with increased bleeding.[46] A review evaluating 29,000 INRs found risk factors for INR ≥ 6 to include: liver disease, alcoholism, drug interactions, warfarin therapy for less than 6 months, and frequent dosage adjustments.[47]

> **Clinical Pearl**
>
> When practicing inpatient anticoagulation, thyroid status is often not a clinical concern unless it is changing. In other words, stable levothyroxine patients in euthyroid status should be treated like patients without thyroid issues. Hypothyroid patients initiated on levothyroxine or having levothyroxine dose increases may require warfarin dose reduction. Patients undergoing hyperthyroid treatment will likely require warfarin dose increases.

Changes in thyroid function cause changes in clotting factor metabolism, necessitating warfarin dose adjustments.[23,40] Hyperthyroidism increases a patient's sensitivity to warfarin by increased catabolism of clotting factors.[23,48] Hyperthyroidism also increases warfarin's binding affinity, further decreasing clotting factor production and warfarin dose requirement.[49] Increased warfarin sensitivity with hyperthyroidism has been observed in at least five human trials.[23,50-53] Published reports show stabilized warfarin patients who subsequently developed hypothyroidism, had a thyroidectomy, or received iodine [131] resulting in hypothyroidism; required a two- to three-fold warfarin dose increase to maintain therapeutic INRs.[54,55]

The mechanism of increased warfarin sensitivity in heart failure is unknown, however, evidence supports lowering warfarin doses, especially during exacerbations. All heart failure patients are not sensitized to warfarin.[47] Sensitization occurs during periods of decompensation or hepatic congestion, possibly due to reduced clotting factor production and plasma volume expansion.[56-58] Seven studies have shown increased sensitivity in heart failure; three of these used increased bleeding to support their conclusion.[56,59-65]

Other disease states have been implicated in difficult warfarin management. Cancer patients are sometimes difficult to manage on warfarin. Factors making these patients difficult to manage include: chemo/warfarin interactions, malnutrition/nausea/vomiting, liver/blood abnormalities, volume changes, and warfarin interruptions due to thrombocytopenia and surgery.[66,67] Fever, commonly present in hospitalized patients, has been shown to reduce metabolism of antipyrine; metabolized through the same pathways as warfarin CYP1A2 and CYP3A4.[25,27,30,68-70] In a small subset of fever patients, increased clotting factor metabolism has also been observed.[48] In practice, many warfarin patients with infections have elevated INRs. Finally, any disease that affects a patient's eating habits or absorption of vitamin K can affect warfarin dosing.

Genetic Issues Affecting Warfarin Dosing

A few genetic polymorphisms decrease warfarin metabolism. Studies have evaluated CYP450 2C9 gene mutations that encode for the enzyme responsible for metabolism of the more potent S-isomer of warfarin. Specific mutations causing increased warfarin sensitivity or bleeding include CYP2C9-2 and CYP2C9-3, with normal metabolism being homozygous CYP2C9-1.[71-80] A gene encoding the CYP450 2C9 enzyme is found on each chromosome. Patients may be normal (CYP2C9-1/1), polymorphic heterozygous (CYP2C9-1/3, -1/2), polymorphic homozygous (CYP2C9-3/3, -2/2) or have mixed polymorphic alleles (i.e., CYP2C9-2/3). Three larger studies of CYP2C9 polymorphism were Herman et al. n = 188,[73] Kamali et al. n = 121,[76] and Scordo et al. n = 93.[79] The most warfarin-sensitive polymorphism in all three trials was the homozygous 3/3 consistently followed by the 2/3, followed by the 1/3 and 2/2, followed by the least affected 1/2 polymorphism, which still required a 30%–40% lower dose than 1/1.[73,76,79] The incidence of specific types of polymorphisms among general populations were similar across the three studies: CYP2C9-1/1 (58%–63%), CYP2C9-1/2 (16%–25%), CYP2C9-1/3 (12%–17%), CYP2C9-2/3 (1%–6%), CYP2C9-3/3 (1%–3%), and CYP2C9-2/2 (0%–2%).[73,76,79] When ethnic groups were studied individually, the incidence differed for each. The incidence of CYP2C9-2 polymorphism was 20% for whites, 1% for African Americans; however, it has

> **Clinical Pearl**
>
> Previously stabilized warfarin patients often have elevated INRs when admitted with decompensated heart failure. This often requires holding or reducing their warfarin dose by about 50% for 1–2 days after admission, but as they diurese and improve, they often require their previous warfarin dose. Pharmacists are often reluctant to resume previous dosing thinking "the dose made them go high" overlooking the acute illness as the cause rather than the dose. As with all warfarin patients, it is important for pharmacists to understand the patient's complete clinical status and not just "treat the numbers."

not been identified in Chinese or Japanese populations.[81] The incidence of the CYP2C9-3 polymorphism was 16.2% for Hispanics, 3.7%–9.2% for whites, 1.7%–2.6% for Asians, and 0.5%–1.25% for African Americans.[81]

Without availability of routine genetic testing, an elevated serum S:R warfarin concentration ratio correlates well with the presence of CYP2C9 polymorphisms. Data from the Herman et al.,[73] Kamali et al.,[76] and Scordo et al.[79] trials show the warfarin S:R concentrations ratios one might expect to find among a sample population: CYP2C9-1/1 (range S:R 0.44–0.63 to 1), CYP2C9-1/2 or 1/3 (range S:R 0.61–0.74 to 1), CYP2C9-2/2 (range S:R 0.8–1.14 to 1), CYP2C9-2/3 (range S:R 0.84–1.47 to 1), and CYP2C9-3/3 (range S:R 2.16–2.65 to 1).[73,76,79] As patients with polymorphisms require lower warfarin doses they often have reduced serum R-isomer concentrations as well. Therefore, an elevated S:R concentration ratio is the distinctive characteristic of probability and may prove to be an inexpensive approach to identify these patients.

Another genetic polymorphism increasing warfarin sensitivity is the vitamin K reductase complex subunit one (VKORC1).[82-86] Warfarin binds the enzyme vitamin K epoxide reductase, the specific protein target being VKORC1 (see Figure 10-1).[87,88] The degree to which these polymorphisms affect warfarin dosing relative to those of the CYP2C9 polymorphisms requires further study as available studies are conflicting, VKORC1 polymorphisms appeared to have a greater impact on dosing by Rieder et al., Wadelius et al., Schalekamp et al., and Bodin et al.[83,86,89,90] However, two studies found CYP2C9 polymorphisms to have a greater impact on warfarin dosing relative to VKORC1 polymorphisms.[82,84] Given multiple variations of these polymorphisms and that both the VKORC1 and CYP2C9 polymorphisms have been identified in the same patient, further study is needed.[90] The study by Reider et al.[83] evaluated the incidence of VKORC1 polymorphisms by specific demographic groups. The specific VKORC1 polymorphisms associated with increased warfarin sensitivity were found in 89%, 37%, and 14% of Asian-Americans, European-Americans, and African Americans, respectively. These findings are consistent with population-based warfarin dosing studies showing Asians often require lower doses, followed by Europeans, who usually require intermediate doses, followed by African descendents requiring larger warfarin doses.[91-94] At least one cause of warfarin resistance is likely associated with mutations of the VKORC1 gene.[95,96] Further investigation is needed to fully understand mutations occurring on VKORC1 gene and their implications on warfarin dosing. In addition to further research on predictors of warfarin sensitivity, more information is needed regarding the development of affordable diagnostic devices that could be selectively used by clinicians to test high-risk patient groups.

Clinical Pearl

Hospitalized patients often have changes in diet causing fluctuating warfarin requirements and dosing that is distinctly different from their outpatient requirements. Further, enteral and parenteral nutritional supplements containing vitamin K further complicate matters. It is important for pharmacists to follow changes in feeding rates and diets as these influence warfarin dosing.

Diet and Vitamin K

The body converts ingested vitamin K1 into a required cofactor (reduced vitamin K, vitamin KH2 used to synthesize coagulation factors: II, VII, IX, X, and proteins C and S (see Figure 10-1). This production process is not sensitive to warfarin and therefore circumvents warfarin's action of causing a partial vitamin K deficient environment.[97] Consistent vitamin K intake is essential to reduce variability in warfarin dosing.[98,99] For new warfarin patients, dietary consistency is a difficult lifestyle adjustment and suggesting a dietary log in the beginning improves stabilization.[98,100,101] Providing patients a list of foods with a high content of vitamin K is helpful in this task. Available are a number of references that describe the vitamin K content of specific foods.[102,103] Vitamin K is often concentrated in green plant materials such as broccoli; herbals such as green tea; certain oils such as canola; and many hospital nutritional supplements, foods, and

Clinical Pearl

The area of pharmacogenomics in relation to warfarin is rapidly evolving. While validated uses of this information to improve direct patient care are not yet available, this may occur in the near future. For example, could genetic genotyping be done on patients to assist in initial warfarin dose selection? Inpatient anticoagulation pharmacists are encouraged to keep up on this cutting edge topic as the information provided is preliminary.

drinks. The message to patients should be to eat the same size and number of servings each week of foods with a high content of vitamin K.

Indications

Given warfarin's long existence, there are many on- and off-label indications supported by clinical trials. Although aspirin is the mainstay for prevention of myocardial infarction (MI), warfarin has generated interesting data. Following MI, patients have a 24% increased DVT risk when not receiving anticoagulation.[104] MI patients occasionally have extended immobility warranting DVT prophylaxis. Warfarin has consistently reduced the risk of pulmonary embolism following MI and less consistently the risk of stroke, recurrent MI, and mortality.[105-107] To quickly summarize, data is best broken down into three evaluated regimens: low intensity (fixed dose 1 and 3 mg or INR < 2), moderate intensity (INR 2–3), and high (INR 2.8–4.8) intensity warfarin. Aspirin plus low-intensity warfarin does not reduce primary outcomes and is associated with a non-statistical increase in bleeding versus aspirin alone.[108-112] Trials comparing aspirin plus moderate-high intensity warfarin show a non-statistically significant reduction of fatal and nonfatal MI versus aspirin alone.[108,113,114] This same regimen showed statistically significant reductions[108,113] and a non-statistically significant reduction[114] favoring combination therapy for the combined endpoint of death, MI, and stroke. Moderate-high intensity warfarin plus aspirin versus aspirin alone has shown an increase risk of bleeding; however, this was often either non-statistically significant increase in major bleeding or a statistically significant increase in minor bleeding.[108,113,114] A review article on warfarin in coronary artery disease showed moderate-high intensity warfarin plus aspirin reduced the combined endpoint of death, MI, and stroke incidence by 54 per 1000 patients at a cost of 16 major bleeds per 1000 patients compared to aspirin alone.[109] The coagulation system remains hyperactive for an extended period following coronary ischemia and MI.[115] There is likely a small population of coronary disease patients who benefit from combination therapy. Patients having atrial fibrillation or possibly those with a significant family history of early coronary disease refractory to usual antiplatelet therapy may benefit from warfarin.

Stroke Prevention in Atrial Fibrillation

Atrial fibrillation (AF) is a growing problem in the United States. Epidemiologic data estimate AF will increase from 2 million in 1995 to over 4 million by 2030.[116] This will have a significant financial and social impact on society due to increased stroke and stroke rehabilitation. U.S. annual incidence of AF induced stroke is approximately 60,000 and growing.[116] Non-valvular AF causes a 5-fold increase stroke risk while valvular AF causes a 17-fold increase in stoke risk (see Table 10-3).[117-122] Strokes resulting from AF are more debilitating than non-cardiogenic strokes. Approximately 71% of first time AF stroke patients either die or have severe permanent neurological impairments.[120] Compounding this problem is underutilization of warfarin providing improved stroke prevention in many patients relative to aspirin. United States data indicate only 20%–44% of AF patients that should receive warfarin actually do.[123-129] Data from a U.S. study site previously involved in an anticoagulation trial for AF, reported 78.8% compliance showing this is a correctable problem.[130] Barriers to appropriate warfarin use in AF include fall risk, inconvenient lab monitoring, interactions, compliance, bleeding risk, and understanding efficacy differences between aspirin and warfarin. Warfarin's superiority over aspirin in moderate to high risk AF has been shown in many studies. Data from two separate meta-analyses have shown the relative risk reduction using warfarin versus aspirin ranges from 36%–46% for all strokes and 46%–52% for ischemic strokes (see Table 10-4).[131-133] Given the variability of stroke rates in AF patients and the apparent reluctance to use warfarin, proper patient selection is important. Patient characteristics with atrial fibrillation and probability of stroke have been evaluated in a number of clinical trials (see Table 10-5).[134-144]

Table 10-3.
Relative Risk of Stroke by Age and Presence of Atrial Fibrillation

STUDY	Mean Age	Stroke Incidence		Relative Risk
		AF	No AF	
Framingham, USA	70 yr	4.1% per year	0.74% per year	5.6
Shibata, Japan	65 yr	5.0% per year	0.90% per year	5.6
Whitehall, UK	60 yr	1.8% per year	0.26% per year	6.9
Reykjavik, Iceland	52 yr	1.6% per year	0.23% per year	7.1

Source: References 120–122.

Table 10-4.
Warfarin vs. Aspirin for Stroke Prophylaxis by Risk Group

Risk Factors	Stroke Incidence with Aspirin	Relative Risk Reduction with Warfarin	NNT☠
Prior Stroke/TIA	10% per year	60% per year	17
High Risk	>4% per year	55% per year	35
Moderate Risk	2%–4% per year	45% per year	75
Low Risk	<2% per year	35% per year	>200

☠ Number treated with warfarin for 1 year instead of aspirin to prevent one stroke
Source: Reference 133.

Table 10-5.
Annual Stroke Rate by the Presence of a Specific Risk Factor

Risk Factor	Percent Range of Annual Stroke Rate	Risk Rating
Prior Stroke/TIA	4%–13% RR 1.9–2.9	High
Women > 75 Years	3.7%–7.1%	High
Systolic BP > 160 mmHg	3.7%–7.1% or RR 2.3	High
Age > 75 Years + History of Hypertension	7.1%	High
Congestive Heart Failure	2.7%–6.8%	High
Age > 75 Years	2.8%	High
History of Hypertension	2.7%–7.6% or RR 1.6–2.2	Moderate-High
Age > 65 Years	2.2%–2.4%	Moderate-High
Diabetes	5.4%–8.6% RR 1.6–1.8	Moderate-High

Source: References 134–144.

Table 10-6.
Antithrombotic Recommendations by Patient and Risk Factor

Patient Type with AF or PAF	Suggested Antithrombotic Without Contraindications	Risk Assessment
Age < 65 years	Aspirin 325 mg daily	No risk factors
Age < 65 years	Warfarin INR 2–3	EF ≤ 35%, history of embolism, hypertension, diabetes, impaired LVH, prior stroke/TIA
Age 65–75	Warfarin INR 2–3 or Aspirin 325 mg daily	No risk factors
Age 65–75	Warfarin INR 2–3	EF ≤ 35%, history of embolism, hypertension, diabetes, impaired LVH, prior stroke/TIA, left atrial enlargement
Age > 75	Warfarin INR 2–3	Without contraindications then regardless

Source: References 141 and 146.

Stroke risk from paroxysmal atrial fibrillation (PAF) or flutter is not much different than chronic AF.[133,135,138,145,146] This is especially true when PAF is accompanied with risk factors such as hypertension, diabetes, mitral stenosis, advanced age, valvular disease, or HF. Sometimes patients are younger and depending on the frequency and duration of irregularity are at lower risk and prophylaxis with aspirin is sufficient. See Table 10-6 for long-term stroke prophylaxis recommendations.

Several strategies exist for cardioversion and how patients are managed is guided by physician/patient preference, time of presentation after onset, and availability of biplane or multiplane transesophageal echocardiography (TEE), and stroke risk factors.[141,146-151] Patients presenting for cardioversion less than 48 hours following onset are considered low risk for left atrial appendage thrombi causing stroke with cardioversion. Patients, however, may not recognize when the AF began and there are other risk factors for stroke to consider. Some studies support early cardioversion in these patients without TEE or prior anticoagulation[144,145] while others enrolling patients with AF less than 72 hours found left atrial thrombi present in 13% of patients, indicating higher than expected risk for stroke.[146] In AF patients presenting less than 48 hours requiring early cardioversion due to hemodynamic instability, cardioversion can be done with or without delay of IV heparin.[141,146] Anticoagulation following cardioversion should be based on patient's stroke risk and certainty of less than 48-hour presentation. If anticoagulation is necessary, warfarin with an INR of 2–3 is recommended for 4 weeks provided patient remains in normal sinus rhythm (NSR).[141,146] AF patients presenting after 48 hours requiring early cardioversion due to hemodynamic instability and without prior anticoagulation (INR 2–3) will require a bolus of IV heparin followed by aPTT-adjusted heparin infusion. These patients also require warfarin INR 2–3 for at least 4 weeks following cardioversion or longer if they revert to atrial fibrillation.[141,146] AF patients presenting after 48 hours or uncertain duration in a stable patient, two options are available. The first being adjusted warfarin INR 2–3 for 3 weeks prior to cardioversion, followed by warfarin INR 2–3 for 4 weeks after cardioversion, assuming NSR is maintained.[141,146] Multiplane TEE allows better visualization of left atrial thrombi predisposing patients to stroke with cardioversion. If high-quality TEE shows no sign of left atrial appendage thrombi, the patient can be placed on IV heparin and cardioverted.[141,146] The presence of left atrial thrombi requires the patient to have 3 weeks of anticoagulation and possibly longer depending on repeat TEE before cardioversion.[141,146] After successful cardioversion, assuming NSR is maintained, patients require warfarin INR 2–3 for 1 month or longer should AF return.[141,146]

DVT Prophylaxis

Warfarin is an effective, inexpensive DVT prophylactic agent at INR 2–3, especially for patients requiring longer durations (i.e., 28–35 days for HIP fracture/replacement or post surgical cancer patients).[152] Slower offset, however, requires earlier coordination for surgical procedures. LMWHs and Xa inhibitors are sometimes cost prohibitive and SC heparin requiring three injections daily for optimal prophylactic effect is uncomfortable. DVT and pulmonary embolism (PE) in hospitalized patients is largely avoidable with prophylaxis, and sometimes these lead to fatality.[153] Surviving DVT patients often have vessel abnormalities causing prolonged symptoms, recurrent DVT, and future increased health costs.[154-158] A hospital's performance on prevention of DVT has the attention of the Joint Commission® and the Agency for Healthcare Research and Quality. Prophylaxis poses only small risk that differs depending on the agent chosen.

Patient risk stratification is important for identifying patients requiring DVT prophylaxis. See Table 10-7 for high-risk patients and DVT incidence by condition. Many inpatient orthopedic procedures, including arthroplasty, require pharmacological VTE prophylaxis regardless of age or risk factors. Warfarin is considered an acceptable

Clinical Pearl

When warfarin is used for DVT prophylaxis, it is typically used in surgical patients requiring longer prophylaxis than routine medical patients. Orthopedics represents an area where warfarin is often used. Why? Orthopedic patients, particularly hip replacement or hip fracture patients, have prolonged DVT risk. The Seventh American College of Chest Physicians Consensus Conference on Antithrombotic Therapy makes a 1A recommendation for extended DVT prophylaxis 28–35 days following hip surgery.[152] Few patients would rather give themselves an injection each day when they could take a pill and have occasional blood draws. Due to delayed warfarin onset, many will bridge high-risk patients (orthopedic surgery with risk factors listed in Table 10-8) with prophylactic doses of heparin or LMWH until the INR is in range.

option for orthopedic surgery DVT prophylaxis.[152] Warfarin's slow onset, even administered the evening before surgery, is unlikely to provide benefit for several days. Studies have shown early anticoagulation, within 12 hours post-op, reduces risk of DVT.[159-167] Initiation of LMWH or fondaparinux before orthopedic surgery or in close proximity 2-6 hours) post operatively is associated with increased bleeding, but this may not apply to SC heparin.[164,165] A review article on DVT prophylaxis duration following various surgeries has been published.[168] Admission types requiring pharmacological DVT prophylaxis with one or no risk factors include: trauma, CHF, bed confinement, critical care, spinal cord injury, and moderate general surgery age 40-60 years. Patients require risk factor assessment as they often have more than one risk factor and each adds cumulative risk for DVT; see Table 10-8 for DVT risk factors.[169] To improve patient safety, institutions may develop a DVT prophylaxis protocol for patient selection.

DVT Treatment

The incidence of DVT and PE is approximately 145 per 100,000 and 69 per 100,000 persons respectively.[170] Complications of untreated DVT include PE, recurrent DVT, subsequent venous valvular dysfunction, residual partial occlusion, and thrombophlebitis.[171,172] The most significant is PE, being the primary cause of death in 100,000 persons/year and a co-morbid contributor of an additional 100,000 deaths.[173] Untreated pulmonary embolism can lead to death, pulmonary hypertension, and right sided heart failure. Goals for treatment include: prevent PE, arrest clot growth, stabilize patients with PE, and prevent recurrent venous thromboembolism (VTE). This requires rapid anticoagulation and on rare occasions a thrombolytic for PE causing hemodynamic compromise. It is important to inquire about recent traumas, surgery, new or changed medications predisposing patients to VTE (i.e., estrogen modifiers) and family history of VTE, as these

Table 10-7.
Risk of DVT From Hospitalization

Risk	Hospitalized Group	Incidence of DVT
Low	Medical patients	10%–20%
Moderate	General surgery Gynecological surgery (major) Neurological Urological surgery (major)	15%–40%
High	HIP or knee (arthroplasty, replacement, fracture) Stroke	20%–60%
Highest	Trauma (major) Spinal cord injury	40%–80%
Variable	Critical care	10%–80%

Source: Reference 152.

Table 10-8.
Cumulative Individual Risk Factors for VTE

Advanced age	Central venous catheter	Acute illness
Contraceptives	COPD/bronchitis/severe pneumonia	Chemotherapy
Immobility	Estrogen replacement	Trauma
Malignancy	Hypercoagulable disease	Heart failure
Obesity	Inflammatory bowel disease	Surgery
Prior VTE	Peripheral vascular disease	Varicose veins
Smoking	Selective estrogen receptor modifiers (SERMS)	Spinal cord injury

Source: Reference 152.

Table 10-9.
Hypercoagulable Conditions

Serum Deficiencies	Gene Mutations	Serum Markers	Other
Antithrombin	Factor V Leiden	⇧ Factor VIII, IX, XI	Activated protein C resistance
Protein C	Prothrombin 20210A	Antiphospholipid antibodies	
Protein S		⇧ Homocysteine	
Plasminogen		⇧ D-dimer after complete anticoagulation course	
		⇧ Lipoprotein (a)	
		⇧ Thrombin-activatable fibrinolysis inhibitor	
		⇧ Thrombin generation > 400 nM after anticoagulation completion	

Source: References 174 and 175.

determine the duration of anticoagulation therapy (idiopathic versus causative insult) and whether patients may benefit from hypercoagulable studies to identify thrombophilias. Approximately 30% of patients with idiopathic DVT or PE have a thrombophilia, especially those presenting younger than 50 years.[174,175] Known hypercoagulable states and at risk serum markers can be found in Table 10-9.

Anticoagulation may be started prior to completion of diagnostic studies in symptomatic patients. Many institutions after baseline labs start a therapeutic dose of an injectable anticoagulant. Using IV heparin versus LMWH or X-a inhibitor during the diagnostic period allows faster offset of action if VTE is ruled out. Once studies confirm VTE, the patient can be started on warfarin. Whether patients continue on IV heparin or are converted to LMWH, Xa-inhibitor, or high dose SC heparin as bridge to therapeutic warfarin is the clinician's choice.[176,177]

Clinical Pearl

Outpatient treatment of VTE is effective and supported by literature as providing significant cost savings and reduced length of stay.[178-186] Pharmacy inpatient anticoagulation services working together with outpatient counterparts can ensure success of this program by providing patient education and follow-up allowing same- or next-day discharge. The financial savings generated by such a program will help justify the need for pharmacists to provide these services.

Recurrent VTE at 2, 5, and 8 years is 17.5%, 25%, and 30% respectively.[170-172,176] Patients with malignancy or hypercoagulable states have a hazard ratio 1.7 and 1.4 for recurrent VTE respectively.[176] Approximately 5% of patients will die as a result of the second VTE event.[187] The duration of anticoagulant therapy should be patient specific and depends on a number of factors including presence of malignancy, idiopathic versus identifiable etiology, first episode versus a recurrent event, and the presence of a known hypercoagulable condition. See Table 10-10 for the recommended duration of anticoagulation based on patient specific criteria. Other considerations in determining duration of treatment may include: elevated D-dimer levels despite usual duration, residual occlusion using compression ultra sonography despite appropriate duration, and elevated (>400 nM) thrombin generation.[176,188-190]

Valvular Heart Disease and Prosthetic Heart Valves

Systemic embolism due to valvular disease has decreased secondary to reduced rheumatic heart disease, improved prosthetic valve technology, improved techniques in valve repair, and increased utilization of anticoagulation.[191] Valvular disease without anticoagulation results in devastating outcomes and these are the most fragile of anticoagulation patients. Without proper anticoagulation, patients are at risk for stroke and may also require valve replacement or repair procedures having survival risks and loss of productivity and quality of life. Therefore, it is important these patients are well managed long-term and during peri-procedural interruptions of anticoagulant therapy. When

Table 10-10.
Recommended Treatment Duration for VTE

DVT/PE Classification and Frequency Group	Suggested Duration of Therapy	Target INR
1st Occurrence–Identified, Modifiable Cause	3 months	2–3
1st Occurrence–with Malignancy	LMWH 3-6 months then warfarin until cancer is resolved	2–3
1st Occurrence–Idiopathic or 1 Thrombophilic Condition	6–12 months	2–3
1st Occurrence–Antiphospholipid Syndrome or ≥ 2 Thrombophilic Conditions	12 months	2–3
Recurrent VTE	Lifetime	2–3
Recurrent VTE + Antiphospholipid Syndrome	Lifetime	2.5–3.5

Source: References 40 and 176.

valvular patients have AF, the risk of systemic emboli increases three to seven times those in normal sinus rhythm.[191] Other risk factors include: heart failure, previous thromboembolism, age (50–69 and ≥70), permanent pacemaker, hypertension, left atrial size ≥ 50 mm, size or severity of valvular lesion, smoking, diabetes, and hyperlipidemia.[191-194] Often, more important is the type and location of the prosthetic heart valve, mechanical valves are more thrombogenic than bioprosthetic valves, yet both are more thrombogenic than native valves.[191-194] Earlier model mechanical valves, like the ball cage, Starr-Edwards, or Bjork-Shiley were highly thrombogenic compared to single tilting disc valves and newer bileaflet valves.[191,192,194] At a goal INR of 2–2.9, incidence of thromboembolism per year was 0.5%, 0.7%, and 2.5% for the bileaflet, tilting disc, and cage ball or cage disc valves, respectively.[195] Prosthetic valves in the mitral position are more thrombogenic than the same valve in the aortic position.[191,192,194] Without anticoagulation, the bileaflet St. Jude valve caused systemic emboli 22% per year in the mitral position versus 12% in the aortic position.[196] Table 10-11 compares the incidence of systemic embolism by valve type and location. Interpret this data carefully as outcomes were extracted from different trials using similar INR ranges with differences in the time patient's spent in range. The same holds true for major bleeding events listed in the final column, these values are best fit estimates.

Patients may receive bioprosthetic or mechanical heart valves; this decision is based on life expectancy and willingness to take life-long warfarin. Bioprosthetic valves have shorter life expectancies (~15 years) but allow patients with no additional risk factors like AF to take aspirin after 3 months of warfarin. Bioprosthetic valves can also be placed in either the aortic or mitral position and are less thrombogenic than mechanical valves. Antithrombotic prophylaxis is the same for the three types of bioprosthetic heart valves; transplanted human, porcine, and pericardial (bovine). Recommendations for anticoagulation are provided in Table 10-12.

Recommendations for antithrombotic therapy in patients with valvular disease, not including prosthetic valves, are covered in Table 10-13. Most patients with valvular disease plus AF require warfarin unless contraindicated. There are other conditions, like septal wall defects, where antithrombotic decisions remain unclear. Exercise caution when labeling treatment failures; adequate doses, therapeutic levels, and dosing compliance must be verified for recent past not just present day. Combination therapy with aspirin is always associated with increased bleeding requiring extra caution when making warfarin dose adjustments. These patients also require additional instruction regarding compliance and changes in medications.

Ischemic Stroke

Stroke prevention with warfarin is limited to patients with AF, hypercoagulable states, or valvular heart disease. Infrequent exceptions may also include septal wall defects or aspirin failures. The majority (85%) of strokes are ischemic and 20% originate within the heart, often secondary to AF.[197] Unfortunately, 30% of ischemic strokes have an unidentifiable origin following a thorough evaluation by neurology and cardiology.[197] While in theory, it seems reasonable to treat patients who present with acute strokes secondary to AF with full dose anticoagulation, randomized trials do not support this practice.[198-204] Other than unquestionable benefits of DVT prophylaxis in acute ischemic

Table 10-11.
Incidence of Systemic Thromboembolism by Valve Type, Location, and INR

Specific Valve Type	Valve Location	Target INR Ranged Desired	Range TE/year	Estimated ❖ Major Bleeding
St. Jude Mechanical Bileaflet	Mitral Position	1.8–2.8	0.4%–6.5%	N/A
		2.5–3.5	3.4%–4.7%	1.2%/year
		2.8–4.5	2.2%–2.9%	0.4%–6.6%/year
	Aortic Position	1.8–2.8	0.7%–3.9%	N/A
		2–3	0.8%–1.9%	4%/year
		2.5–4.5	0.8%–3.0%	2.0%–6.6%/year
Medtronic Hall	Mitral Position	2.0–3.0	N/A	4%/year
		2.5–3.5	2.1%–4.7%	1.2%/year
		3.0–4.5	1.5%	0.4%–6.6%/year
	Aortic Position	2–3	1.3%	4%/year
		2.5–3.5	N/A	1.2%/year
		3.0–4.5	0.7%	0.4%–6.6%/year
Bjork Shiley Spherical Disc	Mitral Position	2.0–4.5	2.6%	1.6%/year
		3.0–4.0	1.5%	N/A
	Aortic Position	2.0–4.5	1%	1.6%/year
		3.0–4.0	0.4%	N/A
Bjork Shiley Convexo Concave	Mitral Position	3.0–4.0	2.1%	N/A
	Aortic Position	3.0–4.0	0.5%	N/A
Sorin Mono	Mitral Position	2.5–4.0	1.7%	N/A
	Aortic Position	2.5–4.0	0.9%	N/A

❖ Each value/range extrapolated/best fit using multiple trials with varying INR compliance.
Source: References 191 and 192.

stroke, guidelines by the American Heart Association and the American Academy of Neurology do not support full dose anticoagulation immediately following due to increased hemorrhagic progression in the early phase.[205,206] The majority of data for non-cardiogenic stroke, including major intracranial artery stenosis, do not support warfarin over aspirin.[207,208] There are small subsets where warfarin has not been evaluated in well-designed trials; however, appear to benefit from warfarin based on nonrandomized, non-comparator trials. These populations include cervical artery dissection, major carotid stenosis awaiting endarterectomy, antiphospholipid antibody, and prothrombotic disorders.[197] Patients with idiopathic stroke and underlying mobile aortic arch thrombi may also benefit from warfarin.[197]

Antiphospholipid Antibody Syndrome (APS)

The autoimmune disorder APS is defined by the presence of antiphospholipid antibodies in a patient with arterial or venous thrombosis or an adverse outcome during pregnancy.[209,210] Generally speaking, there are two types of antiphospholipid antibodies (APLAs); lupus anticoagulants and anticardiolipin antibodies. Lupus anticoagulants are known to prolong phospholipid-dependent clotting assays.[211-213] APLAs are commonly found in approximately 30%–50% of systemic lupus erythematosus (SLE) patients. This is in contrast to 1%–10% of the general population.[214,215] APLAs are found in 4%–21% of the general population presenting with thrombosis.[216,217] During a 6-year follow-up of APS patients, the incidence of VTE was 29%–55% with nearly half being pulmonary embolism.[218] In a study using stricter criteria for APS diagnosis, the incidence of thrombosis was 32%.[219] In patients less than 50 years presenting with stroke, approximately 50% were found to have APLAs.[220] There are a number of theories why APS patients are predisposed to thrombotic events. These include: increased endothelial cell activation, increased oxidative injury of vascular endothelium, interference with phospholipid-binding proteins involved in regulation of the clotting cascade, increased activa-

Table 10-12.
Antithrombotic Recommendations for Patients with Prosthetic Heart Valves

Prosthetic Heart Valve by Type, Location, and Risk Conditions	Antithrombotic Therapy	Duration	INR
Mechanical Valve (except ball cage) Aortic Position	Warfarin + UF/LMWH bridge 2 in range INRs	Indefinite	2–3
Mechanical Valve Mitral Position	Warfarin + UF/LMWH bridge 2 in range INRs	Indefinite	2.5–3.5
Ball Cage Valve (any position)	Warfarin + aspirin 75–100 mg daily	Indefinite	2.5–3.5
Bioprosthetic Valve–No Risk Factors Aortic Position	Aspirin 80–100 mg daily or ↓	3 months	N/A
	Warfarin + UF/LMWH bridge 2 in range INRs	3 months, then aspirin 75–100 mg	2–3
Bioprosthetic Valve–no risk factors Mitral Position	Warfarin + UF/LMWH bridge 2 in range INRs	3 months, then aspirin 75–100 mg	2–3
High Risk Conditions or Treatment Failures with Prosthetic Heart Valve			
Mechanical Valve (Any Position) + AF, MI, Left Atrial Enlargement, Endocardial Damage, Low EF, Systemic Embolism at Goal INR	Warfarin + aspirin 75–100 mg daily	Indefinite	2.5–3.5
Bioprosthetic Valve (Any Position) with History of Systemic Embolism	Warfarin + UF/LMWH bridge 2 in range INRs	3–12 months	2–3
Bioprosthetic Valve (Any Position) Left Atrial Thrombus at Surgery	Warfarin + UF/LMWH bridge 2 in range INRs	Indeterminate	2–3
Bioprosthetic Valve (Any Position) Atrial Fibrillation	Warfarin + UF/LMWH bridge 2 in range INRs	Indefinite	2–3

Source: References 191, 192, and 194.

tion of platelets, and possibly inhibition of protein C and S activity.[221-223]

The presence of APLAs in and of itself is not an indication for warfarin. It is likely patients with SLE and APLAs have higher risk than patients having only APLAs.[224,225] Based on consensus opinion, asymptomatic APLA positive patients without history of thrombosis may benefit from aspirin 81 mg daily.[226] Based on consensus recommendations, pregnant patients with APLAs and one previous late pregnancy loss or ≥ two early pregnancy losses, warrants treatment with aspirin 81 mg daily and prophylactic doses of LMWH or unfractionated heparin.[227] Initiation of aspirin 81 mg daily should begin during trials of conception and prophylactic doses of LMWH or unfractionated heparin should be started when viable pregnancy is confirmed and continued through late into the final trimester.[228] Treatment recommendations for VTE with APS can be found in Table 10-10.

Dose Management

Secondary to warfarin's delayed onset of action, initiation and management of warfarin often requires management of injectable anticoagulants. For many indications it is important that initiation of warfarin be overlapped or bridged with an injectable anticoagulant. Both should be overlapped for at least 4–5 days and the INR should be in range and stable before discontinuation of injectable anticoagulation.[39,40,176,191] Since warfarin has no action on existing clotting factors, this overlap period allows for depletion of existing clotting factors while the injectable anticoagulant immediately inhibits clotting factors currently present in the circulation. Extended overlap with injectable anticoagulants, in theory could increase a patients risk for bleeding. Given an elevated INR reflects a reduced concentration or quantity of functional clotting factors, continuation or initiation of injectable anticoagulants while therapeutic on warfarin, means inhibiting the activity of an already reduced quantity of functional clotting factors.

In patients taking warfarin prior to admission, it is important to obtain patient's dosing history to know warfarin requirements in a healthy state. The patient's indication for warfarin is also important to

Table 10-13.

Antithrombotic Recommendations for Patients with Valvular Heart Disease

Heart Valve Disease and Risk Conditions	Antithrombotic Therapy	Duration	INR
Mitral Valve Disease in Normal Sinus Rhythm with Left Atrial Diameter < 5.5 cm	No warfarin, possibly aspirin 75–100 mg daily	N/A	N/A
Rheumatic Mitral Valve with AF or History of Systemic Embolism	Warfarin without aspirin	Indefinite	2–3
Mitral Valvuloplasty Procedure No Risk Factors or Events	Warfarin	3 wks prior and 4 wks after	2–3
	Then no warfarin or aspirin	Indefinite	N/A
Mitral Annular Calcification Without Systemic Embolism	No warfarin or aspirin	Indefinite	N/A
Aortic Valve/Aortic Arch Disorders Without Embolism or Indication	No warfarin or aspirin	Indefinite	N/A
Endocarditis and Mechanical Valve Without Contraindications — Aortic	Warfarin + UF/LMWH bridge 2 in range INRs	Indefinite	2–3
Endocarditis and Mechanical Valve Without Contraindications — Mitral	Warfarin + UF/LMWH bridge 2 in range INRs	Indefinite	2.5–3.5
Nonbacterial Endocarditis and Systemic or Pulmonary Emboli	IV unfractionated heparin	Unspecified	N/A
Endocarditis with Disseminated Cancer or Debilitating Disease with Aseptic Vegetations	IV unfractionated heparin	Unspecified	N/A
High Risk Conditions or Treatment Failures with Valvular Heart Disease			
Rheumatic Mitral Valve with AF or History of Systemic Embolism <u>and</u> Systemic Embolism at Goal INR	Warfarin + aspirin 75–100 mg daily or dipyridamole/clopidogrel	Indefinite	2–3
Mitral Valve Disease in Normal Sinus Rhythm with Left Atrial Diameter >5.5 cm	Warfarin	Indefinite	2–3
Mitral Valvuloplasty with Unexplained TIA or Stroke	Aspirin 50–162 mg daily or dipyridamole/clopidogrel	Indefinite	N/A
Mitral Valvuloplasty with TIA or Systemic Embolism Despite Antiplatelet Therapy	Warfarin	Indefinite	2–3
Mitral Annular Calcification with Non-Calcific Systemic Embolism	Warfarin	Long-term Unspecified	2–3
Aortic Valve/Aortic Arch Disorder with Mobile Aortic Atheromas and Aortic Plaques > 4 mm by TEE	Warfarin	Unspecified	2–3

Source: References 191–194.

Managing Anticoagulation Patients in the Hospital: The Inpatient Anticoagulation Service

> **Clinical Pearls**
>
> Data on how often INRs are required in the inpatient setting is scarce. Considering the instability of patients in high acuity settings, increased probability of medication interactions, and changes in dietary intake of vitamin K, many hospitals often have policies requiring daily INRs and daily warfarin dosing. This ensures patients, at least in theory, are reassessed daily. This type of policy leads to unnecessary INR checks, however, it is likely better than the alternative which is a lack of proper oversight of this high-risk medication.
>
> Many hospitals standardize their warfarin administration time to the evening so dose adjustments can be made the same day as an INR check and to match when most patients take warfarin at home. When designing these systems, it is important to assure enough time has passed, particularly after the first dose of warfarin, before INR is checked. Most hospitals try to assure at least 12 hours have passed.

determine appropriate therapeutic range. Medication changes occur frequently in hospitalized patients therefore medication interaction screening is required daily. Hospitalized patients are also more likely to experience significant changes in dosing requirements secondary to nutritional feedings and changes in clotting factor metabolism or production related to fever, thyroid, liver disease, decompensated heart failure, or other diseases.

There is much debate regarding the most appropriate way to initiate warfarin and dose selection. The benefits of obtaining an early therapeutic INR include: reduced length of stay; reduced exposure to heparin and possibly HIT; reduced expense of LMWH, and reduced heparin monitoring. Risks that must be weighed against these benefits include: overshooting desired INR, risk of bleeding associated with elevated INR, cost and inconvenience of increased monitoring associated with elevated INRs, delayed discharge secondary to elevated INR, and a clouded picture of patient's maintenance dose when loading doses are used. Use of excessive (20-mg) loading doses is not recommended, even 15-mg doses have not been studied in well-designed clinical trials.[40] The Coumadin® package insert recommends initiation of 2–5 mg per day and adjustment based on INR determinations.[229] The initiation dose should take into consideration acuity of the indication and warfarin sensitizers such as age, gender, weight, ethnic background, bleeding risks (i.e., postoperative), nutritional status, presence of interacting medications, and illnesses such as liver disease or heart failure. In contrast to younger patients, older patients require lower doses, more often become supratherapeutic, and take longer to return to the desired INR.[230-236] In addition, elevated INRs are more likely to cause bleeding in older versus younger patients.[237-240] Garcia evaluated 12,202 patients finding a 0.4-mg decrease in weekly maintenance dose for each additional year of age.[241] Furthermore, for any given age, men required 4.5 mg more warfarin per week than women.[241] The study showed a 5-mg daily dose would exceed the average maintenance for 82% of women and 65% of men older than 70 years.[241] Warfarin dose requirements by patient weight didn't correlate as well as gender or age however, patients greater than 234 pounds required larger maintenance doses.[241]

A number of warfarin dosing nomograms have been evaluated. These studies have important differences when interpreting results including: enrollees' age, inpatient versus outpatient, gender mixes, co-morbidities, and controlling for variables known to affect warfarin sensitivity.[242-249] With the exception of the Gedge study,[243] a summary of trial results are found in Table 10-14. The inpatient study by Gedge (Table 10-15) was interesting in that a single 10-mg dose was compared to initiation with two 10-mg doses. Warfarin loading doses are linked to increased, although non-significant, increases in bleeding.[246, 247] These studies however, were not sufficiently powered to detect statistically significant increases in bleeding.[246, 247] Readers are

> **Clinical Pearl**
>
> Inpatient anticoagulation pharmacists need to identify warfarin sensitization factors when initiating and managing warfarin. Factors include, interacting medications, elderly, malnutrition, and disease states such as heart failure. For these reasons, acutely ill patients starting warfarin should be initiated on 5 mg of warfarin or less per day.

referred to these articles to make their own evaluation regarding the nomograms; however, caution is advised regarding the use of initiation doses greater than 5 mg in high bleeding risk patients.

Initiating 7.5 mg of warfarin in an elderly post operative female may result in major bleeding and over-shoot the desired INR delaying discharge. In patients requiring acute anticoagulation, it is sug-

Table 10-14.
Warfarin High Dose vs. Low Dose Initiation Nomograms

Study	Mean Age	INR	10 mg Nomogram	5 mg Nomogram	p value
Harrison[244]	N/A	2–3 @ 36 h	6 (24%)	1 (4%)	N/A
		> 2 @ 36 h	11 (44%)	2 (8%)	0.005
n = 25 10 mg		> 3 @ 36 h	5 (20%)	1 (4%)	N/A
n = 24 5 mg		2–3 @ 60 h	9 (36%)	10 (42%)	N/A
		> 2 @ 60 h	18 (72%)	10 (42%)	N/A
		> 3 @ 60 h	9 (36%)	0 (0%)	0.002
Kovacs[245]	55.5 years	Mean to INR > 1.9	4.2 days	5.6 days	<0.001
		< 2 or >3 @ 1 week	N/A	N/A	N/A
n = 104 10 mg		Total INRs < 2 or >3 in 4 weeks	186	207	>0.2
n = 97 5 mg		2–3 @ day 5	86 (83%)	45 (46%)	<0.001
Crowther[242]	~ 66 years	<2 @ day 3	43%	44%	N/A
		2–3 @ day 3	33%	50%	N/A
n = 21 10 mg		> 3 @ day 3	24%	6%	N/A
n = 31 5 mg		<2 @ day 5	15%	8%	N/A
		2–3 @ day 5	69%	88%	N/A
		> 3 @ day 5	15%	4%	N/A
O'Connell[246]		<2 @ day 2	88%	84%	N/A
		2–3 @ day 2	0%	6%	N/A
n = 40 *9 mg = 72.4 yr		> 3 @ day 2	5%	0%	N/A
n = 33 *≤ 5 mg = 77.3 yr		Time to INR > 2	3 days	3.4 days	0.38
*doses above are means		<2 @ day 4	60%	48%	N/A
		2–3 @ day 4	10%	24%	N/A
		>3 @ day 4	18%	15%	N/A
		≥1 INR @ ≥ 4	21%	28%	0.54
Quiroz[247]	~ 50.5 years	2 INRs > 1.9	5 days	5 days	N/A
		Mean INR @ day 5	2.2	2	N/A
n = 25 10 mg		>2 @ day 3	favored		<0.01
n = 25 5 mg		>2 @ day 4	favored		<0.01
		2–3 @ day 5	56%	52%	> 0.5
		2–3 @ day 10		favored	<0.01
		2–3 @ day 11		favored	<0.01
		2–3 @ day 14		favored	<0.01
		>3 overall	14.5%	3.7%	<0.001

Table 10-15.
Warfarin High Dose vs. Modified High Dose Initiation Nomograms

Study	Age	INR	10 mg × 2 doses	10 mg × 1 doses	p value
Gedge[243] n = 120	65–75 yr n = 30 10 mg × 2 doses	INR > 4.5 in 8 days	20%	3%	< 0.05
	n = 30 10 mg × 1 doses	Time with INR 2–3	2.7 days	3.0 days	0.03
		Time to INR >2	3.8 days	4.6 days	0.03
	> 75 yr n = 30 10 mg × 2 doses	INR > 4.5 in 8 days	37%	3%	< 0.01
		Time with INR 2–3	2.4 days	2.9 days	0.04
	n = 30 10 mg × 1 doses	Time to INR > 2	3.5 days	4.5 days	0.003
	Combined n = 120	Doses held in 8 days	59 held doses	18 held doses	N/A

gested to bridge with injectable anticoagulant rather than use excessive warfarin doses. The clinician should obtain a thorough patient history to identify drug interactions, nutritional status, liver disease or heart failure, herbal use, history of bleeds or thromboembolic events, and patient's previous warfarin dosing history if available.

Laboratory Monitoring

Warfarin intensity was originally reported in prothrombin time (PT), the seconds increasing corresponding to a reduction in factors II, VII, and X. Although warfarin inhibits factor IX production, the PT does not measure factor IX.[40] The PT is obtained by adding calcium and thromboplastin to the patient's serum in a citrated plasma tube.[40,39] Due to variation in prothrombin time results from different labs using different thromboplastin agents, it became necessary to standardize prothrombin time ratio so a given sample provided reproducible results at different labs. One of these strategies was the INR measurement adjusting for thromboplastin reagent sensitivity as determined by the International Sensitivity Index (ISI). The INR was adopted in 1982 and was the beginning of improvements towards a standardized measurement of warfarin intensity. The INR calculation = (patient prothrombin time/mean prothrombin time)^{ISI}.

Another improvement for warfarin monitoring was improved sensitivity of thromboplastin reagents. The lower the ISI value the more sensitive the thromboplastin. In 1992 the ISI values were 1.4 to 2.8 for most U.S. laboratories.[250-253] Shortly thereafter, recombinant DNA technology allowed for more sensitive thromboplastin reagents with ISI values of 0.9 to 1.[254] Another variable for INR results is the concentration of citrate used in collection tubes and filling the tube with the proper blood volume.[255,256] Citrate concentrations generally range from 3.2%–3.8%; a higher concentration caused by under-filling the tube can cause an elevated INR.[255] The likelihood of this problem may be reduced by using 3.2% citrated plasma tubes and insuring appropriate blood volume is collected in the tube.[40] Automated analyzers and their calibration methods can also affect the reliability and reproducibility of INR results, for a more in-depth review the reader is referred to the following citations.[257-266]

It is important to understand INRs for patients with lupus anticoagulant, particularly those with prothrombin antibodies, can be falsely elevated.[211-213, 267, 268] The degree of false elevation varies according to the reagent used.[211, 212, 268] Variation of INR results may be minimized using standardized plasma samples during calibration and using local analyzer specific ISI values.[269] Other methods for monitoring or validation of usual INR results have been investigated for lupus anticoagulant and include: measuring prothrombin activity or native thrombin, prothrombin and proconvertin test, and measuring chromogenic factor X activity.[40, 211, 270]

> **Clinical Pearl**
>
> Nomograms can be used to develop institution protocols/guidelines; however, nomograms do not take into account the rapid changing status of the hospitalized patient. Pharmacists require the ability to deviate from the nomogram when their clinical judgment deems this necessary to assure they are treating the patient, not the numbers.

Management of Non-Therapeutic INRs

Elevations in INR are broadly categorized as those requiring warfarin dose adjustments versus warfarin reversal and elevations complicated by serious bleeding versus those involving life threatening bleeding.[40] Management is very patient- and case-specific, and controversy also exists given the number of available options and lack of well-designed trials comparing these options.[40] These decisions can be further complicated by supply issues with prothrombin-complex concentrates (PCC).

Among the worst bleeding events secondary to warfarin are intracranial hemorrhages (ICH). ICHs are the most fatal of strokes with a mortality rate of 30%–55% and in warfarin patients this increases to 67%.[271-274] The objective is to stop early expansion occurring in approximately 40%, as continuation of bleeding into the hematoma is a predictor of death.[275,276,277] ICHs with warfarin are at greater risk for expansion; 50% versus 18%–38% in those without anticoagulation.[275,276,278]

Although there is a black box warning for IV vitamin K due to anaphylactic reactions, life threatening bleeding is a justifiable cause to use this route.[40,279-281] Incidence of IV vitamin K anaphylactic reactions is low and is estimated to be as few as three cases per 10,000 doses.[280,282] Vitamin K by the IV route works in less than 4 hours and is both faster and more potent than SC, IM, or oral routes.[281,283,284] In serious and life-threatening bleeding, it is recommended that vitamin K 10 mg by slow (30 minutes) IV piggyback infusion be supplemented with fresh frozen plasma (FFP) or PCC.[40] In urgent cases and/or where there are supply issues with FFP or PCC, recombinant factor VIIa can be considered as an alternative to PCC.[40] In bleeding patients anticoagulated with warfarin, administration of vitamin K is required to maintain sustained reversal and prevent early re-bleeding.[40,285,286]

Fresh frozen plasma (FFP) contains clotting factors and has been used effectively to augment the affects of IV vitamin K in patients with serious bleeding related to warfarin. FFP is commonly ordered as 2–6 units; however, it may also be dosed at 10–15 mL/kg or more for extreme bleeding cases.[287] Newer alternatives have overcome shortcomings of FFP; however, the cost of these alternatives and supply issues are problematic. A disadvantage of FFP is requirement for thawing and compatibility testing; this can delay initiation without early coordination between the physician, unit, and lab. Another FFP disadvantage is the low concentration and content variability of individual clotting factors.[286,288,289] The low concentration of clotting factors in FFP requires large volumes ranging from 800–3500 mL to achieve INRs ≤ 1.4.[288,290-293] For patients with heart failure and other volume-sensitive patients, this may require slower administration and aggressive diuresis. Rare adverse events of FFP include allergic reactions, blood-borne infections, citrate toxicity, and transfusion-related lung injury.[294,295] Nonetheless, FFP when administered with IV vitamin K is effective for management of life threatening bleeding.[40,287,288,290,296] In using this combination, early patient presentation and rapid administration of both improves early reversal of warfarin.[288,290]

Prothrombin-Complex Concentrate (PCC) provides a concentrated supply of vitamin K dependent clotting factors II, VII, IX, and X. PCC does not require compatibility testing or thawing before use.[286,297] Secondary to virus inactivation, PCCs have a lower risk of infection unless available FFPs contain methylene blue or are solvent detergent treated FFPs.[297] There are differing opinions regarding dose of PCCs; the U.K. guidelines for warfarin reversal recommends 50 units/kg.[298] Some studies suggest dose should be based on INR. One study used 25 units/kg for INRs between 2–3.9, 35 units/kg for INRs between 4–5.9, 50 units/kg for INRs > 6.[288,299] Other studies showing successful reversal have used a standard dose of 30 units/kg or even smaller doses such as 500 units were reported effective in elderly patients.[300,301] Dosing differences may partly be explained by varying quantities and type of individual clotting factors in these products. Some contain equal amounts of factors II, VII, IX, and X where others may contain varying quantities II, IX, and X.[297] Package inserts are often helpful in providing detailed information regarding quantities of each factor and dosing. Several trials indicate PCCs more rapidly correct the INR than administration of FFP.[288,302,303] This may be related to the FFP dose or late initiation, slower FFP administration, and varying doses or routes of adjunctive vitamin K. Given these differences, nothing remains crystal clear when selecting an adjunctive agent to IV vitamin K for reversal. Disadvantages of PCCs include: cost, occasional supply issues, DIC development, thrombosis potential in high-risk patients, and lack of standardized dosing.[286,297,304-307]

Recombinant factor VIIa is another adjunctive agent that may be combined with IV vitamin K.

Recombinant VIIa reverses anticoagulation by activating factors IX, X, and II. Concerns whether there are sufficient quantities of these factors in patients receiving warfarin requires further study. Possibly more concerning is the recently published article by O'Connell[308] describing their review of 431 adverse drug events associated with Recombinant VIIa submitted to the FDA March 1999 to December 2004. Of the 431 reports, 185 describe thrombotic events warranting further investigation, given underreporting of ADRs, and the need to determine the actual occurrence rate.[308] In the Mayer trial 309 combined arteriole and venous thrombotic events were 2%, 6%, 4% and 10% for the placebo, 40 mcg/kg, 80 mcg/kg, and 160 mcg/kg groups, respectively. Recombinant VIIa has been studied in hemorrhagic stroke; however, it is important to note these studies excluded patients with history of thrombosis and those taking warfarin.[309, 310] These results, therefore, do not provide support for factor VIIa in warfarin patients with ICH. Sorensen[311] evaluated warfarin patients with CNS bleeds (n = 6) and (n = 1) at risk for ICH. Admission INRs were 2.9 to 4.1 for six patients and greater than 7 for one. All but two patients received IV vitamin-K, 10 mg IV x 4 patients and 1 mg IV x 1 patient. One patient had not received warfarin in the previous 9 days having an INR of 3.6. Three patients received FFP, 2 units each. INRs following above interventions were less than 2.8 for four patients, less than 4 for two patients, and 6.6 for the seventh patient. Six of seven patients underwent neurosurgical drainage of hematomas after receiving a bolus of 10–40 mcg/kg Recombinant VII, for an intended target INR ≤ 1.5. One patient who did not receive vitamin K preoperatively required three bags of FFP to maintain an INR < 2.0 post-operatively. This study indicates recombinant VIIa monotherapy is not sufficient for warfarin patients and must be administered with IV vitamin K given factor VIIa's short half-life of 2.3 hours.[312] Freeman[291] evaluated warfarin patients with acute ICH (n = 7) who required immediate reversal of warfarin. Admission INRs were ≥ 2.9 for six patients and 5.6 for the seventh. All but one received vitamin K; however, three of six patients were given less than the recommended 10-mg dose. Only one vitamin K dose was given IV, two were given SC, and routes on the other three were not stated. Six of seven patients received a mean dose of 7.2 units of FFP. The mean INR prior to recombinant VIIa was 2.7 and decreased to 1.08 after administration of 62 mcg/kg. It is interesting to note the patient presenting with an INR of 5.6 did not reach an INR less than 2 before 18 hours. The reader is referred to other studies investigating the role of recombinant VIIa for patients experiencing serious or life threatening bleeding.[292,313-316] Possible limitations of recombinant VIIa is that it may not completely reverse warfarin effects, especially those with elevated INRs, and also does not appreciably increase the activity level of factors II, IX, and X following administration.[317,291,314] Concerns regarding wide acceptance of recombinant VIIa for warfarin reversal include: limited data of factor VIIa in warfarin patients, emerging risks for thrombosis with added patient experience, and an estimated acquisition cost of $5,714 per dose at 40 mcg/kg in a 70-kg patient.[286,308,318]

> **Clinical Pearl**
>
> Injectable vitamin K can be given orally when doses less than 2.5 mg are desired.

Routine management of moderately elevated INRs requires holding one or more doses and/or small doses of oral vitamin K. Trials show the oral route is less variable, more reliable, and safer than the other routes.[40,279] The daily risk of bleeding secondary to a temporary elevated INR is low and more frequent monitoring is an option.[40]

Elevated INRs less than 5 and without significant bleeding can generally be managed by omitting a single dose and repeating the INR next day. Warfarin can be resumed at a lower dose when the INR is close to or in the desired range. The amount of dose reduction is based on the cause and whether it is reversible, such as a drug interaction, where patients can be switched from ciprofloxacin or sulfamethoxazole to cephalexin for UTI.

INRs greater than 5 but less than 9 and without significant bleeding can be managed by omitting one or two doses guided by daily INRs. Depending on the patient's bleeding risks (i.e., elderly, liver disease, malnourished, CHF) the patient may be given oral vitamin K ≤ 5 mg in addition to one or two held doses. Acutely ill patients are often slower to correct and interactions sometimes involve medications without alternatives.

Patients with elevated INRs ≥ 9 and without significant bleeding should be given vitamin K 5–10 mg orally. This would be expected to drop the INR within 24–48 hours. The warfarin should be placed on hold and resumed based on daily INR determinations.[40] In a hospitalized patient, repeat INRs should be preformed daily to guide subse-

> **Clinical Pearl**
>
> Many inpatient anticoagulation programs develop vitamin K reversal guidelines for their institution. This aids both the pharmacists and the physicians. Another project many departments take on is the development of usage criteria for recombinant factor VIIa to attempt to minimize the thrombotic risk to patients and save institution resources. Figures 5-1 and 5-11 in Chapter 5 are examples of these documents.

quent dosing. In patients with elevated INRs and upcoming procedures, oral vitamin K is useful in reversing many patients within 24–48 hours.[40]

Management of Warfarin for Invasive Procedures

In preparing anticoagulated patients for an invasive surgical procedure, the first step is to identify the patient's risk for thrombotic event without anticoagulation. Patients going for surgical procedures can generally be placed into one of three categories; low, moderate, or high risk for thrombosis. Individual risks are additive; for example, AF with versus without prior stroke or TIA. See Table 10-16 for patient types, risk stratification, and peri-procedural anticoagulation management.[39,40,191,319,320] The decision to use large weight-based doses of SC heparin instead of LMWH seems an acceptable alternative.[39,40] When used for short durations, as in the periprocedural setting, monitoring may not be necessary. At least for short periods in the setting of acute DVT treatment (high risk), weight-based (333 units/kg × 1 dose then 250 units/kg) SC heparin twice daily appears as effective as adjusted IV heparin or weight-based SC LMWH for treatment of VTE.[177,321,322] However, when bridge therapy is required for extended periods in high-risk patients such as those with mechanical heart valves or even short periods in renal dysfunction patients, aPTT monitoring and adjustment of high-dose SC heparin is warranted. Platelet count monitoring is also necessary for HIT.

Another option that has been evaluated to prepare patients for minor to major surgical procedures is lowering the intensity of anticoagulation.[39,40,323] In a small population, this was evaluated in high-risk thromboembolism patients undergoing higher risk bleeding procedures.[323] Other studies have evaluated partial or full-dose anticoag-

Table 10-16.

Risk of Thrombotic Event Without Therapy

Indication for Anticoagulation	Thrombotic Event per Year	Suggested Method for Prophylaxis
Low Risk of Thromboembolism		
Non Valvular AF w/o Risk Factors	5%	■ D/C aspirin if any 7 days prior*
BioProsthetic Valve Mitral or Aortic Position*	0.2%–3.3%	■ D/C warfarin 4 days prior to procedure ■ Optional prophylactic dose UFH or LMWH 2 days prior to surgery
VTE > 3 months	10%	Prophylactic dose UFH or LMWH postoperatively and begin warfarin
Bi-leaflet Aortic Valve	10%–12%	
Moderate Risk of Thromboembolism		
AF with Risk Factors or Previous Embolism	12%	■ D/C aspirin if any 7 days prior ■ D/C warfarin 4 days prior to procedure
Arterial Embolism in the Last Month	15%	■ Prophylactic dose UFH or LMWH 2 days prior to surgery
Recurrent Venous Thromboembolism	15%	■ Prophylactic dose UFH or LMWH postoperatively and begin warfarin ■ Optional weight-based IV UFH or SC LMWH postoperatively and begin warfarin
High Risk of Thromboembolism		
Dual-Leaflet (St. Jude) Mechanical Mitral Valve	22%	■ D/C aspirin if any 7 days prior ■ D/C warfarin 4 days prior to procedure
Single-Leaflet (Bjork-Shiley) Mechanical Aortic Valve	23%	■ Weight-based SC or IV UFH or SC LMWH started ~ 2 days preoperatively. Continue SC agent ~ 12 h pre-op, Continue IV agent ~ 5 h pre-op
VTE < 3 months	40%	
Multiple (St. Jude) Mechanical Valves	91%	■ As soon as safely possible begin weight-based IV UFH or SC LMWH postoperatively and begin warfarin

Source: References 39, 40, 191, 319, and 320.

ulation in orthopedic surgical patients to determine the effectiveness of VTE prophylaxis and bleeding incidence.[324-326] Using this method, patients have their dose reduced to half their usual maintenance dose 5–7 days prior to the procedure. A follow-up INR with possible dose adjustment is scheduled a few days prior to the procedure. The goal is to obtain an INR of 1.3 to 2, depending on bleeding risk of the procedure, on the operative day.[39,40,323]

Other encountered procedures include gastrointestinal (GI) procedures. The American Society of Gastrointestinal Endoscopy divided endoscopic procedures into two groups, those at low and high risk for bleeding; see Table 10-17.[327] In their 2002 guidelines for anticoagulated patients, they do not routinely recommend withholding patient's anticoagulation for low risk procedures.[327] Generally, for high-risk procedures anticoagulation can be withheld for short periods similar to management of patients in Table 10-16.[327]

Other procedures identified as low risk for bleeding, and therefore better to continue anticoagulation in patients at high risk for thromboembolisms, include: arthrocentesis, cataract surgery, minor cutaneous and dermatologic procedures, and joint and soft tissue injections.[1,39,40,319,320,323] Anticoagulation may also be reduced to the lower end of the patient's therapeutic range when the risk for bleeding is higher.

Warfarin and Hemorrhage Risk

Factors associated with increased bleeding on warfarin include: age (>75 years old); warfarin intensity; renal insufficiency or anemia; history of bleeding; hypertension; history of stroke; use of aspirin, NSAIDs, or other medications affecting platelet function or GI irritants; peripheral vascular disease; multiple medications or new interacting medication; and heart failure.[39,40,46,237-240,328-330] Given

> **Clinical Pearl**
>
> Many patients have a comprehensive anticoagulation bridging plan in place prior to elective admissions. Unfortunately, this bridge therapy plan is sometimes overlooked post-procedure. Sometimes, no plan was considered at all pre-procedure. A key role for inpatient anticoagulation pharmacists is to ensure implementation of necessary bridge therapy when planned or when it was not planned yet indicated. For example, anticoagulation pharmacists should carefully evaluate and consider starting injectable anticoagulants post surgery in any patient with a history of mechanical mitral valve replacement.

the very clear association of increased INR and bleeding, anything with the potential to increase INR increases risk of bleeding. Additional bleeding risks may include malnutrition, alcohol intake, herbal use, noncompliance, peptic ulcer disease, and malignancy. Two studies have identified an increased bleeding risk with the first 3 months of warfarin initiation.[328,239] See Table 10-18 for a comparison of bleeding risks by INR and indication.[331-334] A number of studies have shown a steep slope increase in bleeding rates for INRs > 5.[195,237,240,335,336] Warfarin use is a significant predictor of mortality in ICH, specifically the odds ratio of mortality was 1.5, 2, and 3.7 for INRs < 2, 2–3, and > 3, respectively.[274] Warfarin did not appear to adversely affect functional recovery in those that survived relative to control patients.[274]

The effect of age on bleeding events with warfarin remains controversial. Trials controlling for other variables like comorbid conditions, found

Table 10-17.
Bleeding Risks Associated with Endoscopic Procedures

Low Bleed-Risk Endoscopic Procedures	High Bleed-Risk Endoscopic Procedures
Upper endoscopy with or without biopsy	Polypectomy
Flexible sigmoidoscopy with or without biopsy	Laser ablation and coagulation
Colonoscopy with or without biopsy	Endoscopic sphincterotomy
Endoscopic retrograde cannulation of the pancreatic duct without sphincterotomy	Percutaneous endoscopic gastrostomy tube placement
Biliary stent insertion without sphincterotomy	Pneumatic or bougie dilation
Endosonography without fine-needle aspiration	Treatment of varices
Push enteroscopy of the small bowel	

Source: Reference 327.

Table 10-18.
Rates of Clinically Significant Bleeding by Intended INR Range

Indication	# Patients Study	Goal INR Range	Bleeding Incidence	p Value
Mechanical Heart Valve with ASA 300 mg/d and Dipyridamole 75 mg bid	n = 99 Altman et al.[331]	2–2.9	6%	<0.02
		3–4.5	24%	
DVT	n = 96 Hull et al.[332]	2–2.5	4.3%	0.015
		3–4.5	22.4%	
Mechanical Heart Valve	n = 247 Saour et al.[333]	1.9–3.6	21.3%	<0.002
		7.4–10.8	42.4%	
Tissue Prosthetic Heart Valve	n = 210 Turpie et al.[334]	2–2.5	5.9%	<0.002
		2.5–4	13.9%	

that age was not an independent risk factor.[337-340] However, two other trials controlling for intensity of anticoagulation and other variables, showed age was an independent risk factor for bleeding.[237, 341]

The inpatient anticoagulation pharmacist is constantly weighing the risk of thrombosis versus bleeding on a daily basis. The pharmacist should always be aware of risk factors the patient carries for bleeding (covered above) due to warfarin, such as:

- age (>75 years old)
- warfarin intensity (high INR, particularly when >5)
- renal insufficiency
- history of bleeding
- hypertension
- history of stroke
- concomitant medications (examples: aspirin, ibuprofen, etc.)
- peripheral vascular disease
- heart failure

This must be balanced against the risk of thrombosis for each individual patient. For the venous thromboembolism, Tables 10-8, 10-9, and 10-10 allow the reader to easily identify different risks of embolism a patient may have. Table 10-5 likewise portrays embolism risk factors for atrial fibrillation. This table also shows that some risk factors seem greater than others. Key risk factors for embolism for prosthetic heart valves discussed in the text (Table 10-11) include:

Clinical Pearls

Patient education on bleeding, minor nose bleeds, gum bleeding after brushing, and increased bruising is common for warfarin patients. However, these may also indicate an elevated INR in a patient not used to these experiences while therapeutic on warfarin. Patients require education on how to manage these symptoms and advice on specific symptoms requiring medical attention. Patients prone to minor nose bleeds should be informed of nasal moisturizers that reduce this occurrence. Patients tend to bruise easily on warfarin; however, bruises should not continue to grow after several days.

Red or brown urine or red or black tarry stools are often symptoms of more serious bleeding. These require medical attention and INR check. Patients with hemorrhoids or frequent constipation may have blood on toilet paper. Stool softeners can be helpful in this situation. This, however, should also be evaluated by a physician in patients recently starting warfarin or for those not having this problem previously. Positive stool guiacs and red or black tarry stools can be symptoms of a more serious condition such as malignancy or the result of excessive anticoagulation. Warfarin patients who develop occult GI bleeding have a 5%–25% chance of finding a malignant source with further evaluation.[40] Any bleeding regardless of source that doesn't resolve quickly with minor attention requires medical attention and check of the INR.

> **Clinical Pearl**
>
> The inpatient anticoagulation pharmacist must carefully monitor his or her patients for planned invasive procedures and consult directly with affected physicians to determine goal INR to minimize bleeding risk.

- Mechanical prosthetic valves are higher risk than bioprosthetic valves
- "Old" first-generation mechanical valves like ball and cage valves
- Mitral valves are higher risk than aortic valves
- Atrial fibrillation
- Left atrial enlargement (≥50 mm)
- Poor left ventricular function
- Age > 70 years old
- History of prior embolism

The skilled inpatient anticoagulation pharmacist will automatically and intuitively weigh the above thrombosis and bleeding risk factors before making management decisions on patients. Often, the pharmacist will be more aggressive with therapy (use higher doses of warfarin, bridge with injectable anticoagulants, etc.) when a patient has a high risk of thrombosis and a low risk of bleeding. At other times, the pharmacist may be more cautious (use lower doses or hold warfarin, forgo the use of injectable anticoagulants, etc.) when the risk of bleeding is high and thrombosis risk is low. In this situation, the skilled pharmacist may even consider a temporary, lower target INR range until the risk of bleeding subsides.

Warfarin Adverse Effects

A serious adverse effect other than bleeding is warfarin-induced skin necrosis.[39,40] Warfarin-induced skin necrosis is a rare side effect with an incidence of 0.01 to 0.1%.[342] Warfarin skin necrosis may occur in all ages or sexes of warfarin patients, however, seems more common in middle-aged, obese females.[343] A review of the literature indicates it more commonly involves fatty subcutaneous areas of the body including the thigh, buttocks, and breast, and a number of cases have also involved the penis.[343-346] Warfarin skin necrosis often occurs between the third and eighth day of therapy; however, it has been reported at day 10 also.[40,343-346] Warfarin skin necrosis often begins with pain in the affected area followed by erythematous flush. This progresses into petechial hemorrhages, then into red, blue, and/or black necrotic tissue that may hemorrhage.[343-345] There is likely an association between warfarin skin necrosis and protein C deficiency and to a lesser extent protein S. This is supported by earlier reports involving large initial doses of warfarin without using injectable anticoagulant bridge therapy.[343] Warfarin skin necrosis can occur without protein C or S deficiency, however, these patients are at greater risk.[40] Management of warfarin skin necrosis should include warfarin discontinuation and initiation of an injectable anticoagulant. An estimated 50% of patients will require surgical debridement.[344] Warfarin can later be restarted at low doses (i.e., 2 mg) providing the patient is on full dose injectable anticoagulant. Slow upward titration of warfarin over several weeks is recommended in conjunction with full dose injectable anticoagulation.[40,343]

Purple toe syndrome is another rare complication of warfarin that generally occurs during the third to tenth week of therapy.[347-349] Warfarin may enhance the release of cholesterol microemboli from plaques on vessel walls.[347] Purple toe syndrome often manifests as painful, purple, or mottled discoloration of the toes and sides of feet. Discolorations often blanch with pressure and sometimes fade with elevation of the effected extremity.[348,349] Discontinuation of warfarin is recommended because patients sometimes progress to gangrenous necrosis requiring debridement and/or amputation.[347,349] Some patients have later been restarted on warfarin therapy without reoccurrence however, close monitoring and patient education is required.[348]

Precautions and Contraindications

In practice, falls are often cited as a reason to avoid warfarin in patients with AF. One study evaluated this theory; their findings were that a patient would have to fall 295 times in 1 year for the risks of warfarin to outweigh the benefits.[350] The authors' major risk of concern was a subdural hematoma while on warfarin. The authors concluded that falls did not justify avoidance of warfarin; however, they felt it was important to identify and correct the reason for falls. They stated falls were a major cause of orthopedic fractures in elderly patients and fractures rather than bleeding on warfarin causes significant morbidity. It is estimated that one in ten falls will result in major injury in community dwelling elderly patients.[351] Other factors important in this population include numerous medications, multiple prescribing physicians, best price pharmacy shopping, multiple medical conditions, more frequent illnesses, and frequent changes in nutritional status.

There are conditions where warfarin is considered a relative contraindication and the clinician must weight patient's specific risks versus benefits. These include: senility, alcoholism, pregnancy 2nd or 3rd trimester, patient reliability, psychosis, and availability of laboratory testing and coordination of dose adjustment. Absolute contraindications include: blood dyscrasias prone to bleeding; recent or planned neuro, ocular, or traumatic surgery; malignant hypertension; overt bleeding or active ulcerations of the GI or respiratory tract; current or recent cerebrovascular hemorrhage; pericarditis or pericardial effusions; eclampsia or preeclampsia; spinal puncture; first trimester of pregnancy, specifically weeks 6 through 12 of gestation; and threatened abortion.

Warfarin precautions include recent surgery or trauma; heparin-induced thrombocytopenia, specifically initiation prior to platelet recovery greater than 100,000 or ideally more than 150,000; altered intestinal flora; IM injections; protein C or S deficiency; thrombocytopenia; liver dysfunction; debilitated patients; elderly; and children. The latter four with regard to reduced dosing and increased monitoring.

The limited studies on children taking warfarin indicate these are difficult to manage patients.[352-355] Plausible factors include: complicated medical problems, non-compliance, developing gut flora, corticosteroids, dietary compliance, enteral feedings, and difficult venous access. Children can be divided into three groups less than 1 year, age 1 to 6 years, and 7 to 18 years.[353] Children less than 1 year require larger doses, longer bridge therapy, and take longer to therapeutic INR.[353,356] Children aged 1 to 6 years often require larger doses than their teenage counterparts.[353,356] A child-based warfarin nomogram has been evaluated in two separate trials.[353,356] Children were initiated at a dose of 0.2 mg/kg with subsequent dosing adjusted by nomogram.[353,356] The largest study enrolling 262 infants and children found the average dose for infants and teenagers to be 0.32 mg/kg and 0.09 mg/kg respectively.[353] Corticosteroids were an independent predictor of time outside therapeutic range.[353] Enteral feedings, phenobarbital, and carbamazepine were found to cause increased warfarin dose requirements.[353] Adverse events in children receiving warfarin appear to be similar to the incidence in adults. In newborn and breast-feeding infants being treated with warfarin, consistent vitamin K intake is problematic. Breast milk should be supplemented with 1–2 ounces of infant formula per day due to the low vitamin K content of breast milk.[357] Children receiving long-term warfarin therapy should have periodic bone density scans.[358,359] Although there is not much data guiding practice, bone development is important during childhood and children with mechanical heart valves receive longer durations of warfarin therapy than most other populations. A case control study compared 17 children having received an average 8.2 years of warfarin to 321 random control patients. They found reduced bone density in the lumbar spine measured by Z-score after controlling for age and body size.[358]

Warfarin and Pregnancy

Warfarin patients attempting pregnancy require frequent pregnancy tests.[360] Warfarin is teratogenic, mostly during the first trimester, weeks 6 through 12 being the most critical.[360, 361] Unlike heparin and LMWH, warfarin crosses the placenta causing fetal warfarin syndrome (FWS).[360,362] Common characteristics of FWS include: nasal hypoplasia, blindness, retardation, seizures, congenital heart disease, scoliosis, low birth weight, deafness, and death.[362] Warfarin use up to the 6th week of gestation is likely safe.[361] Warfarin during the 2nd and 3rd trimester may also be safe although one study reported neurodevelopmental problems may be more likely in offspring exposed to warfarin during the 2nd and 3rd trimester of pregnancy.[363]

VTE treatment during pregnancy may be done with IV heparin, LMWH, or high dose adjusted SC heparin after an IV bolus. Given the risk of heparin-induced thrombocytopenia, frequent aPTT monitoring, and osteoporosis; LMWH with a category B pregnancy rating should be given higher priority as a treatment alternative.[360] Anticoagulation must be discontinued 24 hours prior to delivery or induction of labor. Pregnancy with prior history of single VTE due to a transient condition no longer present may only require careful monitoring and patient education. If the prior VTE was due to pregnancy or related to estrogen and/or risk factors such as extended immobility or obesity are present, prophylactic anticoagulation (enoxaparin 40 mg SC daily, dalteparin 5000 units SC daily, or heparin 5000 units SC q 8–12 h) up to delivery is appropriate.[360] Recommendations for anticoagulation in other clinical scenarios of pregnancy can be found in Table 10-19. In all pregnant patients with history of prior VTE, elastic compression stockings are recommended during and 4-6 weeks after delivery.[360]

Generic Versus Brand Warfarin

Access to generic medications has saved consumers eight to ten billion dollars.[364] The 1984 Drug Competition and Patent Term Restoration Act, improved patient's access to generic medications and

Table 10-19.

Clinical Scenarios Requiring Anticoagulation During Pregnancy

Patient Type	Recommended Anticoagulation Regimens
No VTE hx with Laboratory-Confirmed Thrombophilia (Listed in Table 10-11)	▪ Prophylactic LMWH (i.e., enoxaparin 40 mg SC daily) ▪ UFH 5000 units SC q12h
Single Idiopathic DVT - not currently on anticoagulation	▪ Prophylactic LMWH (i.e., dalteparin 5000 U SC daily) ▪ UFH 5000 units SC q12h ▪ UFH SC q12h adjusted to anti-Xa 0.1–0.3 U/mL ▪ Also during postpartum period for 4–6 weeks
Single Idiopathic DVT with Thrombophilia (Listed in Table 10-11) - not currently on anticoagulation	▪ Intermediated-dose LMWH (enoxaparin 40 mg SC q 12 h or dalteparin 5000 U SC q12h) ▪ UFH SC q12h adjusted to anti-Xa 0.1–0.3 U/mL ▪ Also during postpartum period for 4–6 weeks
Multiple DVT or Single with Thrombophilia (Listed in Table 10-11) - currently on anticoagulation	▪ Full adjusted dose LMWH ▪ Full adjusted dose UFH, to anti-Xa 0.3–0.7 U/mL (after IV bolus, dosing may be adjusted SC bid)
Pregnancy with APLAs and One Previous Late Pregnancy Loss or ≥ Two Early Pregnancy Losses, Preeclampsia, Intrauterine Growth Restriction - not currently on anticoagulation	▪ Aspirin 81 mg po daily <u>plus</u> one from below: • Prophylactic LMWH (i.e., dalteparin 5000 U SC daily) • UFH 5000 units SC q12h • UFH SC q12h adjusted to anti-Xa 0.1–0.3 U/mL D/C aspirin ~ 5 days before delivery D/C LMWH or UFH ~ 24 h before delivery
Pregnancy with Congenital Thrombophilic Deficit and Recurrent Miscarriages, 2nd or 3rd Trimester Loss, Severe or Recurrent Preeclampsia, or Abruption - not currently on anticoagulation	▪ Aspirin 81 mg po daily <u>plus</u> one from below: • Prophylactic LMWH (i.e., dalteparin 5000 U SC daily) • UFH 5000 units SC q 12h • UFH SC q12h adjusted to anti-Xa 0.1–0.3 U/mL D/C aspirin ~ 5 days before delivery D/C LMWH or UFH ~ 24 h before delivery Restart proph LMWH or UFH post delivery x 4–6 weeks
Pregnancy with Mechanical Heart Valve	▪ Full dose LMWH adjusted to anti-Xa 1–1.2 U/mL measured 4 hours post injection till <u>or</u> ▪ Full adjusted dose UFH, to anti-Xa 0.35–0.7 U/mL (after IV bolus, dosing may be adjusted SC bid) <u>or</u> ▪ AFTER 13th week of gestation, either of the above therapies may be converted to warfarin adjusted according to Table 10-14. Halfway through the third trimester patient must be switched back to adjusted UFH or LMWH. ▪ High-risk conditions also require addition of aspirin, see Table 10-14.

Source: Reference 360.

cost savings. This act also established a method for determining a generic drug's bioequivalence to a branded product.[364] Generic products are considered bioequivalent after passing a single dose two way crossover study in 24 to 36 healthy subjects. A passing analysis requires peak serum concentration (Cmax) and area under the curve (AUC) to fall within 80%–125% of the branded product with a 90% confidence interval.[365,366] Unlike aminoglycosides, therapeutic warfarin is not determined by serum concentrations but rather INR measurements. Two concerns arise from this. First total concentrations are measured not concentrations of the specific isomers (reminder that the S isomer is more potent than the R isomer). The second is that intraindividual variability has been identified when looking at warfarin plasma concentrations versus anticoagulant response.[367] These are merely observations and whether there is a clinically important change after switching to generic can only be determined from well designed clinical trials.

The FDA conducts approximately 3,500 inspections per year in manufacturing facilities and brand name manufacturers produce approximately 50% of generic products.[364] Generic warfarin was previously available; however, after litigation was withdrawn in 1992 and then became available again in 1997.[368,369] In addition to Bristol Meyers Squibb Coumadin®, the electronic orange book lists seven AB rated generic warfarins.[370] Given the number of generics, it is difficult to determine the variability if any, one might find with a specific generic. Available data evaluating some of these generics, indicates a clinically significant problem is unlikely and variability is more likely from other causes.

Given warfarin's narrow therapeutic window, increased monitoring following a change in brand is reasonable. However, the FDA in January 1998 regarding narrow therapeutic index generics stated, "It is not necessary for the health care provider to approach any one therapeutic class of drug products differently from any other class, when there has been a determination of therapeutic equivalence by FDA for the drug products under consideration."[371] In this letter they further stated the "FDA approved product labeling does not recommend that any additional tests need to be performed by the health care provider when a switch occurs from a brand-name drug product to a generic equivalent drug product, from a generic equivalent to a brand-name product drug, or from one generic product to another when both are deemed equivalent to a brand-name drug product."[371] Available data supports allowing patients wanting to switch to generic, the opportunity to do so with temporary increased monitoring. See Table 10-20 for a summary of published clinical trials.[372-375]

Conclusion

Warfarin is an extremely effective anticoagulation medication that has been in use over fifty years. Despite that long track record of efficacy, it remains one of the most inherently dangerous medications used in clinical medicine. Its complicated pharmacodynamic profile and numerous factors make it an excellent target for an inpatient anticoagulation service to manage. Inpatient anticoagulation pharmacists face a daunting, but surmountable, task in mastering the management of this medication. Inpatient pharmacists who learn to manage warfarin well will tremendously improve care to the patients they serve.

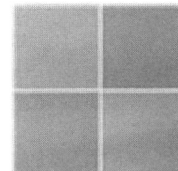

Patient Cases

Case 1

MJ is a 56-yo female admitted to the hospital with shortness of breath and chest pain. Her past medical history includes atrial fibrillation, hypertension, and chronic heart failure. Social history includes smoking 1 ppd and she denies ethanol intake. She reports taking the following medications at home: warfarin 5 mg daily, other medications include losartan 50 mg po daily, digoxin 0.25 mg po daily, furosemide 40 mg po daily, conjugated estrogens 0.625 mg po daily, and metoprolol XL 50 mg po daily. She also reports starting doxycycline 100 mg twice daily which was prescribed 6 days ago by her primary care physician for community acquired pneumonia. She denies any signs/symptoms of stroke, thromboembolic complications, or bleeding. She reports eating less than her usual over the past several days since she began feeling sick and nauseous. She has been on her current dose of warfarin for over 6 months with INRs ranging from 2.1–3.3. Her INR on admission was 4.7 (goal 2–3) and has been placed on hold pending a consult from the pharmacy anticoagulation service team. She denies any missed doses of warfarin. You speak with the physician who feels the patient has not improved on the current antibiotics after reviewing chest X-ray, vitals, and lung sounds. It is also noted that the patient has a heart rate of 50. Her serum creatinine is also elevated at 1.4 which her physician feels may be due to reduced fluid intake and possibly worsening heart failure. Blood and sputum cultures were drawn and antibiotics have been changed to levofloxacin 500 mg daily po daily and the doxycycline has been discontinued.

Q: How should the warfarin be managed upon hospital admission?

A: The best course of action is to hold warfarin and draw daily INRs. The elevated INR is likely due to numerous reasons including doxycycline therapy, reduced PO intake, and a possible heart failure exacerbation. Due to the elevation in serum creatinine, use of doxycycline, low heart rate, and poor appetite, you also ask the physician to consider the possibility of digoxin toxicity.

Day 2. The next morning's labs reveal a digoxin level of 2.9 and an INR of 4.1 following one held dose. The physician holds the digoxin, thanks you for your insight, and asks you to continue to manage the anticoagulation.

Table 10-20.
Observations Following Changes Between Branded and Generic Warfarin

Author/Study Design/Brand	Subjects	Outcomes Evaluated	Conclusion
Milligan[368] Prospective, non-blinded, non-randomized observational study Brand 8 months control vs. Barr for 10 months after	n = 182 Mean age 75 y AF: 60% Valve: 13% Stroke/TIA: 11% DVT/PE: 9% Other: > 6%	Bleeding req. med. care	No difference
		Dose changes/Pt days	No difference
		Required INRs/Pt days	No difference
		Thrombotic events	No difference
		INRs in therapeutic range	75.6% vs. 78.4% $P = 0.3$
Witt[369] Retrospective, uncontrolled, Brand 90 days control vs. Barr for 90 days thereafter	n = 2299 Mean age 69 y AF: 41% Valve: 12% Stroke/TIA: 8% DVT/PE: 27% Other: >12%	# INR tests per patient	3.92 brand vs. 3.89 Barr $p < 0.05$
		Warfarin dose (mg)	4.54 brand vs. 4.49 Barr $p < 0.05$
		INRs within therapeutic range	65.9% brand vs. 63.3% Barr $p = 0.0002$
		INR control after Barr switch change by > 10%	33.1% improved 38.9% worsened
		Complication rate per 100 patient years	NS
		% patients > 1 dose change	NS
Swenson[372] Prospective, non-blinded, non-randomized observational study, Brand 4 weeks vs. Barr/Brand for 8 weeks thereafter	n = 105 Converted to Barr n = 105 Stay Brand Mean age 76–78 y AF: 64%–70%	INR Brand pre/post	2.6/2.8
		INR Brand/Barr post change	2.6/2.7
		Required dose changes	31 Barr/63 Brand
		INR change > 1	10 Barr/14 Brand
Weibert[373] Randomized, prospective, single-blind, multi-center, crossover trial. All 4 weeks Brand then 4 weeks either Brand/Apothecon (Sandoz) then crossover 4 weeks	n = 113 Mean age 70 y AF: 100%	Number INRs < 1.8	Brand: 9 Apothecon: 9
		Number INRs > 3.2	Brand: 9 Apothecon: 10
		Dose change ≥ 20%	Brand: 7 Apothecon: 7
		Significant bleed/thromb	NS
Lee[374] Randomized, prospective, observer-blind, crossover trial. 3 x 28d periods Brand x 28d > Generic 56d Generic x 28d > Brand 56d	n=34 Mean age 52 y Mech valve 100%	Pooled mean INR	2.28 vs. 2.27
		Adverse events	NS
Pereira[375] Randomized, prospective, triple-blind, crossover trial. Brand versus Apo-warfarin	n=7 Mean age 63 y Mech valve 100%	Mean INR results	NS
		INR variation	NS

Q: How should the warfarin be managed at this point?

A: Although the INR has improved, the INR is still > 4. The risks of thrombosis this patient has are history of hypertension and heart failure. Since the patient continues to appear sensitive to warfarin, it would be wise to hold warfarin and continue daily INRs.

Day 3. The next morning's labs reveal an INR of 3 following two held doses. The patient is afebrile, feeling better, and has resumed her previous appetite. She wants to be discharged from the hospital and her physician agrees. He requests from you warfarin discharge instructions, the patient will be discharged on levofloxacin 500 mg po daily, digoxin 0.125 mg po daily, and her previous meds excluding doxycycline.

Q: How should the warfarin be handled at this point?

A: Resume warfarin 5 mg daily po daily and have an INR drawn 2–3 days following discharge.

Case 2

DJ is a 64-yo female admitted to the hospital after 5 days of dizziness spells, pounding in her chest, and new onset chest pain. Her past medical history includes hypertension, unstable angina with no previous heart attack, and chronic heart failure. She reports having familiar episodes of a racing heart in the past but that it has always gone away before now and that it had never made her feel dizzy. Social history includes previous smoker but quit 7 years ago and occasional ethanol ingestion of two drinks four times per week. She reports taking the following medications at home: aspirin 81 mg po daily, lisinopril 20 mg po daily, digoxin 0.125 mg po daily, furosemide 40 mg po daily, KCL 20 mEq po daily, nitroglycerin SL spray prn, and carvedilol 12.5 mg bid. She denies any symptoms of weakness in her arms or legs, headache, visual or hearing disturbances, or other stroke symptoms. EKG reveals no ST segment changes only atrial fibrillation. Her heart rate is 140 beats per minute. Cardiac enzymes are also noted to be negative. The patient is admitted to the telemetry floor and started on a diltiazem drip which resolves the patient's symptoms. Pharmacy is consulted for anticoagulation management in preparation for cardioversion.

Q: What are the acceptable options for anticoagulation to facilitate cardioversion in this patient?

A: Given the duration of atrial fibrillation > 48 hr and that the patient is hemodynamically stable, cardioversion should be postponed. She will require 3 weeks of warfarin INR 2–3 before elective cardioversion. The patient should be started on warfarin 4 mg daily and an INR drawn in 2 days. The patient has two risk factors for stroke due to atrial fibrillation (risk factors of history of hypertension and chronic heart failure) may or may not be started on an injectable anticoagulant as bridge therapy. The aspirin should likely be discontinued due lower bleeding risk, but it would be reasonable to wait until the INR is in range if an injectable anticoagulant is not used (offers some stroke protection).

Although the above strategy was chosen in this case, one other strategy could have been implemented. If high quality TEE was performed and showed no sign of left atrial appendage thrombi, the patient could be placed on IV heparin and cardioverted.

Day 3. The morning labs reveal an INR of 1.6 following two 4-mg doses of warfarin.

Q: How should the warfarin be managed at this point?

A: Continue warfarin 4 mg daily and draw daily INRs if the patient remains hospitalized. The patient may also be discharged on warfarin 4 mg daily having an INR drawn in 2 days and instructions not to take her warfarin until the INR results are returned. The maintenance dose for this patient will likely be around 24 mg/week. Once the patient is therapeutic on warfarin, it may be best to discontinue aspirin if it was continued initially. The aspirin may be resumed once the patient has been converted and the 4 weeks of warfarin after conversion is complete provided the patient does not have a recurrence of atrial fibrillation, which is quite common.

Case 3

AM is a 27-yo female who presents to the emergency department with unexplained shortness of breath, cough, and chest pain × 2 weeks. She teaches physical education and coaches' volleyball and basketball at the local high school. In addition, AM usually runs 3 miles about 3 days per week. She visited her primary care physician 10 days ago complaining of shortness of breath and exercise intolerance. She stated that she had difficulty walking up the stairs. AM is well known to her physician, he has been her physician for 5 years. She admits to being overly concerned about her health sometimes. Her physician could not find obvious causes of her symptoms and thought she was worrying for no reason given her great physical condition. Prior to admission AA was in excellent health and appears very conscious about her health. Her only medication is birth control. She was previously taking ethinyl estradiol (20 mcg)/norethindrone (1 mg) (Loestrin 21 1/20) for 7 years but switched to ethinyl estradiol (35 mcg)/norgestimate (0.18, 0.215, 0.25 mg, Ortho Tri-Cyclen) 3 months ago to help with her acne. Patient appears moderately distressed and anxious. Vital signs: T: 98.9°F, BP: 129/78, HR: 109 bpm, RR: 22/min. Labs are normal except for elevated d-dimer. CBC, PT, PTT baseline labs are also normal. A CT identifies a large PE although the patient appears stable. Due to the patient's age and excellent physical condition hematology is consulted along with pharmacy for anticoagulation management.

Q: How should this patient initially be managed?

A: An excellent strategy would be to start the patient on a heparin drip with an 80 units/kg bolus then followed by an 18 units/kg/hr infusion. An a aPTT should be drawn in 6 hours and adjust per hospital protocol. Administer warfarin 7.5 mg daily and start daily INRs.

Day 3. The INR is 1.7 after two 7.5-mg doses of warfarin and the patient remains therapeutic on IV heparin. The patient just started a new job at the local high school and does not have very many sick days and wishes to go home.

Q: You are asked for advice by the physician who feels the patient is stabilized clinically and feels she is reliable for follow-up as an outpatient. Hematology also reports a hypercoagulable panel found she has a heterozygous Factor V Leiden gene mutation.

A: As long as the patient is hemodynamically stable and appears reliable for education and follow-up the patient can be discharged. Case management will need to confirm the patient or the insurance is willing and able to pay for outpatient LMWH. Ideally, the hospital has LMWH outpatient discharge kits. These usually have a sharps container, instructional video, alcohol swabs, and an educational booklet. Once payment arrangements are confirmed and availability at the local pharmacy is established, patient education and switch to a therapeutically dosed (i.e., enoxaparin 1 mg/kg sc twice daily) LMWH can be made. The IV heparin can be shut off at the time of LMWH administration. It is best if the patient gives this injection herself. This way the patient is observed, and shows she is willing to administer the injections on her own following discharge. The patient should be discharged on warfarin 7.5 mg daily and also LMWH therapy. Overlap should be for 5 days total assuming there have been two therapeutic INRs on warfarin. An INR should be drawn on the second morning following discharge with instructions not to take her warfarin until the INR results are returned. Given the patient's Factor V Leiden gene mutation, she will require warfarin for 6–12 months, even though the birth control pill change may have contributed to the event. Non-hormonal forms of birth control should now be used in this patient to minimize risk of venous thromboembolism and to avoid pregnancy while on warfarin.

References

1. Ansell J, Hirsh J, Dalen J, et al. Managing oral anticoagulant therapy. *Chest.* 2001;119(suppl):22S-38S.
2. ISMP:Institute for Safe Medication Practices. High Alert Medication List 2005. Available at:www.ismp.org Accessed August 19th, 2006
3. Marketos M. The top 200 generic drugs in 2003 (by units). *Drug Topics.* 2004;148:76.
4. Nutescu EA, Bauman JL. New developments in anticoagulation therapy: oral direct thrombin inhibitors. *Pharmacotherapy.* 2004;24(10) part 2:165S.
5. Nutescu EA, Spinler SA, Dager WE, et al. Transitioning from traditional to novel anticoagulants:the impact of oral direct thrombin inhibitors on anticoagulation management. *Pharmacotherapy.* 2004;24(10) part 2:199S-202S.
6. Hirsh J, Dalen JE, Anderson DR, et al. Managing oral anticoagulant therapy. *Chest.* 2001;119(suppl):8S-21S.
7. Friedman PA, Rosenberg RD, Hauschta PV, Fitz-James A. A spectrum of partially carboxylated prothrombins in the plasmas of coumarin-treated patients. *Biochim Biophys Acta.* 1977;494:271-76.
8. Malhotra OP, Nesheim ME, Mann KG, et al. The kinetics of activation of normal and gamma-carboxylated prothrombins. *J Biol Chem.* 1985;260:279-87.
9. Malhotra OP. Dicumarol-induced prothrombins containing 6, 7, and 8 gamma carboxyglutamic acid residues: isolation and characterization. *Biochem Cell Biol.* 1989;67:411-21.
10. Malhotra OP. Dicumarol-induced 9 gamma carboxyglutamic acid prothrombIn: isolation and comparison with 6, 7, 8, and 10 gamma carboxyglutamic acid isomers. *Biochem Cell Biol.* 1990;68:705-15.
11. Friedman PA, Przysiecki CT. Vitamin K-dependent carboxylation. *Int J Biochem Biophys Acta.* 1977;494:271-76.
12. Lian JB, Hauschka PV, Gallop PM. Properties and biosynthesis of a vitamin K-dependent calcium binding protein in bone. *Fed Proc.* 1978;37:2615-20.
13. O'Reilly RA. Warfarin metabolism and drug-drug interactions. In: Wessler S, Becker CG, Nemerson Y, eds. The new dimensions of warfarin prophylaxis (vol. 214): Advances in experimental medicine and biology. New York, NY: Plenum, 1986;205-12.
14. O'Reilly RA. Vitamin K and other oral anticoagulant drugs. *Annu Rev Med.* 1976;27:245-261.
15. Kelly JG, O'Malley K. Clinical pharmacokinetics of oral anticoagulants. *Clin Pharmacokinet.* 1979;4:1-15.
16. Sutcliffe FA, MacNicoll AD, Gibson GG. Aspects of

anticoagulant action: a review of the pharmacology, metabolism, and toxicity of warfarin and cogeners. *Rev Drug Metabol Drug Interactions.* 1987;5:225-72.
17. Hirsh J. Oral anticoagulant drugs. *N Engl J Med.* 1991;324(26):1829-98.
18. Robinson DS, Benjamin DM, McCormack JJ. Interaction of warfarin and nonsystemic gastrointestinal drugs. *Clin Pharmacol Ther.* 1971;12:491-95.
19. Holbrook AM, Wells PS, Crowther NR. Pharmacokinetics and drug interactions with warfarin. In: Poller L, Hirsh J, eds. Oral Anticoagulants. Dunton Green, England: Hodder and Stoughton;1996.
20. Bechtold H, Andrassy K, Jahnchen E, et al. Evidence for impaired hepatic vitamin K1 metabolism in patients treated with N-methylthiotetrazole cephalosporins. *Thromb Haemost.* 1984;51:358-61.
21. Weitekamp MR, Aber RC. Prolonged bleeding times and bleeding diathesis associated with moxalactam administration. *JAMA.* 1983;249:69-71.
22. Angaran DM, Dias VC, Arom KV, et al. The comparative influence of prophylactic antibiotics on the prothrombin response to warfarin in the postoperative prosthetic cardiac valve patient:cefamandole, cefazolin, vancomycin. *Ann Surg.* 1987;206:155-61.
23. Owens JC, Neely WB, Owen WR. Effect of sodium dextrothyroxine in patients receiving anticoagulants. *N Engl J Med.* 1962;266:76-9.
24. Busenbark LA, Cushnie SA. Effect of Graves' disease and methimazole on warfarin anticoagulation. *Ann Pharmacother.* 2006;40(6):1200-3.
25. Rettie AE, Korzekwa KR, Kunze KL, et al. Hydroxylation of warfarin by human cDNA-expressed cytochrome P-450: a role for P-4502C9 in the etiology of (S)- warfarin-drug interactions. *Chem Res Toxicol.* 1992;5:54-9.
26. O'Reilly RA. The stereoselective interaction of warfarin and metronidazole in man. *N Engl J Med.* 1976:295:354-7.
27. Cupp MJ, Tracy S. Cytochrome P450: New nomenclature and clinical implications. *Am Fam Phys.* 1998;57(1):107-15.
28. Toon S, Low LK, Gibaldi M, et al. The warfarin-sulfinpyrazone interaction: stereochemical considerations. *Clin Pharmacol Ther.* 1986;39:15-24.
29. O'Reilly RA. Stereoselective interaction of trimethoprimsulfamethoxazole with the separated enantiomorphs of racemic warfarin in man. *N Engl J Med.* 1980;302:33-35.
30. Holbrook AM, Pereira JA, Labiris R, et al. Systematic overview of warfarin and its drug and food interactions. *Arch Inter Med.* 2005;165:1095-106.
31. Israel DS, Stotka J, Rock W, et al. Effect of ciprofloxacin on the pharmacokinetics and pharmacodynamics of warfarin. *Clin Infect Dis.* 1996;22:251-56.
32. Arnold LM, Nisen LR, Ng TM. Moxifloxacin and warfarin: additional evidence for a clinically relevant interaction. *Pharmacotherapy.* 2005 Jun;25(6):904-7.
33. Ravnan SL, Locke C. Levofloxacin and warfarin interaction. *Pharmacotherapy.* 2001;21:884-85.
34. O'Reilly, RA. Studies on the optical enantiomorphs of warfarin in man. *Clin Pharmacol Ther.* 1974;16:348-54.
35. Wood GD, Deeble T. Warfarin: dangers with antibiotics. *Dent Update.* 1993;20:350-53.
36. Foster DR, Milan NL. Potential interaction between azithromycin and warfarin. *Pharmacotherapy.* 1999;19:902-08.
37. Byers M. Clarithromycin-warfarin interaction resulting in an elevated INR. *Can J Hosp Pharm.* 1997;50:285-87.
38. Breckenridge A, Orme M, Wesseling H, et al. Pharmacokinetics and pharmacodynamics of the enantiomers of warfarin in man. *Clin Pharmacol Ther.* 1974;15,424-30
39. Hirsh J, Fuster V, Ansell J, et al. American Heart Association/American College of Cardiology Foundation guide to warfarin therapy. *Circulation.* 2003;107;1692-711.
40. Ansell J, Hirsh J, Poller L, et al. The pharmacology and management of the vitamin K antagonists. The Seventh ACCP Conference on Antithrombotic and Thrombolytic Therapy. *Chest.* 2004;123 (3):204S-33S.
41. Donaldson GWK, Kavies SH, Darg A, et al. Coagulation factors in chronic liver disease. *J Clin Pathol.* 1969;22:199-204.
42. Gallus AS, Lucas CR, Hirsh J. Coagulation studies in patients with acute infectious hepatitis. *Br J Haematol.* 1972;22:761-71.
43. Koller F. Theory and experience behind the use of coagulation tests in diagnosis and prognosis of liver disease. *Scand J Gastroenterol.* 1973;8(suppl 19):51-61.
44. Kovacs MJ, Wong A, MacKinnon K, et al. Assessment of the validity of the INR system for patients with liver impairment. *Thromb Haemost.* 1994;71:727-30.
45. Mammen EF. Coagulation abnormalities in liver disease. *Hematol Oncol Clin North Am.* 1992;6:1247-57.
46. Landefeld CS, Cook EF, Flatley M, et al. Identification and preliminary validation of predictors of major bleeding in hospitalized patients starting anticoagulant therapy. *Am J Med.* 1987;82:703-13.
47. Brigden ML, Kay C, Le A, et al. Audit frequency and clinical response to excessive oral anticoagulation in an outpatient population. *Am J Hematol.* 1998;59:22-27.
48. Loeliger EA, Van Der Esch B, Mattern MJ, et al. The biological disappearance rate of prothrombin, factors VII, IX, and X from plasma in hypothyroidism, hyperthyroidism, and during fever. *Thromb Diath Haemorrh.* 1964;10:267-77.
49. Solomon HM, Schrogie JJ. Change in receptor site affinity: a proposed explanation for the potentiating effect of D-thyroxine on the anticoagulant response to warfarin. *Clin Pharmacol Ther.* 1967;8:797-99.
50. McIntosh TJ, Brunk SF, Kolln I, et al. Increased sensitivity to warfarin in thyrotoxicosis. *J Clin Invest.* 1970;49:63a.
51. Vagenakis AG, Cote R, Miller ME, et al. Enhancement of warfarin-induced hypoprothrombinemia by thyrotoxicosis. *Hopkins Med J.* 1972;131:69-73.
52. Self TH, Weisburst M, Wooten F, et al. Warfarin-induced hypoprothrombinemia; potentiation by hypothyroidism. *JAMA.* 1975;231:1165-66.
53. Kellett HA, Sawers JSA, Boulton FE, et al. Problems of anticoagulation with warfarin in hyperthyroidism. *Q J Med.* 1986;58:43-51.
54. Walters MB. The relationship between thyroid function and anticoagulation therapy. *Am J Cardiol.* 1963;11:112-14.
55. Stephens MA, Self TH, Lancaster D et al. Hypothyroidism: effect on warfarin anticoagulation. *South*

56. Stats D, Davison S. The increased hypoprothrombinemic effect of small doses of dicumarol in congestive heart failure. *Am J Med Sci.* 1949;21:318-23.
57. O'Reilly, RA. Interaction of spironolactone and racemic warfarin in man. *Clin Pharmacol Ther.* 1980;27:198-201.
58. O'Reilly, RA, Sahud MA, Aggeler PM. Impact of aspirin and chlorthalidone on the pharmacodynamics of oral anticoagulant drugs on man. *Ann NY Acad Sci.* 1971;179:173-86.
59. Doecke CJ, Cosh DG, Gallus AS. Standardization initial warfarin treatment: evaluation of initial treatment response and maintenance dose prediction by randomized trial, and risk factors for an excessive warfarin response. *Aust NZ J Med.* 1991;21:319-24.
60. Killip T, Payne MA. High serum transaminase activity in heart disease. *Circulation.* 1960;21:646-60.
61. Oates A, Jackson PR, Austin CA et al. A new regimen for starting warfarin therapy in out-patients. *Br J Clin Pharmacol.* 1998;46:157-61.
62. O'Reilly RA, Aggeler PA. Determinants of the response to oral anticoagulant drugs in man. *Pharmacol Rev.* 1970;22:35-96.
63. Petitti DB, Storm BL, Melmon KL. Prothrombin time ratio and other factors associated with bleeding in patients treated with warfarin. *J Clin Epidemiol.* 1989;42:759-64.
64. Peyman MA. The significance of hemorrhage during the treatment of patients with coumarin anticoagulants. *Acta Med Scand.* 1958;162(suppl):1-62
65. Anderson FA, Spencer FA. Risk factors for venous thromboembolism. *Circulation.* 2003;107;9-16.
66. Bona RD, Sivjee KY, Hickey AD, et al. The efficacy and safety of oral anticoagulation in patients with cancer. *Thromb Haemost.* 1995;74:1055-58.
67. Munter G, Hershko C. Increased warfarin sensitivity as an early manifestation of occult prostate cancer with chronic disseminated intravascular coagulation. *Acta Haematol.* 2001;105(2):97-9.
68. Shedlofsky SI, Israel BC, McClain CJ, et al. Endotoxin administration to humans inhibits hepatic cytochrome P450-mediated drug metabolism. *J Clin Invest.* 1994;94:2114-209.
69. Sonne J, Dossing M, Loft S, et al. Antipyrine clearance in pneumonia. *Clin Pharmacol Ther.* 1985;37:701-4.
70. Sharer JE, Wrighton SA. Identification of the human hepatic cytochromes P450 involved in the in vitro oxidation of antipyrine. *Drug Metab Dispo.* 1996;24:487-94.
71. Aithal GP, Day CP, Kesteven PJ, et al. Association of polymorphisms in the cytochrome P450 CYP2C9 with warfarin dose requirement and risk of bleeding complications. *Lancet.* 1999;353:717-9.
72. Freeman BD, Zehnbauer BA, McGrath S, et al. Cytochrome P450 polymorphisms are associated with reduced warfarin dose. *Surgery.* 2000;128:281-5.
73. Herman D, Locatelli I, Grabnar I, et al. Influence of CYP2C9 polymorphisms, demographic factors and concomitant drug therapy on warfarin metabolism and maintenance dose. *Pharmacogenomics J.* 2005;5:193-202.
74. Higashi MK, Veenstra DL, Midori Konto L, et al. Association between CYP2C9 genetic variants and anticoagulation related outcomes during warfarin therapy. *JAMA.* 2002;287:1690-8.
75. Hillman MA, Wilke RA, Caldwell MD, et al. Relative impact of covariates in prescribing warfarin according to CYP2C9-genotype. *Pharmacogenetics.* 2004;14:539-47.
76. Kamali F, Khan TI, King BP, Frearson R, Kesteven PJ, Wood P, et al. Contribution of age, body size, and CYP2C9 genotype to anticoagulant response to warfarin. *Clin Pharmacol Ther.* 2004;75:204-12
77. Lindh JD, Lundgren S, Holm L, et al. Severalfold increase in risk of over anticoagulation by CYP2C9 mutations. *Clin Pharmacol Ther.* 2005 Nov;78(5):540-50.
78. Margaglione M, Colaizzo D, D'Andrea G, et al. Genetic modulation of oral anticoagulation with warfarin. *Thromb Haemost.* 2000;84:775-8.
79. Scordo MG, Pengo V, Spina E, et al. Influence of CYP2C9 and CYP2C19 genetic polymorphisms on warfarin maintenance dose and metabolic clearance. *Clin Pharmacol Ther.* 2002;72:702-10.
80. Taube J, Halsall D, Baglin T. Influence of cytochrome P-450 CYP2C9 polymorphisms on warfarin sensitivity and risk of over-anticoagulation in patients on long-term treatment. *Blood.* 2000;96:1816-9.
81. Dang MN, Hambleton J, Kayser SR. The influence of ethnicity on warfarin dosage requirement. *Ann Pharmacother.* 2005;39:1008-12.
82. D'Andrea G, D'Ambrosio RL, Di Perna P, et al. A polymorphism in the VKORC1 gene is associated with an interindividual variability in the dose-anticoagulant effect of warfarin. *Blood.* 2005;105:645-9.
83. Rieder MJ, Reiner AP, Gage BF, et al. Effect of VKORC1 haplotypes on transcriptional regulation and warfarin dose. *N Engl J Med.* 2005;352:2285-93.
84. Sconce EA, Khan TI, Wynne HA, et al. The impact of CYP2C9 and VKORC1 genetic polymorphism and patient characteristics upon *Clin Pharmacol Ther.* 2005;77:479-85.
85. Veenstra DL, You JH, Rieder MJ, et al. Association of vitamin K epoxide reductase complex 1 (VKORC1) variants with warfarin dose in a Hong Kong Chinese patient population. *Pharmacogenet Genomics.* 2005;15:687-91.
86. Wadelius M, Chen LY, Downes K, et al. Common VKORC1 and GGCX polymorphisms associated with warfarin dose. *Pharmacogenomics J.* 2005;5:262-70.
87. Li T, Chang CY, Jin DY, et al. Identification of the gene for vitamin K epoxide reductase. *Nature.* 2004;427:541-45.
88. Rost S, Fregin A, Ivaskevicius V, et al. Mutations in VKORC1 cause warfarin resistance and multiple coagulation factor deficiency type 2. *Nature.* 2004;427:537-41.
89. Bodin L, Verstuyft C, Tregouet DA, et al. Cytochrome P450 (CYP2C9) and vitamin K epoxide reductase (VKORC1) genotypes as determinants of acenocoumarol sensitivity. *Blood.* 2005;106:135-40.
90. Schalekamp T, Brasse BP, Roijers JF, et al. VKORC1 and CYP2C9 genotypes and acenocoumarol anticoagulation status: interaction between both genotypes affects over anticoagulation. *Clin Pharmacol Ther.* 2006;80(1):13-22.
91. Absher RK, Moore ME, Parker MH. Patient-specific

factors predictive of warfarin dosage requirements. *Ann Pharmacother.* 2002;36:1512-7.
92. Chenhsu RY, Chiang SC, Chou MH, et al. Long-term treatment with warfarin in Chinese population. *Ann Pharmacother.* 2000;34:1395-401.
93. Gage BF, Eby C, Milligan PE, et al. Use of pharmacogenetics and clinical factors to predict the maintenance dose of warfarin. *Thromb Haemost.* 2004;91:87-94.
94. Yu HC, Chan TY, Critchley JA, et al. Factors determining the maintenance dose of warfarin in Chinese patients. *QJM.* 1996;89:127-35.
95. Rost S, Fregin A, Ivaskevicius V, et al. Mutations in VKORC1 cause warfarin resistance and multiple coagulation factor deficiency type 2. *Nature.* 2004;427:537-41.
96. Yuan HY, Chen JJ, Lee MM et al. A novel functional VKORC1 promoter polymorphism is associated with inter-individual and inter-ethnic differences in warfarin sensitivity. *Hum Mol Genet.* 2005;14:1745-51.
97. Bovill EG, Lawson J, Sadowski J, et al. Mechanisms of vitamin k metabolism and vitamin k-dependent hemostasis: implications for warfarin therapy. In: Ezekowitz MD, ed. *The Heart as a Source of Systemic Embolization.* New York, NY: Marcel Dekker;1992.
98. Booth SL, Charnley JM, Sadowski JA, et al. Dietary vitamin K1 and stability of oral anticoagulation: proposal of a diet with constant vitamin K1 content. *Thromb Haemost.* 1997;3:504-09.
99. O'Reilly R, Rytand D. "Resistance" to warfarin due to unrecognized vitamin K supplementation. *N Engl J Med.* 1980;303:160-61.
100. Suttie JW, Mummah-Schendel LL, Shah DV, et al. Vitamin K deficiency from dietary vitamin K restriction in humans. *Am J Clin Nutr.* 1988;47:475-80.
101. Couris RR, Tataronis GR, Booth SL, et al Development of a self-assessment instrument to determine daily intake and variability of dietary vitamin K. *J Am Coll Nutr.* 2000;19(6):801-06.
102. Bolton-Smith C, Price RJ, Fenton ST, et al. Compilation of a provisional UK database for the phylloquinone (vitamin K1) content of foods. *Br J Nutr.* 2000;83:389-99.
103. Sadowski JA, Booth SL, Mann KG, et al. Structure and mechanism of activation of vitamin K antagonists. In: Poller L, Hirsh J, eds. *Oral Anticoagulants.* London, UK:Arnold;1996:9-29.
104. Warlow C, Beattie AG, Terry G, et al. A double blind trial of low doses of subcutaneous heparin in the prevention of deep vein thrombosis after myocardial infarction. *Lancet.* 1973;2:934-36.
105. Cairns JA, Hirsh J, Lewis HD Jr, et al. Antithrombotic agents in coronary artery disease. *Chest.* 1992;102(suppl):456s-81s.
106. Drapkin A, Merskey C. Anticoagulant therapy after acute myocardial infarction: relation of therapeutic benefit to patient's age, sex, and severity of infarction. JAMA. 1972;222:541-48.
107. Medical Research Council Group. Assessment of short-term anticoagulant administration after cardiac infarction: report of the Working Party on Anticoagulant Therapy in Coronary Thrombosis. *BMJ.* 1969;1:335-42.
108. Anand SS, Yusuf S, Pogue J, et al. OASIS Investigators- Long-term oral anticoagulant therapy in patients with unstable angina or suspected non-Q-wave myocardial infarction. *Circulation.* 1998;98:1064-70.
109. Anand SS, Yusuf S, Pogue J, et al. Oral anticoagulant therapy in patients with coronary artery disease: a meta analysis. *JAMA.* 1999;282: 2058-67.
110. Anand SS, Yusuf S, Pogue J, et al. Oral anticoagulant therapy in patients with coronary artery disease. *J Am Coll Cardiol.* 2003;41:62S-69S.
111. Coumadin Aspirin Reinfarction Study (CARS) Investigators. Randomized double-blind trial of fixed low-dose warfarin with aspirin after myocardial infarction. *Lancet.* 1997;350:389-96.
112. Post Coronary Artery Bypass Graft Trial Investigators. The effect of aggressive lowering of low density lipoprotein cholesterol levels and low dose anticoagulation on obstructive changes in saphenous vein coronary artery bypass grafts. *N Engl J Med.* 1997;336:153-62.
113. Cohen M, Adams C, Hawkins L, et al. Usefulness of antithrombotic therapy in resting angina pectoris or non-Q-wave myocardial infarction (a pilot study from the Antithrombotic Therapy in Acute Coronary Syndromes Group). *Am J Cardiol.* 1990;66:1287-92.
114. Cohen M, Adams C, Perry G, et al. Combination antithrombotic therapy in unstable rest angina and non-Q-wave myocardial infarction in non-prior aspirin users. *Circulation.* 1994;89:81-8.
115. Merlini PA, Bauer KA, Oltrona L, et al. Persistent activation of coagulation mechanism in unstable angina and myocardial infarction. *Circulation.* 1994;90:61-8.
116. Go AS, Hylek EM, Phillips KA Prevalence of Diagnosed Atrial Fibrillation in Adults National Implications for Rhythm Management and Stroke Prevention: the Anticoagulation and Risk Factors In Atrial Fibrillation (ATRIA) Study. *JAMA.* 2001;285:2370-75.
117. Albers GW, Atwood JE, Hirsh J, et al. Stroke prevention in non-valvular atrial fibrillation. *Ann Intern Med.* 1991;115:727-36.
118. Cerebral Embolism Task Force. Cardiogenic brain embolism: the second report of the Cerebral Embolism Task Force. *Arch Neurol.* 1989;46:727-43.
119. Wolf PA, Abbott RD, Kannel WB. Atrial fibrillation as an independent risk factor for stroke: the Framingham study. *Stroke.* 1991;22:983-88.
120. Wolf PA, Abbott RD, Kannel WB. Atrial fibrillation: a major contributor to stroke in the elderly. The Framingham study. *Arch Intern Med.* 1987;147:1561-64.
121. Nakayama T, Date C, Yokoyama T. 15.5-Year follow-up study of stroke in a Japanese provincial city: the Shibata study. *Stroke.* 1997 28:45-52.
122. Flegel KM, Shipley MJ, Rose G. Risk of stroke in non-rheumatic atrial fibrillation. *Lancet.* 1987;1(8532):526-9.
123. Albers GW, Bittar N, Young L, et al. Clinical characteristics and management of acute stroke in patients with atrial fibrillation admitted to U.S. university hospitals. *Neurology.* 1997;48:1598-04.
124. Antani MR, Beyth RJ, Covinsky KE, et al. Failure to prescribe warfarin to patients with nonrheumatic atrial fibrillation. *J Gen Intern Med.* 1996;11:713-20.

125. Beyth RJ, Antani MR, Covinsky KE, et al. Why isn't warfarin prescribe to patients with nonrheumatic atrial fibrillation. *J Gen Intern Med.* 1996;11:721-28.
126. Brass LM, Krurnholz HM, Scinto JM, et al. Warfarin use among patients with atrial fibrillation. *Stroke.* 1997;28:2382-89.
127. Gurwitz JH, Monette J, Rochon PA, et al. Atrial fibrillation and stroke prevention with warfarin in the long term-care setting. *Arch Intern Med.* 1997;157:978-84.
128. Munschauer FE, Priore RL, Hens M, et al. Thromboembolism prophylaxis in chronic atrial fibrillation: practice patterns in community and tertiary-care hospitals. *Stroke.* 1997;28:72-6.
129. Whittle J, Wickenheiser L, Venditti LN. Is warfarin underused in the treatment of elderly persons with atrial fibrillation? *Arch Intern Med.* 1997;157:441-5.
130. Gottlieb LK, Salem-Schatz S. Anticoagulation in atrial fibrillation: does efficacy in clinical trials translate into effectiveness in practice? *Arch Intern Med.* 1994;154:1945-53.
131. Hart RG, Benavente O, McBride R, et al. Antithrombotic therapy to prevent stroke in patients with atrial fibrillation: a meta-analysis. *Ann Intern Med.* 1999;131:492-501.
132. van Walraven C, Hart RG, Singer DE, et al. Oral anticoagulants vs. aspirin in nonvalvular atrial fibrillation-an individual patient recta-analysis. *JAMA.* 2002;288:2441-48.
133. Hart RG, Halperin JL, Pearce LA, et al. Lessons from the stroke prevention in atrial fibrillation trials. *Ann Intern Med.* 2003;138(10):831-38.
134. Albers GW, Dalen JE, Laupacis A, et al. Antithrombotic therapy in atrial fibrillation. *Chest.* 2001;119:194S-206S
135. Atrial Fibrillation Investigators. Risk factors for stroke and efficacy of antithrombotic therapy in atrial fibrillation: analysis of pooled data from five randomized controlled trials. *Arch Intern Med.* 1994;154:1449-57.
136. Feinberg WM, Kronmal RA, Newman AB, et al. Stroke risk in an elderly population with atrial fibrillation. *J Gen Intern Med.* 1999;14:56-59
137. Gage BF, Waterman AD, Shannon W, et al. Validation of clinical classification schemes for predicting stroke: results from the National Registry of Atrial Fibrillation. *JAMA.* 2001;285:2864-70.
138. Hart RG, Pearce LA, McBride R, et al. Factors associated with ischemic stroke during aspirin therapy in atrial fibrillation: analysis of 2012 participants in the SPAF I-III clinical trials. *Stroke.* 1999;30:1223-29.
139. Predictors of thromboembolism in atrial fibrillation: I. Clinical features of patients at risk. The Stroke Prevention in Atrial Fibrillation Investigators. *Ann Intern Med.* 1992;116:1-5.
140. The Stroke Prevention in Atrial Fibrillation Investigators. Predictors of thromboembolism in atrial fibrillation: II. Echocardiographic features of patients at risk. *Ann Intern Med.* 1992;116:16-12.
141. Singer DE, Albers GW, Dalen JE, et al. Antithrombotic therapy in atrial fibrillation. *Chest.* 2004;126:429-56S.
142. Stroke Prevention in Atrial Fibrillation Investigators. Risk factors for thromboembolism during aspirin therapy in patients with atrial fibrillation: the Stroke Prevention in Atrial Fibrillation Study. *J Stroke Cerebrovasc Dis.* 1995;5:147-57.
143. Stroke Prevention in Atrial Fibrillation Investigators. Predictors of thromboembolism in atrial fibrillation: I. Clinical features of patients at risk. *Ann Intern Med.* 1992;116:1-5.
144. Wang TJ, Massaro JM, Levy D, et al. A risk score for predicting stroke or death in individuals with new-onset atrial fibrillation in the community: the Framingham Heart Study. *JAMA.* 2003;290:1049-56.
145. Hart RG, Pearce LA, Rothbart RM, et al. Stroke with intermittent atrial fibrillation: incidence and predictors during aspirin therapy. *J Am Coll Cardiol.* 2000;35:183-7.
146. ACC/AHA/ESC 2006 Guidelines for the Management of Patients with Atrial Fibrillation-Executive Summary. *Circulation.* 2006;114:700-52.
147. Fatkin D, Scalia G, Jacobs N, et al. Accuracy of biplane transesophageal echocardiography in detecting left atrial thrombus. *Am J Cardiol.* 1996;77:321-3.
148. Manning WJ, Weintraub RM, Waksmonski CA, et al. Accuracy of transesophageal echocardiography for identifying left atrial thrombi: a prospective, intraoperative study. *Arch Intern Med.* 1995;123:817-22.
149. Gallagher MM, Hennessy BJ, Edvardsson N. Embolic complications of direct current cardioversion of atrial arrhythmias: association with low intensity of anticoagulation at the time of cardioversion. *J Am Coll Cardiol.* 2002;40:926-33.
150. Weigner MJ, Caulfield TA, Danias PG, et al. Risk for clinical thromboembolism associated with conversion to sinus rhythm in patients with atrial fibrillation lasting less than 48 hours. *Ann Intern Med.* 1997;126:615-20.
151. Mitchell MA, Hughes GS, Ellenbogen KA, et al. Cardioversion-related stroke rates in atrial fibrillation and atrial flutter [abstract]. *Circulation.* 1997;96:1-453.
152. Geerts WH, Pineo GF, Heit JA et al. Prevention of venous thromboembolism. The Seventh ACCP Conference on Antithrombotic and Thrombolytic Therapy. *Chest.* 2004;126(3):338-400S.
153. Stein PD, Henry JW. Prevalence of acute pulmonary embolism among patients in a general hospital and at autopsy. *Chest.* 1995;108:978-81.
154. Caprini JA, Botteman MF, Stephens JM, et al. Economic burden of long-term complications of deep vein thrombosis after total hip replacement surgery in the United States. *Value Health.* 2003;6:59-74
155. Heit JA, Rooke TW, Silverstein MD, et al. Trends in the incidence of venous stasis syndrome and venous ulcer: a 25-year population-based study. *J Vasc Surg.* 2001;33:1022-27.
156. Kahn SR, Hirsch A, Shrier I. Effect of post-thrombotic syndrome on health-related quality of life after deep venous thrombosis. *Arch Intern Med.* 2002;162:1144-48.
157. Lindner DJ, Edwards JM, Phinney ES, et al. Long-term hemodynamic and clinical sequellae of lower extremity deep vein thrombosis. *J Vasc Surg.* 1986;4:436-42.
158. Prandoni P, Lensing AW, Cogo A, et al. The long-term clinical course of acute deep venous thrombosis. *Ann Intern Med.* 1996;125:1-7.
159. Eriksson BI, Wille-Jorgensen P, Kalebo P, et al. A

comparison of recombinant hirudin with a low-molecular-weight heparin to prevent thromboembolic complications after total hip replacement. *N Engl J Med.* 1997;337:1329-35.

160. Hull RD, Pineo GF, Francis C, et al. Low-molecular-weight heparin prophylaxis using dalteparin extended nut-of-hospital vs. in-hospital warfarin/out-of-hospital placebo in hip arthroplasty patients: a double-blind, randomized comparison. *Arch Intern Med.* 2000;160:2208-15.

161. Hull RD, Pineo GF, Francis C, et al. Low-molecular-weight heparin prophylaxis using dalteparin in close proximity to surgery vs. warfarin in hip arthroplasty patients: a double-blind, randomized comparison. *Arch Intern Med.* 2000;160:2199-207.

162. Hull RD, Pineo GF, Stein PD, et al. Timing of initial administration of low-molecular-weight heparin prophylaxis against deep vein thrombosis in patients following elective hip arthroplasty: a systematic review. *Arch Intern Med.* 2001;161:1952-60.

163. Hull RD, Burke N, Mah AF, et al. Timing of initial administration of prophylaxis against deep vein thrombosis in patients following hip or knee surgery [abstract]. *J Thromb Haemost.* 2003;1:P2043.

164. Raskob GE, Hirsh J. Controversies in timing of the first dose of anticoagulant prophylaxis against venous thromboembolism after major orthopedic surgery. *Chest.* 2003;124 (suppl):379S-85S.

165. Strebel N, Prins M, Agnelli G, et al. Preoperative or postoperative start of prophylaxis for venous thromboembolism with low-molecular-weight heparin in elective hip surgery? *Arch Intern Med.* 2002;162:1451-56.

166. Turpie A, Bauer K, Eriksson B, et al. Efficacy and safety of fondaparinux in major orthopedic surgery according to the timing of its first administration. *Thromb Haemost.* 2003;90:364-66.

167. Turpie AGG, Bauer KA, Eriksson BI, et al. Fondaparinux vs. enoxaparin for the prevention of venous thromboembolism in major orthopedic surgery: a meta-analysis of 4 randomized double-blind studies. *Arch Intern Med.* 2002;162:1833-40.

168. Kearon C. Duration of venous thromboembolism prophylaxis after surgery. *Chest.* 2003;124 (suppl):386S-92S.

169. Rosendaal FR. Venous thrombosis: a multi-causal disease. *Lancet.* 1999;353:1167-73.

170. Silverstein, MD, Heit, JA, Mohr, DN, et al Trends in the incidence of deep vein thrombosis and pulmonary embolism: a 25-year population-based study. *Arch Intern Med.* 1998;158:585-93.

171. Prandoni, P, Lensing, AW, Cogo, A, et al The long-term clinical course of acute deep venous thrombosis. *Ann Intern Med.* 1996;125:1-7.

172. Prandoni, P, Villalta, S, Bagatella, P, et al The clinical course of deep-vein thrombosis: prospective long-term follow-up of 528 symptomatic patients. *Haematologica.* 1997;82:423-28.

173. Anderson, FA, Wheeler, HB, Goldberg, RJ, et al. A population-based perspective of the hospital incidence and case-fatality rates of deep vein thrombosis and pulmonary embolism: The Worcester DVT Study. *Arch Intern Med.* 1991;151:933-8.

174. Crowther MA, Kelton JG. Congenital thrombophilic states associated with venous thrombosis: a qualitative overview and proposed classification system. *Ann Intern Med.* 2003;138:128-34.

175. Bauer KA. The thrombophilias: well-defined risk factors with uncertain therapeutic implications. *Ann Intern Med.* 2001;135:367-73.

176. Buller HR, Agnelli G, Hull RD, et al. Antithrombotic therapy for venous thromboembolic disease. The Seventh ACCP Conference on Antithrombotic and Thrombolytic Therapy. *Chest.* 2004;126(3):338-400S.

177. Kearon C, Ginsberg JS, Julian JA, et al. Comparison of fixed dose weight adjusted unfractionated heparin and low molecular weight heparin for acute treatment of venous thromboembolism. *JAMA.* 2006;296:935-42.

178. ASHP therapeutic position statement on the use of low-molecular-weight heparins for adult outpatient treatment of acute deep-vein thrombosis. *Am J Health-Syst Pharm.* 2004;61(18):1950-5.

179. Chong BH, Brighton TA, Baker RI, et al. Once-daily enoxaparin in the outpatient setting versus unfractionated heparin in hospital for the treatment of symptomatic deep-vein thrombosis. *J Thromb Thrombolysis.* 2005 Jun;19(3):173-81.

180. Dager WE, King JH, Branch JM, et al. Tinzaparin in outpatients with pulmonary embolism or deep vein thrombosis. *Ann Pharmacother.* 2005;39(7-8):1182-7.

181. Shapiro N, Spear J, Sheehy S, et al. Barriers to the use of outpatient enoxaparin therapy in patients with deep venous thrombosis. *Am J Emerg Med.* 2005;23(1):30-4.

182. Lee M, Pao D, Hsu T, et al. Cost savings and effectiveness of outpatient treatment with low molecular weight heparin of deep vein thrombosis in a community hospital. *Can J Clin Pharmacol.* 2004;11(1):17-27.

183. Boucher M, Rodger M, Johnson JA, et al. Shifting from inpatient to outpatient treatment of deep vein thrombosis in a tertiary care center: a cost-minimization analysis. *Pharmacotherapy.* 2003;23(3):301-9.

184. Spyropoulos AC, Hurley JS, Ciesla GN, et al. Management of acute proximal deep vein thrombosis: pharmacoeconomic evaluation of outpatient treatment with enoxaparin vs. inpatient treatment with unfractionated heparin. *Chest.* 2002;122(1):108-14.

185. Baron RM, Goldhaber SZ. Deep venous thrombosis: early discharge strategies and outpatient management. *J Thromb Thrombolysis.* 1999;7(2):113-22.

186. Yusen RD, Haraden BM, Gage BF, et al. Criteria for outpatient management of proximal lower extremity deep venous thrombosis. *Chest.* 1999;115(4):972-9.

187. Douketis JD, Kearon C, Bates S, et al. Risk of fatal pulmonary embolism in patients with treated venous thromboembolism. *JAMA.* 1998;279:458-62.

188. Eichinger S, Minar E, Bialonczyk C et al. D-dimer levels and risk of recurrent venous thromboembolism. *JAMA.* 2003;290:1071-4.

189. Hron G, Kollers M, Binder BR, et al. Identification of patients at low risk for recurrent venous thromboembolism by measuring thrombin generation. *JAMA.* 2006;296(4):397-402.

190. Prandoni P, Lensing AW, Prins MH, et al. Residual venous thrombosis as a predictive factor of recurrent venous thromboembolism. *Ann Intern Med.* 2002;137:955-60.

191. Salem DN, Stein PD, Ahmad AA, et al. Antithrom-

192. Stein PD, Alpert JS, Bussey HI, et al. Antithrombotic therapy in patients with mechanical and biological prosthetic heart valves. The Sixth ACCP Conference on Antithrombotic and Thrombolytic Therapy. *Chest.* 2001;119(1):220S-27S.
193. Salem DN, Daudelin DH, Levine HJ, et al. Antithrombotic therapy in valvular heart disease. The Sixth ACCP Conference on Antithrombotic and Thrombolytic Therapy. *Chest.* 2001;119(1):207S-19S.
194. Goldsmith I, Turpie AG, Lip GY. Clinical review: ABC of antithrombotic therapy: Valvar heart disease and prosthetic heart valves *BMJ.* 2002;325:1228-31.
195. Cannegieter SC, Rosendaal FB, Wintzen AII, et al. Optimal oral anticoagulant therapy in patients with mechanical heart valves. *N Engl J Med.* 1995;333:11-17.
196. Baudet EM, Puel V, McBride JT, et al. Long-term results of valve replacement with the St. Jude Medical prosthesis. *J Thorac Cardiovasc Surg.* 1995;109:858-70.
197. Albers GW, Amarenco P, Easton JD, et al. Antithrombotic and thrombolytic therapy for ischemic stroke. The Seventh ACCP Conference on Antithrombotic and Thrombolytic Therapy. *Chest.* 2004;126 (3):483S-512S.
198. Berge E, Abdelnoor M, Nakstad PH, et al. Low molecular-weight heparin versus aspirin in patients with acute ischemic stroke and atrial fibrillation: a double-blind randomized study. HAEST Study Group. Heparin in Acute Embolic Stroke Trial. *Lancet.* 2000;355:1205-10.
199. Low molecular weight heparinoid, ORG 10172 (danaparoid), and outcome after acute ischemic stroke: a randomized controlled trial. The Publications Committee for the Trial of ORG 10172 in Acute Stroke Treatment (TOAST) Investigators. *JAMA.* 1998;279:1265-72.
200. Swanson RA. Intravenous heparin for acute stroke: what can we learn from the mega-trials? *Neurology.* 1999;52:1746-50.
201. Grau AJ, Hacke W. Is there still a role for intravenous heparin in acute stroke? Yes. *Arch Neurol.* 1999;56:1159-60.
202. Sandercock P. Is there still a role for intravenous heparin in acute stroke? No. *Arch Neurol.* 1999;56:1160-1.
203. Moonis M, Fisher M. Considering the role of heparin and low-molecular-weight heparins in acute ischemic stroke. *Stroke.* 2002;33:1927-33.
204. Counsell C, Sandercock P. Low-molecular-weight heparins or heparinoids versus standard unfractionated heparin for acute ischemic stroke (Cochrane review). *Stroke.* 2002;33:1925-6.
205. Adams H, Adams R, Zoppo GD, et al. AHA/ASA scientific statement: guidelines for early management of patients with ischemic stroke—2005 guidelines update. *Stroke.* 2005;36:916-21.
206. Coull BM, Williams LS, Goldstein LB, et al. American Academy of Neurology; American Stroke Association. Anticoagulants and antiplatelet agents in acute ischemic stroke: report of the joint stroke development committee of the American Academy of Neurology and the American Stroke Association. *Neurology.* 2002:59:13-22.
207. Mohr JP, Thompson JLP, Lazar RM, et al. A comparison of warfarin and aspirin for the prevention of recurrent ischemic stroke. *N Engl J Med.* 2001;345:1444-51.
208. Chimowitz MI. Warfarin vs. aspirin for symptomatic intracranial disease (WASID) [abstract]. *Stroke.* 2000;31:562.
209. Lim W, Crowther MA, Eikelboom JW. Management of antiphospholipid antibody syndrome: a systematic review. *JAMA.* 2006;295(9):1050-7.
210. Wilson WA, Gharavi AE, Piette JC. International classification criteria for antiphospholipid syndrome: synopsis of a post-conference workshop held at the ninth international (tours) aPL Symposium. *Lupus.* 2001;10(7):457-60.
211. Moll S, Ortel TL. Monitoring warfarin therapy in patients with lupus anticoagulants. *Ann Intern Med.* 1997;127:177-85.
212. Della Valle P, Crippa L, Safa O, et al. Potential failure of the international normalized ratio (INR) system in the monitoring of oral anticoagulation in patients with lupus anticoagulants. *Ann Med Interne.* (Paris). 1996;147(suppl):10-4.
213. Triplett DA. Antiphospholipid antibodies. *Arch Pathol Lab Med.* 2002;126:1424-9.
214. Long AA, Ginsberg JS, Brill-Edwards P, et al. The relationship of antiphospholipid antibodies to thromboembolic disease in systemic lupus erythematosus: a cross-sectional study. *Thromb Haemost.* 1991;66:520-4.
215. Petri M. Epidemiology of the antiphospholipid antibody syndrome. *J Autoimmunity.* 2000;15:145-51.
216. Ginsberg JS, Wells PS, Brill-Edwards P, et al. Antiphospholipid antibodies and venous thromboembolism. *Blood.* 1995;86:3685-91.
217. Mateo J, Oliver A, Borrell M, et al. Laboratory evaluation and clinical characteristics of 2,132 consecutive unselected patients with venous thromboembolism: results of the Spanish Multicentric Study on Thrombophilia (EMET-Study). *Thromb Haemost.* 1997;77:444-51.
218. Levine JS, Branch DW, Rauch J. The antiphospholipid syndrome. *N Engl J Med.* 2002;346(10):752-63.
219. Cervera R, Piette JC, Font J, et al. Antiphospholipid syndrome: clinical and immunologic manifestations and patterns of disease expression in a cohort of 1,000 patients. *Arthritis Rheum.* 2002;46:1019-27.
220. Brey RL, Hart RG, Sherman DG, et al. Antiphospholipid antibodies and cerebral ischemia in young people. *Neurology.* 1990;40(8):1190-6.
221. Mackworth-Young CG, Antiphospholipid syndrome: multiple mechanisms. *Clin Exp Immunol.* 2004;136:393-401.
222. De Groot PG, Derksen RHWM. Pathophysiology of the antiphospholipid syndrome. *J Thromb Haemost.* 2005;3(8):1854-60.
223. Shapiro SS. The lupus anticoagulant/antiphospholipid syndrome. *Annu Rev Med.* 1996;47(1):533-53.
224. Somers E, Magder LS, Petri M. Antiphospholipid antibodies and incidence of venous thrombosis in a cohort of patients with systemic lupus erythematosus. *J Rheumatol.* 2002;29:2531-6.

225. Petri M. Thrombosis and systemic lupus erythematosus: the Hopkins Lupus Cohort perspective. *Scand J Rheumatol.* 1996;25:191-3.
226. Alarcon-Segovia D, Boffa MC, Branch W, et al. Prophylaxis of the antiphospholipid syndrome: a consensus report. *Lupus.* 2003;12:499-503.
227. Bates SM, Greer IA, Hirsh J, Ginsberg JS. Use of antithrombotic agents during pregnancy: the Seventh ACCP Conference on Antithrombotic and Thrombolytic Therapy. *Chest.* 2004;126(3):627S-44S.
228. Tincani A, Branch W, Levy RA, et al. Treatment of pregnant patients with antiphospholipid syndrome. Lupus. 2003;12:524-9.
229. Coumadin® [package insert]. Wilmington, DE: DuPont Pharma; January 2001.
230. Fihn SD, Callahan CM, Martin DC, et al. The risk for and severity of bleeding complications in elderly patients treated with warfarin: the National Consortium of Anticoagulation Clinics. *Ann Intern Med.* 1996;124:970-9
231. Gurwitz JH, Avorn J, Ross-Degnan D, et al. Aging and the anticoagulant response to warfarin therapy. *Ann Intern Med.* 1992;116:901-4
232. Hylek EM, Regan S, Go AS, et al. Clinical predictors of prolonged delay in return of the international normalized ratio to within the therapeutic range after excessive anticoagulation with warfarin. *Ann Intern Med.* 2001;135:393-400.
233. James AH, Britt RP, Raskino CL, et al. Factors affecting the maintenance dose of warfarin. *J Clin Pathol.* 1992;45:704-6.
234. Redwood M, Taylor C, Bain BJ, et al. The association of age with dosage requirement for warfarin. *Age Ageing.* 1991;20:217-20.
235. Wynne H, Cope L, Kelly P, et al. The influence of age, liver size and enantiomer concentrations on warfarin requirements. *Br J Clin Pharmacol.* 1995;40:203-7.
236. Wynne HA, Kamali F, Edwards C, et al. Effect of ageing upon warfarin dose requirements: a longitudinal study. *Age Ageing.* 1996;25:429-31.
237. Hylek EM, Singer DE. Risk factors for intracranial hemorrhage in outpatients taking warfarin. *Ann Intern Med.* 1994;120:897-902.
238. Landefeld CS, Goldman L. Major bleeding in outpatients treated with warfarin: incidence and prediction by factors known at the start of outpatient therapy. *Am J Med.* 1989;87:144-52.
239. Palareti G, Leali N, Coccheri S, et al. Bleeding complications of oral anticoagulant treatment: an inception-cohort, prospective collaborative study (ISCOAT); Italian Study on Complications of Oral Anticoagulant Therapy. *Lancet.* 1996;348:423-8.
240. Van der Meer FJ, Rosendaal FR, Vandenbroucke JP, et al. Bleeding complications in oral anticoagulant therapy: an analysis of risk factors. *Arch Intern Med.* 1993;153:1557-62.
241. Garcia D, Regan S, Crowther M, et al. Warfarin maintenance dosing patterns in clinical practice: implications for safer anticoagulation in the elderly population. *Chest.* 2005;127;2049-56.
242. Crowther MA, Ginsberg JB, Kearon C, et al. A randomized trial comparing 5-mg and 10-mg warfarin loading doses *Arch Intern Med.* 1999;159:46-8.
243. Gedge J, Orme S, Hampton KK, et al. A comparison of a low dose warfarin induction regimen with a modified Fennerty regimen in elderly inpatients. *Age Ageing.* 2000;29:31-4.
244. Harison L, Johnston M, Massicotte MP, et al. Comparison of 5-mg and 10-mg loading doses in initiation of warfarin therapy. *Ann Intern Med.* 1997;126(2):133-6.
245. Kovacs MJ, Rodger M, Anderson DR, et al. Comparison of 10-mg and 5-mg warfarin initiation nomograms together with low-molecular-weight heparin for outpatient treatment of acute venous thromboembolism. *Ann Intern Med.* 2003;138:714-9.
246. O'Connell MB, Kowal PR, Allivato CJ, et al. Evaluation of warfarin initiation regimens in elderly inpatients. *Pharmacotherapy.* 2000;20(8):923-30.
247. Quiroz R, Gerhard-Herman M, Kosowsky JM, et al. Comparison of a single end point to determine optimal initial warfarin dosing (5 mg versus 10 mg) for venous thromboembolism. *Am J Cardiol.* 2006;98:535-7.
248. Ramzi DW, Leeper KV. DVT and pulmonary embolism: part II treatment and prevention. *Am Fam Physician.* 2004;69:2841-8.
249. Roberts GW, Druskeit T, Jorgensen LE, et al. Comparison of an age adjusted warfarin loading protocol with empirical dosing and Fennerty's protocol. *Aust N Z J Med.* 1999;29(5):731-6.
250. Poller L, Taberner DA. Dosage and control of oral anticoagulants: an international survey. *Br J Haematol.* 1982;51:479-85.
251. Bussey HI, Force RW, Bianco TM, et al. Reliance on prothrombin time ratios causes significant errors in anticoagulation therapy. *Arch Intern Med.* 1992;152:278-82.
252. Kirkwood TBL. Calibration of reference thromboplastins and standardization of the prothrombin time ratio. *Thromb Haemost.* 1983;49:238-44.
253. Poller L. Progress in standardization in anticoagulant control. *Hematol Rev.* 1987;1:225-41.
254. Tripodi A, Chantarangkul V, Braga M, et al. Results of a multicenter study assessing the status of a recombinant thromboplastin for the control of oral anticoagulant therapy. *Thromb Haemost.* 1994;72:261-7.
255. Duncan EM, Casey CR, Duncan BM, et al. Effect of concentration of trisodium citrate anticoagulant on calculation of the international normalized ratio and the international sensitivity index of thromboplastin. *Thromb Haemost.* 1994;72:84-8.
256. Adcock DM, Kressen DC, Marlar RA. Effect of 3.2% vs. 3.8% sodium citrate on routine coagulation testing. *Am J Clin Pathol.* 1997;107:105-10.
257. Horsti J, Uppa H, Vilpo J. Poor agreement among prothrombin time international normalized ratio methods: comparison of seven commercial reagents. *Clinical Chemistry.* 2005;51(3):553-60.
258. Jacobson AK, Ruybalid RL, Johnston M, et al. Significant variation in the reporting of prothrombin time results despite utilization of the INR method of reporting [abstract]. *Circulation.* 1999;100:I-620.
259. Kinck KM, Doetkott C, Miller DR. Clinical impact of interlaboratory variation in international normalized ratio determinations. *Am J Health-Syst Pharm.* 2001;58:684-8.
260. Poller L, Thomson JM, Taberner DA. Effect of au-

tomation on the prothrombin time test in NEQAS surveys. *J Clin Pathol.* 1989;42:97-100.
261. Thomson JM, Taberner DA, Poller L. Automation and prothrombin time: a United Kingdom field study of two widely used coagulometers. *J Clin Pathol.* 1990;43:679-84.
262. Van Den Besselaar AM, Barrowcliffe TW, Houbouyan-Reveillard LL, et al. Guidelines on preparation, certification, and use of certified plasmas for ISI calibration and INR determination. *J Thromb Haemost.* 2004;2:1946-53.
263. Van Rijn JL, Sehmidt NA, Rutten W. Correction of instrument and reagent based differences in determination of the international normalized ratio (INR) for monitoring anticoagulant therapy. *Clin Chem.* 1989;355:840-3.
264. Kazama M, Suzuki S, Abe T, et al. Evaluation of international normalized ratios by a controlled field survey with 4 different thromboplastin reagents. *Thromb Haemost.* 1990;64:535-41.
265. Ng VL, Levin J, Corash L, et al. Failure of the international normalized ratio to generate consistent results within a local medical community. *Am J Clin Pathol.* 1993;99:689-94.
266. Poller L. Laboratory control of oral anticoagulants [editorial]. *BMJ.* 1987;294:1184.
267. Sanfelippo MJ, Sennet J, McMahon EJ. Falsely elevated INRs in warfarin-treated patients with the lupus anticoagulant. *Wis Med J.* 2000;99:62-4.
268. Robert A, LeQuerrec A, Delahousse B, et al. Control of oral anticoagulation in patients with the antiphospholipid syndrome: influence of the lupus anticoagulant on international normalized ratio. *Thromb Haemost.* 1998;80:99-103.
269. Lawrie AS, Purdy G, Mackie IJ, et al. Monitoring of oral anticoagulant therapy in lupus anticoagulant positive patients with the anti-phospholipid syndrome. *Br J Haematol.* 1997;98:887-92.
270. Rosborough TK, Shepherd MF. Unreliability of international normalized ratio for monitoring warfarin therapy in patients with lupus anticoagulant. *Pharmacotherapy.* 2004;24 (7):838-42.
271. Brott T, Broderick J, Kothari R, et al. Early hemorrhage growth in patients with intracerebral hemorrhage. *Stroke.* 1997;28:1-5.
272. Juvela S. Risk factors for impaired outcome after spontaneous intracerebral hemorrhage. *Arch Neurol.* 1995 ;52:1193-200.
273. Franke CL, de Jonge J, van Swieten JC, et al. J. Intracerebral hematomas during anticoagulant treatment. *Stroke.* 1990;21:726-30.
274. Rosand J, Eckman MH, Knudsen KA, et al. The effect of warfarin and intensity of anticoagulation on outcome of intracerebral hemorrhage. *Arch Intern Med.* 2004;164:880-4.
275. Brott T, Broderick J, Kothari R, et al. Early hemorrhage growth in patients with intracerebral hemorrhage. *Stroke.* 1997;28:1-5.
276. Kazui S, Naritomi H, Yamamoto H, et al. Enlargement of spontaneous intracerebral hemorrhage. Incidence and time course. *Stroke.* 1996;27:1783-7.
277. Becker KJ, Baxter AB, Bybee HM, et al. Extravasation of radiographic contrast is an independent predictor of death in primary intracerebral hemorrhage. *Stroke.* 1999;30:2025-32.
278. Flibotte JJ, Hagan N, O'Donnell J, et al. Warfarin, hematoma expansion, and outcome of intracerebral hemorrhage. *Neurology.* 2004;63:1059-64.
279. Vitamin K [package insert]. Lake Forest, IL: Hospira Inc; November 2004.
280. Fiore LD, Scola MA, Cantillon CE, et al. Anaphylactoid reactions to vitamin K. *J Thromb Thromholysis.* 2001;11:175-83.
281. Watson HG, Baglin T, Laidlaw SL, et al. A comparison of the efficacy and rate of response to oral and intravenous vitamin K in reversal of over-anticoagulation with warfarin. *Br J Haematol.* 2001;115:145-9.
282. Riegert-Johnson DL, Volcheck GW. The incidence of anaphylaxis following intravenous phytonadione (vitamin K1): a 5-year retrospective review. *Ann Allergy Asthma Immunol.* 2002;89:400-6.
283. Whitling AM, Bussey HI, Lyons RM. Comparing different routes and doses of phytonadione for reversing excessive anticoagulation. *Arch Intern Med.* 1998;158:2136-40.
284. Raj G, Kumar R, McKinney P. Time course of reversal of anticoagulant effect of warfarin by intravenous and subcutaneous phytonadione. *Arch Intern Med.* 1999;159:2721-4.
285. Hanley JP. Warfarin reversal. *J Clin Pathol.* 2004;57:1132-9.
286. Steiner T, Rosand J, Diringer M. Intracerebral hemorrhage associated with oral anticoagulant therapy current practices and unresolved questions. *Stroke.* 2006;37:256-62.
287. O'Shaughnessy DF, Atterbury C, Bolton Maggs P, et al. Guidelines for the use of fresh-frozen plasma, cryoprecipitate and cryosupernatant. *Br J Haematol.* 2004;126:11-28.
288. Makris M, Greaves M, Phillips WS, et al. Emergency oral anticoagulant reversal: the relative efficacy of infusions of fresh frozen plasma and clotting factor concentrate on correction of the coagulopathy. *Thromb Haemost.* 1997;77:477-80.
289. Makris M, Watson HG. The management of coumarin-induced over anticoagulation annotation. *Br J Haematol.* 2001;114:271-80.
290. Goldstein JN, Thomas SH, Frontiero V, et al. Timing of fresh frozen plasma administration and rapid correction of coagulopathy in warfarin-related intracerebral hemorrhage. *Stroke.* 2006;37:151-5.
291. Freeman WD, Brott TG, Barrett KM, et al. Recombinant factor VIIa for rapid reversal of warfarin anticoagulation in acute intracranial hemorrhage. *Mayo Clin Proc.* 2004;79:1495-500.
292. Brody DL, Aiyagari V, Shakleford AM, et al. Use of recombinant factor VIIa in patients with warfarin-associated intracranial hemorrhage. *Neurocritical Care.* 2005;2:263-7.
293. Pindur G, Morsdorf S, Schenk JF, et al. The overdosed patient and bleedings with oral anticoagulation. *Semin Thromb Hemost.* 1999;25:85-8.
294. Gilstad CW. Anaphylactic transfusion reactions. *Curr Opin Hematol.* 2003;10:419-23.
295. Pomper GJ, Wu Y, Snyder EL. Risks of transfusion-transmitted infections. *Curr Opin Hematol.* 2003;10:412-8.
296. Hellstern P, Muntean W, Schramm W, et al. Practical guidelines for the clinical use of plasma. *Thromb Res.* 2002;107(supp 1):S53-7.

297. Hanley JP. Warfarin reversal. *J Clin Pathol.* 2004;57:1132-9.
298. British Committee for Standards in Haematology. Guidelines on oral anticoagulation. 3rd ed. *Br J Haematol.* 1998;101:374-87.
299. Preston FE, Laidlaw ST, Sampson B, et al. Rapid reversal of oral anticoagulation with warfarin by a prothrombin complex concentrate (Beriplex): efficacy and safety in 42 patients. *Br J Haematol.* 2002;116:619-24.
300. Evans G, Luddington R, Baglin T. Beriplex P/N reverses severe warfarin-induced over anticoagulation immediately and completely in patients presenting with major bleeding. *Br J Haematol.* 2001;115:998-1001.
301. Yasaka M, Oomura M, Ikeno K, et al. Effect of prothrombin complex concentrate on INR and blood coagulation system in emergency patients treated with warfarin over dose. *Ann Hematol.* 2003;82:121-3.
302. Nitu IC, Perry DC, Lee CA. Clinical experience with the use of clotting factor concentrates in oral anticoagulation reversal. *Clin Lab Haematol.* 1998;20:363-7.
303. Fredriksson K, Norrving B, Stromblad LG. Emergency reversal of anticoagulation after intracerebral hemorrhage. *Stroke.* 1992;23:972-7.
304. Roddie PH, Stirling C, Mayne EE, et al. Thrombosis and disseminated intravascular coagulation following treatment with the prothrombin complex concentrate, DEFIX. *Thromb Haemost.* 1999;81:667.
305. Kohler M, Hellstern P, Lechler E, et al. Thromboembolic complications associated with the use of prothrombin complex and factor IX concentrates. *Thromb Haemost.* 1998;80:399-402.
306. Hellstern P. Production and composition of prothrombin complex concentrates: correlation between composition and therapeutic efficiency. *Thromb Res.* 1999(supp);95:S7-12.
307. Kohler M, Habauer G, Miyashita C, et al. Quality control of prothrombin complex preparations: in vivo and in vitro findings. *Beitr Infusionsther.* 1990;26:186-9.
308. O'Connell KA, Wood JJ, Wise RP, et al. Thromboembolic adverse events after use of recombinant human coagulation factor VIIa. *JAMA.* 2006;295:293-8.
309. Mayer SA, Brun NC, Begtrup K, et al. Recombinant activated factor VII for acute intracerebral hemorrhage. *N Engl J Med.* 2005;352(8):777-85.
310. Mayer SA, Brun NC, Broderick J, et al. Safety and feasibility of recombinant factor VIIa for acute intracerebral hemorrhage. *Stroke.* 2005;36;74-9.
311. Sorensen B, Johansen P, Nielsen GL et al. Reversal of the international normalized ratio with recombinant activated factor VII in central nervous system bleeding during warfarin thromboprophylaxis: clinical and biochemical aspects. *Blood Coagul Fibrinolysis.* 2003;14(5):469-77.
312. NovoSeven [package insert]. Princeton, NJ: Novo Nordisk Pharmaceuticals Inc; 2003.
313. Fewel ME, Park P. The emerging role of recombinant-activated factor VII in neurocritical care. *Neurocritical Care.* 2004;1:19-30.
314. Deveras RAE, Kessler CM. Reversal of warfarin-induced excessive anticoagulation with recombinant human factor VIIa concentrate. *Ann Intern Med.* 2002;137:884-8.
315. Veshchev I, Elran H, Salame K. Recombinant coagulation factor VIIa for rapid preoperative correction of warfarin-related coagulopathy in patients with acute subdural hematoma. *Med Sci Monit.* 2002;8:98-100.
316. Lin J, Hanigan WC, Tarantino M, et al. The use of recombinant activated factor VII to reverse warfarin induced anticoagulation in patients with hemorrhages in the central nervous system: preliminary findings. *J Neurosurg.* 2003;98:737-40.
317. Makris M, Watson HG. Reversal of coumarin-induced over anticoagulation: reply to Escobar. *Br J Haematol.* 2002;118:926.
318. Rudisill CN, Hockman RH, Degregory KA, et al. Implementing guidelines for the institutional use of factor VIIa (recombinant): a multidisciplinary solution. *Am J Health-Syst Pharm.* 2006;63:1641-6.
319. Dunn AS, Turpie AG. Perioperative management of patients receiving oral anticoagulants. *Arch Intern Med.* 2003;163:901-8.
320. Kearon C, Hirsh J. Management of anticoagulation before and after elective surgery. *N Engl J Med.* 1997;336:1506-11.
321. Hommes DW, Bura A, Mazzolai L, et al. Subcutaneous heparin compared with continuous intravenous heparin administration in the initial treatment of deep vein thrombosis. *Ann Intern Med.* 1992;116:279-84.
322. Prandoni P, Carnovali M, Marchiori A. Subcutaneous adjusted-dose unfractionated heparin vs fixed-dose low-molecular-weight heparin in the initial treatment of venous thromboembolism. *Arch Intern Med.* 2004;164:1077-83.
323. Larson BJG, Zumberg MS, Kitchens CS, et al. A feasibility study of continuing dose-reduced warfarin for invasive procedures in patients with high thromboembolic risk. *Chest.* 2005;127:922-7.
324. Francis, CW, Marder, VJ, Evarts, CM, et al Two-step warfarin therapy. *JAMA.* 1983;249:374-8.
325. Morris GK, Mitchell JR. Warfarin sodium in prevention of deep venous thrombosis and pulmonary embolism in patients with fractured neck of femur. *Lancet.* 1976;2:869-72.
326. Salzman EW, Harris WH, DeSanctis RW. Reduction in venous thromboembolism by agents affecting platelet function. *N Engl J Med.* 1971;284:1287-92.
327. Eisen GM, Baron TH, Dominitz JA, et al. Guidelines on the management of anticoagulation and antiplatelet therapy for endoscopic procedures. *Gastrointest Endosc.* 2002;55(7):775-9.
328. Landefeld CS, Beyth RJ. Anticoagulant-related bleeding: clinical, epidemiology, prediction, prevention. *Am J Med.* 1993;95:315-28.
329. Bleeding during antithrombotic therapy in patients with atrial fibrillation. The Stroke Prevention in Atrial Fibrillation Investigators. *Arch Intern Med.* 1996;156:409-16.
330. Fitzmaurice DA, Blann AD, Lip GY. Bleeding risks of antithrombotic therapy. *BMJ.* 2002;325(7368):828-31.
331. Altman R, Rouvier J, Gurfinkel E, et al. Comparison of two levels of anticoagulant therapy in patients with substitute heart valves. *J Thorac Cardiovasc*

Surg. 1991;101:427-31.
332. Hull R, Hirsh J, Jay R, et al. Different intensities of oral anticoagulant therapy in the treatment of proximal-vein thrombosis. *N Engl J Med.* 1982;307:1676-81.
333. Saour JN, Sieck JO, Mamo LAR, et al. Trial of different intensities of anticoagulation in patients with prosthetic heart valves. *N Engl J Med.* 1990;322:428-32.
334. Turpie AGG, Gunstensen J, Hirsh J, et al. Randomized comparison of two intensities of oral anticoagulant therapy after tissue heart valve replacement. *Lancet.* 1988;1:1242-5.
335. European Atrial Fibrillation Trial Study Group. Optimal oral anticoagulant therapy in patients with nonrheumatic atrial fibrillation and recent cerebral ischemia. *N Engl J Med.* 1995;333:5-10.
336. Oden A, Fahlen M. Oral anticoagulation and risk of death: a medical record linkage study. *BMJ.* 2002;325(7372):1073-5.
337. Fihn SD, McDonell M, Martin D, et al. Risk factors for complications of chronic anticoagulation, a multi-center study; Warfarin Optimized Outpatient Follow-Up Study Group. *Ann Intern Med.* 1993;118:511-20.
338. Gurwitz JH, Avorn J, Ross-Degnan D, et al. Aging and the anticoagulant response to warfarin therapy. *Ann Intern Med.* 1992;116:901-4.
339. Pettiti DB, Strom BL, Melmon KL. Duration of warfarin anticoagulation therapy and the probabilities of recurrent thromboembolism and hemorrhage. *Am J Med.* 1986;81:255-9.
340. Petty GW, Lennihan L, Mohr JP, et al. Complications of long-term anticoagulation. *Ann Neurol.* 1988;23:570-4.
341. Landefeld CS, Rosenblatt MW, Goldman L. Bleeding in outpatients treated with warfarin: relation to the prothrombin time and important remedial lesions. *Am J Med.* 1989;87:153-9.
342. Koch-Weser J. Coumadin necrosis. *Ann Intern Med.* 1968;68:1365-6.
343. McKnight JT, Maxwell AJ, Anderson RL. Warfarin necrosis. *Arch Fam Med.* 1992;1:105-8.
344. Cole MS, Minifee PK, Wolma FJ. Coumarin necrosis: a review of the literature. *Surgery.* 1988;103:271-7.
345. Renick AM. Anticoagulant-induced necrosis of skin and subcutaneous tissues: report of two cases and review of the literature. *South Med J.* 1976;69:775-8.
346. Horn JR, Danziger LH, Davis RJ. Warfarin-induced skin necrosis: report of four cases. *Am J Health-Syst Pharm.* 1981;38:1763-8.
347. Hyman BT, Landas SK, Ashman RF, et al. Warfarin-related purple toes syndrome and cholesterol microembolization. *Am J Med.* 1987;82(6):1233-7.
348. Talmadge DB, Spyropoulos AC. Purple toes syndrome associated with warfarin therapy in a patient with antiphospholipid syndrome. *Pharmacotherapy.* 2003;23(5):674-7.
349. Lebsack CS, Weibert RT. Purple toes syndrome. *Postgrad Med.* 1982;71(5):81-4.
350. Man-Son-Hing M, Nichol G, Lau A, et al. Choosing antithrombotic therapy for elderly patients with atrial fibrillation who are at risk for falls. *Arch Intern Med.* 1999;159:677-85.
351. Campbell AJ, Borrie MJ, Spears GF, et al. Circumstances and consequences of falls experienced by a community population 70 years and over during a prospective study. *Age Ageing.* 1990;19:136-41.
352. Hrada Y, Imai Y, Kurosawa H, et al. Ten-year follow-up after valve replacement with the St Jude medical prosthesis in children. *J Thorac Cardiovasc Surg.* 1990;100:175-80.
353. Streif W, Andrew M, Marzinotto V, et al. Analysis of warfarin therapy in pediatric patients: a prospective cohort study of 319 patients. *Blood.* 1999;94(9):3007-14.
354. Stewart S, Cianciotta D, Alexson C, et al. The long-term risk of warfarin sodium therapy and the incidence of thromboembolism in children after prosthetic cardiac heart valves. *J Thorac Cardiovasc Surg.* 1987;93:80-5.
355. Woods A, Vargas J, Berri G et al. Antithrombotic therapy in children and adolescent. *Thromb Res.* 1986;42:289-301.
356. Andrew M, Marzinotto V, Brooker L, et al. Oral anticoagulation in pediatric patients: a prospective cohort study. *Thromb Haemost.* 1994;71:265-9.
357. Andrew M, Moanagle P, Brooker L. Oral anticoagulant therapy in pediatric patients. In: Thromboembolic Complications during Infancy and Childhood. Hamilton. BC: Decker Inc; 2000:278-356.
358. Barnes C, Newall F, Ignjatovic V, et al. Reduced bone density in children on long-term warfarin. *Pediatr Res.* 2005;57(4):578-81.
359. Massicotte P, Julian J, Weber C, et al. Osteoporosis: a potential complication of long-term warfarin therapy [abstract]. *Thromb Haemost.* 1999;(suppl):1333a.
360. Bates SM, Greer IA, Hirsh J, et al. Use of antithrombotic agents during pregnancy. The Seventh ACCP Conference on Antithrombotic and Thrombolytic Therapy. *Chest.* 2004;126(3):p627S-44S.
361. Hall JAG, Paul RM, Wilson KM. Maternal and fetal sequelae of anticoagulation during pregnancy. *Am J Med.* 1980;68:122-40.
362. Briggs GG, Freeman RK, Yaffe SJ. *Drugs in Pregnancy and Lactation.* 5th ed. Baltimore, MD: Lippincott Williams & Wilkins; 1998.
363. Wesseling J, van Driel D, Heymans HAS, et al. Coumarins during pregnancy: long term effects on growth and development in school age children. *Thromb Haemost.* 2001;85:609-13.
364. US Food & Drug Administration, Equivalence of Generic Drugs. September, 1999. Available at: http://www.fda.gov/cder/consumerinfo/generic_equivalence.htm. Accessed September 29, 2006.
365. Henderson JD, Esham RH. Generic substitution: issues for problematic drugs. *SMJ.* 2001;94(1):16-21.
366. Benet LZ, Goyan JE. Bioequivalence and narrow therapeutic drugs. *Pharmacotherapy.* 1995;15:433-40.
367. Sawyer W. Warfarin. In: Mungall DR, ed. *Applied Clinical Pharmacokinetics.* New York: Raven Press; 1983:187-222.
368. Milligan PE, Banet GA, Waterman AD, et al. Substitution of generic warfarin for coumadin in an HMO setting. *Ann Pharmacother.* 2002;36(5):764-78.
369. Witt DM, Tillman DJ, Evans CM, et al, Evaluation of the clinical and economic impact of a brand name to generic warfarin sodium conversion pro-

gram. *Pharmacotherapy.* 2003;23(3):360-8.
370. US Food & Drug Administration, Electronic Orange Book. August, 2006. Available at: http://www.fda.gov/cder/ob/htm. Accessed September 29, 2006.
371. US Food & Drug Administration, Letter to Health Practitioners, Therapeutic Equivalence of Generic Drugs. January 28, 1998. Available at: http://www.fda.gov/cder/news/nightenlett.htm. Accessed September 29, 2006.
372. Swenson CN, Fundak G. Observational cohort study of switching warfarin sodium products in a managed care organization. *Am J Health-Syst Pharm.* 2000;57:452-5.
373. Weibert RT, Yeager BF, Wittkowsky AK, et al. A randomized, crossover comparison of warfarin products in the treatment of chronic atrial fibrillation. *Ann Pharmacother.* 2000;34:981-8.
374. Lee HL, Kan CD, Yang YJ. Efficacy and tolerability of the switch from a branded to a generic warfarin sodium product: an observer-blinded, randomized, crossover study. *Clinical Therapeutics.* 2005;27(3):309-19.
375. Pereira JA, Holbrook AM, Dolovich L, et al. Are brand name and generic warfarin interchangeable? Multiple N-of-1 randomized, crossover trials. *Ann Pharmacother.* 2005;39(7):1188-93.

Chapter 11

Heparin, Low Molecular Weight Heparin, and Fondaparinux

Edith Nutescu, William Dager

Chapter Outline

- Introduction
- Unfractionated heparin
  - Pharmacology
  - Pharmacokinetics/pharmacodynamics
  - Indications
  - Dosing and administration
  - Monitoring
  - Side effects, precautions, and contraindications
- Low molecular weight heparin
  - Pharmacology
  - Pharmacokinetics/pharmacodynamics
  - Indications
  - Dosing and administration
  - Monitoring
  - Side effects, precautions, and contraindications
- Fondaparinux
  - Pharmacology
  - Pharmacokinetics/pharmacodynamics
  - Indications
  - Dosing and administration
  - Monitoring
  - Side effects, precautions, and contraindications
- Reversal of anticoagulant effect
  - Unfractionated heparin
  - LMWH
  - Fondaparinux
- Special patient populations
  - Renal impairment
  - Extremes of body weight
  - Pregnancy
  - Pediatric patients
- Conclusion
- Patient case
- References

Introduction

Historically, unfractionated heparin (UFH) represented the mainstay parenteral anticoagulant used in the prevention or treatment of arterial and venous thrombosis. In recent years, agents with improved pharmacologic properties such as the low molecular weight heparins (LMWHs) and the pentasaccharide (fondaparinux) have been added to the armamentarium of antithrombotic agents used for these indications.[1,2] Pharmacists and health-care providers involved in managing antithrombotic therapies need to be familiar with the pharmacologic and pharmacokinetic differences between these agents, and also with the variety of clinical nuances for appropriate and safe use.

The goal of this chapter is to provide a practical overview on essential clinical knowledge that will facilitate appropriate and safe use of UFH, LMWH, and fondaparinux in daily clinical practice.

Unfractionated Heparin

Unfractionated heparin has been one of the most commonly used anticoagulants for the prevention and treatment of thrombosis. Commercially available UFH preparations are isolated from porcine intestinal mucosa or bovine lung. Bovine derived heparin, however, is no longer available in the United States. No differences in antithrombotic activity have been demonstrated between the various UFH preparations.[1,3,4]

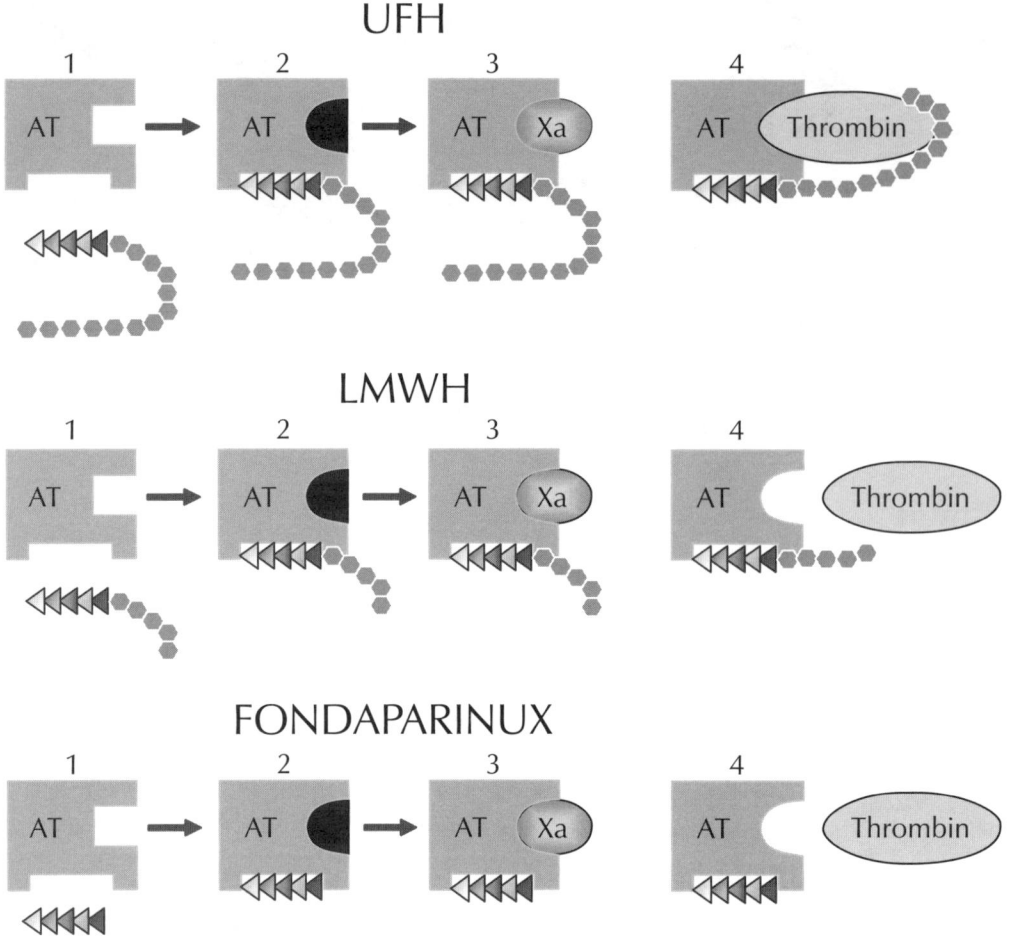

Figure 11-1. Mechanism of action of UFH, LMWH, and fondaparinux. Abbreviations: UFH = unfractionated heparin; LMWH = low molecular weight heparin; AT = antithrombin; Xa = activated factor X.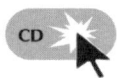

Pharmacology

Heparin is composed of a heterogeneous mixture of glycosaminoglycans with variable chain lengths and pharmacological properties. The mean molecular weight of UFH is 15,000 daltons (range of 3,000 to 30,000 daltons). The length of each UFH molecule confers its anticoagulant and elimination profile. Longer UFH chains are cleared more rapidly, generally by hepatic elimination than shorter chains which tend to be cleared renally.[1,5]

Heparin exerts its anticoagulant effect by augmenting the natural anticoagulant antithrombin (AT) (see Figure 11-1).[1] A specific pentasaccharide sequence on the heparin molecule binds to AT and causes a conformational change which greatly accelerates its enzymatic activity. This complex inhibits thrombin (factor IIa) as well as factors Xa, IXa, XIa, and XIIa. Thrombin and factor Xa are most sensitive to this inhibition and are inactivated in an equal 1:1 ratio. In order to inactivate thrombin, the UFH molecule needs to form a ternary complex by binding to both AT and thrombin. Only UFH molecules that are at least 18 saccharide units long are able to form this bridge between AT and thrombin. In contrast, inhibition of factor-Xa does not require the formation of a ternary complex. Heparin molecules as short as 5 saccharide units can catalyze the inactivation of factor-Xa. Unlike thrombolytics, UFH will not dissolve a formed clot but prevent its propagation and growth.[1,3,5,6]

After it has produced its effect, UFH detaches from AT and re-attaches with another AT molecule. Because of its large size, the UFH-AT complex is unable to inactivate clot-bound thrombin or factor Xa. UFH binds to platelets and has an inhibitory effect on platelet aggregation. In addition, when used in higher doses, UFH also binds to heparin cofactor II, further enhancing the inhibition of thrombin activity.[1,5,6]

> **Clinical Pearl**
>
> Patients with acute thrombosis may frequently have higher UFH dose requirements to attain therapeutic effect as these patients have been noted to eliminate UFH more rapidly, possibly because of increased binding to acute phase reactants.

Pharmacokinetics/Pharmacodynamics

The half-life of UFH is dose-dependent. The typical half-life ranges between 30 to 90 minutes, but it can be longer (~150 minutes) when UFH is given in high doses (see Table 11-1). Unfractionated heparin is eliminated by two mechanisms: (1) enzymatic degradation via a rapid, saturable zero-order process, and (2) renally via a first-order, non-saturable slower process. At lower concentrations, UFH is primarily cleared via enzymatic processes while at higher concentrations it may be subject to renal elimination. The contribution of each mechanism to the total clearance of UFH is related to the dose and size of the heparin molecules. The rate of clearance of UFH is reduced in patients with renal and hepatic dysfunction.[1, 5-7]

Due to its nonspecific binding to various cellular proteins, UFH has several limitations including poor bioavailability when given subcutaneously (SC) and significant intra- and inter-patient variability in

> **Clinical Pearl**
>
> Due to its lower and variable bioavailability if the SC route of administration is used, higher doses of UFH should be initiated in order to attain therapeutic anticoagulation effect quickly. The initial SC UFH dose should be approximately 10% to 20% higher than the usual IV dose required to maintain therapeutic effect (see Table 11-2).

Table 11-1.

Pharmacologic and Clinical Properties of UFH, LMWH, and Fondaparinux

Property	UFH	LMWH	Fondaparinux
Source	Extracted from porcine intestinal mucosa or beef lung	Chemical or enzymatic depolymerization of UFH	Chemical synthesis
Molecular weight (Daltons)	Mean 15,000	Mean 5000	1728
SC bioavailability	30% to 70% (dose dependent)	~90%	100%
Activated clotting factors reduced	Multiple: factors IIa, IXa, Xa, XIIa	Factors Xa > IIa	Factor Xa
Binding to proteins other than target	Yes	Limited	Limited
Anti-Xa:anti-IIa	1:1	2:1 to 4:1	100% anti-Xa
Primary route of elimination	Enzymatic degradation at low doses and renal at higher dose	Renal primarily	Renal
Half-life (SC route)	30–150 min (dose dependent)	3–4 hours	17–21 hours
Effects of protamine	Complete neutralization	Partial neutralization	No effect

SC = subcutaneous; UFH = unfractionated heparin; LMWH = low molecular weight heparin anticoagulant response.[3,8] When given via the SC route, the bioavailability of UFH ranges from 30% when given in low doses to as much as 70% when given in high doses.[1,5]

After SC administration, the onset of anticoagulant effect is usually achieved 1 to 2 hours and peak effect is achieved at 3 hours.[9] Several days may be required to reach steady-state pharmacodynamic assessment values when SC UFH is given in full therapeutic doses. Intramuscular administration is not recommended due to erratic absorption and risk of hematoma formation. When UFH is given via the intravenous (IV) route, continuous IV infusion is preferred over intermittent IV boluses. Intermittent bolus injections result in high peak anticoagulant levels and have been associated with a higher risk of major bleeding.[1,4,5]

Clinical Pearl

When transitioning from UFH to an alternative parenteral anticoagulant agent with rapid onset of activity, it may be preferable to wait a selected period of time before initiating the alternative therapy. However, in the setting of multiple distractions to the health-care staff, delay in initiating the ordered anticoagulant can occur, resulting in an undesired lapse in anticoagulation therapy. Thus, unless an atypical clinical situation is present, it is suggested to stop the UFH at the same time as initiating any new anticoagulant that has a rapid onset of action (also see Table 11-3).

Indications

The use of UFH has been investigated for the prevention and treatment of thrombosis in several arterial and venous indications. The most commonly used indications for UFH include the prophylaxis and treatment of venous thromboembolism (VTE), prevention of stroke in atrial fibrillation, disseminated intravascular coagulation, prophylaxis and treatment of peripheral arterial embolism, prevention of clotting in arterial and cardiac surgeries, and as an anticoagulant in blood transfusions, extracorporeal circulation, dialysis procedures, and in blood samples for laboratory purposes.[1,4]

Dosing and Administration

For systemic anticoagulation effects, UFH is typically administered via the IV or SC route.[1,4] The actual dose and route of administration for UFH will be dependent on the indication for therapy, the therapeutic goals, and the patient's individual response to therapy (see Tables 11-2, 11-4, and 11-5). For the prevention of VTE, UFH is usually given by SC injection. The typical dose for prophylaxis ranges from 5,000 units given every 12 hours in moderate risk patients to 5,000 units given every 8 hours in higher risk patients.[1,10] In order to improve compliance and to avoid missed doses, standard dosing times should be developed especially when SC UFH is given as an every 8-hour regimen. In certain clinical situations when there is a need for rapid reversal of anticoagulation, such as increased bleeding risk, or the need to rapidly reverse anticoagulation for an invasive procedure, or when there are bioavailability concerns (critical care setting)

Table 11-2.

Sample Dosing and Monitoring Nomogram for Adjusted-Dose Subcutaneous UFH
As an alternative to IV administration, UFH can be administered SC twice daily. The recommended initial dose is 250 units/kg SC given q12 hours (or 17,500 IU SC every 12 hours). aPTT should be drawn at 6 hours (mid-interval) after the dose. Subsequent doses should be adjusted based on aPTT response (see dosing chart below).

aPTT (sec)	Dose Adjustment	Time of Next aPTT
<40	Increase by 36 to 48 units/kg q 12 hours	6 hours post-dose
40–59	Increase by 24 to 36 units/kg q 12 hours	6 hours post-dose
60–90 (institution-specific therapeutic range)*	No change	Next AM, then daily (less frequent monitoring may be required with long-term use)
91–103	Decrease by 6 to 12 units/kg q 12 hours	6 hours post-dose
104–124	Decrease by 12 to 24 units/kg q 12 hours	6 hours post-dose
>124	Decrease by 24 to 36 units/kg q 12 hours	6 hours post-dose

*Institution specific therapeutic aPTT range of 60–90 seconds is equivalent to a plasma heparin concentration of 0.3–0.7 anti-Xa units/mL or 0.2–0.4 units/mL by protamine titration. Range may vary depending on the assay sensitivity to heparin for a particular reagent.
aPTT = activated partial thromboplastin time; IV = intravenous; SC = subcutaneous; UFH = unfractionated heparin; AM = morning.

Table 11-3.
Practical Considerations for Transitioning Between Various Anticoagulant Agents

Conversion from IV UFH infusion to adjusted-dose SC UFH	• Calculate the 24-hour IV UFH dose requirement needed to maintain therapeutic aPTT • Increase the total 24-hour UFH dose requirement by 10% to 20% (SC dosage requirements are higher then IV) • Divide the dose calculated above by 2 to determine the initial q12 hours SC dosing requirement • Discontinue IV UFH and initiate the 1st SC UFH dose (as calculated above) within 1 hour • Check aPTT at 6-hours after 1st SC dose • Adjust further SC UFH doses based on aPTT and dosing nomogram from Table 11-2
Conversion from IV UFH infusion to SC LMWH (or SC fondaparinux)	• Calculate the appropriate LMWH (or fondaparinux) dose based on the specific indication for use and patient weight • Discontinue IV UFH and initiate the 1st SC LMWH (or fondaparinux) dose within 1 hour

Conversion from SC LMWH or SC fondaparinux to IV UFH infusion	• Calculate the appropriate IV UFH dose based on indication for use and patient weight (see Table 11-4)
	• Discontinue SC LMWH or SC fondaparinux and initiate IV UFH 1–2 hours (no bolus) before the next SC LMWH or fondaparinux dose would have been administered:
	  a. When switching from SC LMWH given q12 hours, initiate IV UFH at 10 to 11 hours after last LMWH dose
	  b. When switching from SC LMWH given q24 hours, initiate IV UFH at 22 to 23 hours after last LMWH dose
	  c. When switching from SC fondaparinux given q24 hours, initiate IV UFH at 22 to 23 hours after last fondaparinux dose
	  d. Check patient's renal status and if impaired, the IV UFH dosing initiation intervals suggested in a–c above need to be extended accordingly
	• Check aPTT at 6 hours after initiating the IV UFH infusion
	• Adjust further UFH doses based on aPTT and dosing nomogram from Table 11-5

Conversion from SC LMWH or SC fondaparinux to adjusted-dose SC UFH	• Calculate the adjusted-dose SC UFH dosing requirements: the recommended initial dose is 250 units/kg SC given q12 hours
	• Discontinue SC LMWH or SC fondaparinux and initiate SC UFH at the time the next SC LMWH or fondaparinux dose is scheduled to be administered:
	  a. When switching from SC LMWH given q12 hours, initiate SC UFH at 12 hours after last LMWH dose
	  b. When switching from SC LMWH given q24 hours, initiate SC UFH at 24 hours after last LMWH dose
	  c. When switching from SC fondaparinux given q24 hours, initiate SC UFH at 24 hours after last fondaparinux dose
	  d. Check patient's renal status and if impaired, the SC UFH dosing initiation intervals suggested in a–c above need to be extended accordingly
	• aPTT should be drawn at 6 hours (mid-interval) after the 1st SC UFH dose
	• Subsequent SC UFH doses should be adjusted based on aPTT and dosing nomogram from Table 11-2

with the SC dose, a continuous IV UFH infusion may be considered targeting a limited (10–20 seconds) rise in the activated partial thromboplastin time (aPTT). The dose of UFH required to achieve a therapeutic anticoagulant response is correlated to the patient's weight.[11, 12] Thus, when immediate and full anticoagulation is required, a weight-based IV bolus dose followed by a continuous infusion is recommended (see Tables 11-4 and 11-5).[1, 5, 11-13] In addition to weight as a predictor for UFH dosing, recent reports support the use of dosing protocols that are based on sex, age and height.[14] Improved initial UFH heparin dosing estimations have also been reported with protocols based on patient age and plasma volume.[15]

The initial recommended weight-based UFH dose in the treatment of VTE is 80 units/kg bolus and 18 units/kg/hour infusion.[11] In the treatment of acute coronary syndromes, the recommended UFH initiation doses are usually lower then the doses used in the treatment of VTE.[1] For patients with unstable angina and non-ST-segment elevation myocardial infarction the recommended UFH bolus is 60–70 units/kg (maximum dose 5,000 units) and the infusion is 12–15 units/kg/hour (maximum dose 1,000 units/hour).[1, 16, 17] In patients with ST-elevation myocardial infarction also receiving thrombolytics, the recommended UFH bolus dose is 60 units/kg (maximum dose 4,000 units) and the infusion is 12 units/kg/hour (maximum dose 1,000 units/hour).[1, 18] In patients undergoing percutaneous coronary intervention, when UFH is administered without the use of glycoprotein IIb/IIIa inhibitors, the recommended UFH bolus dose is 70–100 units/kg, with additional boluses of 2,000–5,000 units if target activated clotting times (ACT)

Table 11-4.
Sample Weight-based Dosing Nomogram for IV UFH in Acute Thrombosis

Initial Loading Dose	Initial Infusion Rate
60–80 units/kg	12–18 units/kg/h
ACS: 60 units/kg (maximum 5000 units; 4000 units if concurrent GPIIbIIIa inhibitor or thrombolytic) Ischemic stroke: No bolus VTE: 80 units/kg (maximum 10,000 units)	ACS: 12 units/kg/h (maximum start rate 1,000 units/h) Ischemic stroke: 12 units/kg/h (maximum start rate 1,000 units/h) VTE: 18 units/kg/h (maximum start rate 1,500 units/h)

Abbreviations: UFH = unfractionated heparin; VTE = venous thrombosis; ACS = acute coronary syndromes; GP IIb/IIIa = glycoprotein IIb/IIIa inhibitors; h = hour; IV = intravenous.

Table 11-5.
Sample Monitoring Nomogram for IV UFH

aPTT (sec)	Maintenance Infusion Rate Dose Adjustment	Time of Next aPTT
Less than 35	80 units/kg bolus then increase infusion by 3 units/kg/h	6 hours
35–49	40 units/kg bolus then increase infusion by 2 units/kg/h	6 hours
50–59	No bolus. Increase infusion by 1 units/kg/h	6 hours
60–90 (institution-specific therapeutic range)*	No change	Next AM, then daily
91–103	Decrease infusion by 1 units/kg/h	6 hours
104–124	Hold infusion for 30 minutes then decrease by 2 units/kg/h	6 hours after resuming infusion
> 124	Hold infusion for 1 hour then decrease by 3 units/kg/h	6 hours after resuming infusion

*Institution specific therapeutic aPTT range of 60–90 seconds is equivalent to a plasma heparin concentration of 0.3–0.7 anti-Xa units/mL or 0.2–0.4 units/mL by protamine titration. Range may vary depending on the assay sensitivity to heparin for a particular reagent.

kg = kilograms; h = hours; AM = morning; aPTT = activated partial thromboplastin time.

> **Clinical Pearl**
>
> In cases of acute thrombosis, or when there is a need to rapidly establish anticoagulation, a bolus dose of UFH may be necessary. If emergent anticoagulation is not necessary, then starting the UFH infusion without a bolus dose will make it easier to assess the response to the infusion alone, titrate to the desired therapeutic effect, and minimize dosing errors (such as under adjusting the infusion rate) associated with administering a bolus dose.

are not achieved. The initial UFH bolus is reduced to 50–70 units/kg when glycoprotein IIb/IIIa inhibitors are also given.[1, 19] In selected populations, such as stroke or atrial fibrillation (non-ablation), a bolus dose may not be necessary. Policies for such selected populations should be determined in advance, and included as options in standardized ordering and monitoring protocols.

Weight-based UFH dosing regimens are more likely to exceed the therapeutic aPTT threshold in the first 24 hours after initiating treatment compared to more traditional dosing regimens such as 5,000 unit bolus dose followed by an infusion administered at 1,000 units/hour.[11] Achieving a therapeutic aPTT in the first 24 hours after initiating UFH has been shown to lower the risk of recurrent VTE.[20, 21]

The SC route of administration can also be employed when treating an acute venous thrombotic event.[1, 22, 23] If the SC route is selected for the treatment of VTE, an initial 5000 unit IV bolus should be given followed by 17,500 units given SC every 12 hours.[1, 23] Subsequent doses of SC UFH need to be adjusted based on the patient's aPTT response (see Table 11-2). However, recent data also supports the efficacy of weight based, unmonitored SC UFH (initial dose of 333 units/kg followed by 250 units/kg every 12 hours) for the treatment of acute VTE, while transitioning to warfarin over a short period of time. The use of weight-based, unmonitored SC UFH has the potential to change the paradigm of VTE treatment and anticoagulant monitoring with UFH.[24] For non-obese patients, the actual body weight should be used to calculate the initial UFH dose.[1, 5, 25] For obese patients, using the actual body weight to calculate the initial dose is controversial. Some experts recommend using an adjusted body weight or a modified dosing weight instead.[26] The infusion rate is then adjusted based on laboratory monitoring of the patient's response.

Higher UFH dose requirements have been reported in patients with acute thrombosis, AT deficiency, and elevated factor VIII levels. The requirement of these higher unfractionated heparin doses is termed *heparin resistance*, and it should be suspected in patients who require more than 35,000–40,000 units (~25 units/kg/hour) of UFH in a 24-hour period.[1, 27]

> **Clinical Pearl**
>
> Lack of a measured response to heparin at rates > 25 units/kg/hour (resistance) can occur when lower antithrombin levels (<70%), or elevated factor VIII or fibrinogen levels are present. When heparin resistance is suspected, a non-antithrombin dependent anticoagulant agent such as a direct thrombin inhibitor can be considered as an alternative treatment option. If a LMWH is used in this setting, heparin resistance may not be recognized potentially resulting in subtherapeutic anticoagulation.

Monitoring

When used in full therapeutic doses, the administration of UFH requires frequent monitoring and subsequent dose adjustments due to intra and inter-patient variability of its anticoagulant response.[1, 28, 29] A variety of laboratory tests can be used to monitor the anticoagulant response to UFH, including the aPTT, ACT, anti-factor Xa activity, and plasma heparin concentrations measured by anti-factor-Xa inhibition or protamine titration assays.[1, 5, 30]

Despite its limitations, the aPTT is still the most widely used laboratory test in clinical practice to monitor the anticoagulant response to UFH. Historically, the therapeutic range of aPTT was con-

> **Clinical Pearl**
>
> Heparin is available in multiple strengths. To avoid potential medication errors, standardization of a bag concentration or identification of different strengths should be considered. Premixed heparin bags (25,000 units/250 mL D5W) are available to reduce potential compounding errors or delays in initiating therapy.

> **Clinical Pearl**
>
> Any time new reagents are purchased for determining the aPTT, the laboratory will need to recalibrate the aPTT target range. If a significant change in the sensitivity for a reagent batch occurs, there may be a notable change in the reported aPTT target ranges, which may be different than the ones listed on pre-established dosing and monitoring protocols. A process should be in place at each institution where any changes in the aPTT reagents are evaluated, and any necessary alteration in the therapeutic range is coordinated with all current heparin dosing protocols in advance of the reagent change.

sidered appropriate if maintained between 1.5 to 2.5 times the mean normal control value. However, due to variations in the reagents and instruments used to measure the aPTT in different laboratories, many reagents do not accurately measure the response to UFH within this fixed therapeutic range. Thus, each institution should establish its own specific therapeutic aPTT range for UFH calibrated for each instrument and reagent lot. This institution-specific aPTT therapeutic range needs to be correlated with a plasma heparin concentration of 0.3 to 0.7 units/mL by an amidolytic anti-factor Xa assay or with a plasma heparin concentration of 0.2 to 0.4 units/mL by protamine titration for the treatment of VTE. The exact therapeutic range for patients with acute coronary syndromes is not well established but it has been suggested at an upper limit of 0.6 units/mL.[1, 31]

The aPTT should be obtained at baseline, 6 hours after initiating the UFH infusion, and 6 hours after each dose change as this is the time required to reach steady-state. The UFH dose is then adjusted based on the specific aPTT measurement and the institutional-specific designated therapeutic range (see Table 11-5).[1, 30, 31]

When interpreting a given aPTT value, it is important to verify that the infusion rate was correct, and that there were no recent interruptions in the UFH infusion. It should also be noted that as the INR increases during concurrent warfarin therapy initiation, a corresponding rise in the aPTT may occur independent of any alterations in the heparin infusion. When "heparin resistance" is suspected, the use of anti-factor Xa concentrations by an assay process that does not incorporate the addition of AT may be an alternative option to the aPTT for UFH monitoring. In addition, the aPTT is not suitable to monitor heparin therapy in patients requiring doses of heparin that will produce serum concentrations > 1 unit/mL. The ACT is the recommended assay when high doses of heparin are used especially during coronary angioplasty or coronary bypass surgery.[1, 19, 27]

> **Clinical Pearl**
>
> In selected surgical procedures such as coronary bypass surgery, vascular surgery, extra corporeal membranous oxygenation (ECMO) or coronary interventions, higher amounts of UFH and ACT monitoring may be used. If the UFH is continued post procedure, it is important to confirm that the rate was appropriately reduced. Any subsequent aPTT measurements, if no reversal was used, may still be influenced by the higher infusion for 8 hours or so after adjusting the infusion rate downwards.

> **Clinical Pearl**
>
> Checking aPTT values earlier than 6 hours after initiating the UFH infusion may be considered, in order to determine if an adequate infusion rate is present (aPTT value close to baseline.) When interpreting this "early" aPTT value, it has to be noted that the bolus dose may artificially increase this reading. UFH bolus doses of > 5000 units can also have an effect on aPTT values drawn 8 hours later.

Several studies have demonstrated that the anti-factor Xa assay can be successfully used instead of the aPTT for UFH anticoagulant effect and dosage monitoring.[14, 15, 27] Levine et al. reported that heparin levels by protamine titration of 0.2 to 0.4 units/mL were equivalent to chromogenic heparin anti-factor Xa levels of 0.35 to 0.67 units/mL.[27] As some institutions have been transitioning to this alternative monitoring parameter for UFH, great care should be taken as recent reports showed variations in the equivalency between heparin levels by protamine titration and levels by anti-factor Xa activity that are instrument and laboratory assay dependent.[32-35] In one study, the average chromogenic anti-factor Xa levels that were equivalent to a heparin level of 0.2 units/mL and 0.4 units/mL by protamine sulfate titration were 0.27 units/mL and 0.44 units/mL[33] which is different than the ranges reported by Levine et al.[27] Significant differences in heparin anti-factor Xa levels were also reported when heparin levels were compared between different instruments and between different commercially available assays, suggesting that the therapeutic range for heparin anti-factor Xa analysis may need to be specific for the specific instrument and laboratory assay used.[35] In addition, adjusting UFH doses based on measured anti-Xa activity has not been validated nor correlated to improved clinical outcomes. More so, the anti-Xa activity assays may not measure some of the other anticoagulant effects of heparin.

Side Effects, Precautions, and Contraindications

Similar to other anticoagulant agents, bleeding is the most commonly associated side effect with UFH. The incidence of UFH associated bleeding complications is minimal with SC prophylactic doses, but higher (2% to 4%) with treatment doses given via IV infusion.[1, 5, 36, 37] The incidence of UFH associated bleeding increases with concurrent use of thrombolytics, glycoprotein IIb-IIIa inhibitors, and other antithrombotic agents. In addition, higher UFH doses have been linked to increased bleeding complications. The risk of UFH-induced bleeding is also increased in surgical or trauma patients, elderly, after invasive procedures, in patients with thrombocytopenia, heavy alcohol consumption, renal failure, neoplasms, and in cases where there is a pre-existing source of bleeding.[1, 4, 5, 37, 38] Patients receiving UFH should be closely monitored for signs and symptoms of bleeding complications. Symptoms will vary depending on the location of bleeding, and may include joint pain, chest pain, abdominal pain, severe headache, black tarry stools, blunt hematuria, and the passage of bright red blood per rectum. In cases of major bleeding complications, therapy should be stopped immediately and appropriate treatment and reversal measures provided. Minor bleeding complications include bruising, epistaxis, gingival bleeding, and prolonged bleeding from cuts.[4-6, 37] Interestingly, the evidence of linking elevated aPTT results and the risk of bleeding in patients treated with UFH is weak at best.[1, 19] As the risk of bleeding is closely related to the presence of underlying risk factors, before initiation of therapy, patients should be carefully screened for any contraindications to UFH.

Local irritation, pain at the injection site, erythema, histamine-like reactions (most commonly

> **Clinical Pearl**
>
> Patients with pork allergy cannot be treated with UFH derived from pork intestines. Fondaparinux, a factor-Xa inhibitor that is a synthetic molecule, can be used as an alternative therapeutic approach in patients with pork allergy and also patients who develop an allergic reaction from either UFH or an LMWH.

itching and burning on plantar side of the feet) and hematoma has been associated with SC UFH administration.[1, 4, 5, 8] In addition, hypersensitivity reactions with chills, fever, and urticaria have also been associated with UFH therapy.[4]

Alopecia, priapism, hyperkalemia, elevated ALT/AST levels, and osteoporosis have been reported with long-term use of UFH.[1, 4-6, 38] Drug interactions are limited with UFH, however, care should be used when given concurrently with other antithrombotic agents due to the increased potential for bleeding complications. Digitalis, nicotine, and antihistamines may counteract the anticoagulant effect of UFH.[4]

Heparin-associated thrombocytopenia (HAT) is a benign, transient, and mild non-immune mediated phenomena, generally occurring within the first few days of treatment in the heparin naïve patient. Platelet counts rarely drop below 100,000 in patients with HAT and recover with continued therapy. In contrast, heparin-induced thrombocytopenia (HIT) is a rare but extremely severe immune-mediated, drug-induced complication associated with UFH use. Once HIT is diagnosed or strongly suspected, prompt discontinuation of all heparin sources (including heparin flushes) and initiation of an alternative anticoagulant therapy is imperative.[39-41]

> **Clinical Pearl**
>
> In patients with HIT who are managed only by discontinuation of UFH, the risk of symptomatic thrombosis is 25% to 50%, and fatal thrombosis is 5%. Thus, in cases where there is a strong clinical suspicion of HIT, in addition to stopping UFH immediately, a direct thrombin inhibitor should be initiated even while waiting for laboratory confirmation for the diagnosis.

The drugs of choice for the treatment of HIT with or without thrombosis are the direct-thrombin inhibitors (DTIs; refer to Chapter 10 for more information on DTIs). Future use of UFH, especially within 3 to 6 months following the diagnosis of HIT, should be avoided. As PF4-heparin antibodies are transient and usually cleared within 3 months, patients with a history of HIT should be tested for HIT antibodies prior to any future use of UFH. Although there are limited data regarding the use of UFH in patients with a remote history of HIT, these patients should receive alternative anticoagulant agents for most indications until more rigorous data will be available.[42, 43]

In cases of typical-onset HIT, platelet counts begin to fall 5 to 10 days after exposure to UFH in heparin naïve individuals, and reach a threshold by days 7 to 14. In delayed-onset HIT, the development of thrombocytopenia can be delayed up to 20 to 40 days, and begin several days after heparin has been stopped in patients naive to heparin therapy. In contrast, rapid-onset HIT can occur very quickly (within 24 hours following UFH initiation), especially in patients with a recent exposure to heparin (i.e., previous 3 months).[40, 42, 44]

Platelet counts less then 150,000 mm^3 or a drop in platelet count greater than 50% from baseline is considered indicative of HIT. In addition to clinical findings, the diagnosis of HIT must be supplemented by laboratory tests confirming the presence of antibodies to heparin or platelet activation induced by heparin. Thrombosis development shortly after documenting thrombocytopenia is a characteristic finding in almost half of all the patients with HIT. Platelet count monitoring should be performed in patients receiving UFH. Before treatment is initiated a baseline platelet count should be documented, then followed by monitoring of platelet counts every other day for 14 days or until UFH therapy is discontinued, whichever occurs first.[40, 42, 43] If HIT occurs, it is crucial to document the occurrence of this reaction in the patient's medical record and educate the patient on this adverse effect so that future heparin use may be appropriately avoided.

> **Clinical Pearl**
>
> In some patients with documented HIT, the platelet count will drop 50% or more from the baseline value, but may not necessarily be less then 150,000. It is important to recognize this > 50% drop in platelet count as indicative of HIT. Development of thrombosis may occur well before the laboratory diagnosis of HIT is made. Thus, acute thrombosis in any patient receiving heparin therapy should be a red flag and these patients should be immediately evaluated for the presence of HIT.

> **Clinical Pearl**
>
> Delayed onset HIT has been reported with the use of heparin (UFH and LMWH.) In individuals who have been recently exposed to heparin and present with a new thrombotic event, a platelet count should be immediately done to assess the presence of HIT prior to initiating any form of heparin.

Low Molecular Weight Heparin

Developed in the 1980s, the LMWHs are smaller molecular weight fragments obtained by chemical or enzymatic depolymerization techniques of UFH.[1, 29] Three LMWH products are commercially available in the U.S.: dalteparin, enoxaparin, and tinzaparin. LMWHs are composed of a heterogeneous mixture of glycosaminoglycans, and vary slightly in their molecular weight distributions and pharmacologic properties (Table 11-1). LMWHs have improved pharmacodynamic and pharmacokinetic properties in comparison to UFH.[1, 6] The introduction of the LMWHs had a significant impact on how we administer anticoagulant therapy, particularly in the acute phase. Due to their convenience of use, these agents have been replacing the use of UFH in many clinical situations.

Pharmacology

Similar to UFH, LMWHs preclude the propagation and extension of formed thrombi.[1] Their anticoagulant effect is mediated through a specific pentasaccharide sequence that binds to AT and potentiates its activity. The smaller molecular weight (< 18 saccharide units in length) fragments cannot bind AT and thrombin simultaneously (see Figure 11-1). Less than 50% of the LMWH molecules have the 18 saccharide units chain length required for simultaneous binding of antithrombin and thrombin. Thus, LMWHs are more specific to inhibiting factor Xa than for inhibiting the activity of thrombin (factor IIa). Their anti-factor Xa:IIa activity ratio, which can vary between agents, ranges from 2:1 to approximately 4:1. In contrast, UFH has an antifactor Xa:IIa activity ratio of 1:1 (Table 11-1).[1, 3, 6, 45]

> **Clinical Pearl**
>
> The aPTT test is not an appropriate laboratory parameter to measure the effect of LMWH. LMWH have minimal effect on factor IIa, thus limited prolongation of aPTT may only be seen in cases of LMWH overdoses.

Pharmacokinetics/Pharmacodynamics

LMWHs have potentially desirable pharmacodynamic and pharmacokinetic properties compared to UFH.[1, 28] Due to a lower extent of binding to certain plasma and cellular proteins, LMWHs have a more predictable anticoagulant response. Therefore, routine dosage adjustments and monitoring of anticoagulation activity are not required in the majority of patients. Low molecular weight heparins have longer plasma half-lives, allowing once or twice daily administration, improved subcutaneous bioavailability, and dose-independent renal clearance.[1, 6, 29] While the absorption of SC UFH is poor and fairly unpredictable, the bioavailability of SC LMWHs is greater than 90%. After a SC LMWH dose, peak anticoagulant effect will occur within 3 to 5 hours. The elimination half-life varies slightly between the various LMWHs and is typically between 3 to 6 hours (see Table 11-1). The primary route of elimination for LMWHs is renal, thus in patients with renal impairment the half-life maybe prolonged.[1, 23, 46]

Indications

The use of LMWHs has been evaluated for several arterial and venous indications, including the treatment of acute coronary syndromes, treatment of VTE in the inpatient and outpatient settings, prevention of VTE in high-risk surgical and medical populations.[1, 6] The FDA-approved indications and recommended dosages vary between the available LMWHs (see Table 11-6). In addition to the FDA labeled indications, LMWHs have been evaluated for many off-label uses such as peri-procedure bridge therapy, prevention and treatment of thrombosis in pregnancy, prevention of VTE in stroke patients, acute spinal cord injury, neurosurgery, multiple trauma, critical illness, etc. LMWHs can also be used as a reasonable alternative to warfarin therapy in circumstances when warfarin therapy fails or is contraindicated, or when a prothrombin time/international normalized ratio (PT/INR) for warfarin, or aPTT for heparin therapy cannot be routinely obtained.[1]

Dosing and Administration

Dosing of the LMWHs will depend on the specific product and also on the indication for use (Table 11-6). Fixed dosages are generally used for prophylactic indications and weight-based dosing regimens are administered in cases of acute thrombotic complications such as for treatment of VTE and ACS.[6, 10, 23] The actual body weight should be used for dosing of LMWHs. Restricting the doses to a certain maximum limit, or "dose capping," is not recommended.[47-50] Pharmacokinetic studies in obese patients support dosing of LMWHs based on the actual body weight and do not show accumulation of LMWH concentrations in these patients

> **Clinical Pearl**
>
> Due to their quick onset of action, LMWH can be initiated and administered via the SC route, obviating the need for an initial IV bolus dose in cases of acute venous thrombosis.

> **Clinical Pearl**
>
> In patients with acute thrombosis, the practice of dose capping or setting a limit of the maximum amount of LMWH administered independent of patient weight is not recommended. The practice of dose-capping can lead to under-dosing in heavy weight patients and a potential increase in recurrent VTE.

when compared to average weight patients.[51, 52]

LMWHs are usually administered by SC injection in the abdominal wall area or the upper outer part of the thighs.[53] IV bolus doses (enoxaparin 30 mg IV along with the first SC dose or if > 8 hours after the initial SC dose and going for percutaneous coronary intervention) have also been evaluated in the setting of ACS.[16] After an SC injection, LMWHs result in sustained antithrombotic activity allowing a dosing interval of every 12 or 24 hours depending on the indication and the specific agent (Table 11-6).

When given as larger (once-daily) doses, a significantly higher peak plasma concentration will occur.[51] The dose for enoxaparin is expressed

Table 11-6.
Indications and Recommended Doses for LMWHs and Fondaparinux

Indications	Enoxaparin	Dalteparin	Tinzaparin	Fondaparinux
VTE Prophylaxis after Hip-Replacement Surgery	30 mg SC Q12 h initiated 12–24 h after surgery OR 40 mg SC Q24 h initiated 10–12 h prior to surgery.	2500 units SC given 6–8 h after surgery, then 5,000 units SC Q24 h OR 5000 units SC Q 24 h initiated the evening prior to surgery	75 units/kg SC Q24 h initiated the evening prior to surgery or 12–24 h after surgery* OR 4500 units SC Q 24 h initiated 12 h prior to surgery*	2.5 mg SC Q24 h initiated 6–8 h after surgery
VTE Prophylaxis after Hip-Fracture Surgery	30 mg SC Q12 h initiated 12–24 h after surgery*	NA	NA	2.5 mg SC Q24 h initiated 6–8 h after surgery
VTE Prophylaxis after Knee-Replacement Surgery	30 mg SC Q12 h initiated 12–24 h after surgery	2500 units SC given 6–8 h after surgery, then 5,000 units SC Q24*	75 units/kg SC Q24 h initiated the evening prior to surgery or 12–24 h after surgery*	2.5 mg SC Q24 h initiated 6–8 h after surgery
VTE Prophylaxis after Abdominal Surgery	40 mg SC Q24 h initiated 1–2 h prior to surgery	2500 units SC 1–2 h prior to surgery, then 2500 units 12 h after surgery followed by 5000 units SC Q24 h	3500 units SC Q 24 h initiated 1–2 h prior to surgery*	2.5 mg SC Q24 h initiated 6–8 h after surgery
VTE Prophylaxis in Acute Medical Illness	40 mg SC Q24 h	5000 units SC Q 24 h	NA	2.5 mg SC Q24 h*
Treatment of VTE (DVT +/- PE)	1 mg/kg SC Q12 h OR 1.5 mg/kg SC Q24 h	100 units/kg SC Q12 h[b] OR 200 units/kg SC Q24 h[b]	175 units/kg SC Q24 h	5 mg SC Q 24 h if weight < 50 kg 7.5 mg SC Q 24 h if weight 50–100 kg 10 mg SC Q 24 h if weight > 100 kg
Unstable Angina or Non-Q-Wave MI	1 mg/kg SC Q12 h[a]	120 units/kg SC Q12 h[b] (maximum dose 10,000 units)	NA	2.5 mg SC Q 24 h*

*Non-FDA approved for indication.

[a]An additional 30-mg IV bolus with the first SC dose has been studied in clinical trials. NA = date not available.

[b]Dalteparin is now FDA approved for the extended treatment of VTE in cancer patients at a dose of 200 units/kg daily given SC for one month, then 150 units/kg daily SC for 5 months. Dalteparin, at doses of 200 units/kg daily SC OR 100 units/kg twice daily SC, has also been evaluated in the treatment of acute VTE (DVT ± PE).

> **Clinical Pearl**
>
> Intermittent dosing regimens for LMWH or fondaparinux should be written as Q 24 hours instead of Q day, or Q 12 hours instead of BID, in order to avoid overlapping therapy (overdosing) secondary to pre-established institutional dosing times. For example, a first dose of a once-daily regimen may be initially given at 0400, and then repeated at 0900 at the daily-established medication administration time.

in milligrams, while dalteparin and tinzaparin are expressed in units of antifactor Xa activity.[1, 6, 46] Pre-filled syringes are available for enoxaparin (treatment and prophylaxis) and dalteparin (prophylaxis). For treatment doses of enoxaparin, the extent of rounding to the nearest 5-mg, 10-mg, or syringe size (or nearest 1–2000 units for dalteparin and tinzaparin for treatment) is unclear. Considering that this class of agents has a therapeutic range wide enough to not necessitate routine monitoring, rounding to the nearest syringe size (weight > 50 kg) is probably feasible in most situations.

Monitoring

Due to the predictable dose-response of LMWHs, routine monitoring of their anticoagulant effect is not necessary in patients whose condition is stable and uncomplicated.[1, 54] The PT, aPTT, and ACT are inappropriate laboratory markers to monitor the anticoagulant effect, as they are only minimally affected by LMWHs. Prior to initiation of LMWH, a baseline PT/INR, aPTT, CBC with platelet count, and serum creatinine should be obtained and documented. Renal function should be periodically assessed during the course of therapy. As HIT is also a concern with LMWH, albeit at a lower incidence than with UFH, platelet counts should be monitored every few (2 to 3) days during the first 2 weeks of therapy, and then periodically thereafter.[1, 6, 29, 40, 42]

While not routinely recommended, measuring a patient's response to LMWH may be warranted in certain high-risk situations such as patients with morbid obesity (weigh more than 150 kg or body mass index more than 50 kg/m^2), very low body weight (less than 50 kg), significant renal impairment (CrCl less than 30 mL/min), neonates and pediatric patients, and pregnant women.[1, 47, 50, 54] In addition, monitoring can also be considered in patients who receive extended therapy (> 1 month) with LMWHs such as cancer patients. Although controversial, measurement of the chromogenic anti factor-Xa activity has been the most widely used method in clinical practice to measure a patient's response to LMWH and is the method recommended by the College of American Pathologists and the 7th ACCP Conference on Antithrombotic and Thrombolytic Therapy.[1, 54] In the setting of major renal failure, it should be noted that other anticoagulant effects may become predomi-

> **Clinical Pearl**
>
> Although an absolute correlation between LMWH anti-Xa activity and patient efficacy and safety outcomes have not been clearly established and its use is highly controversial, until better markers for LMWH monitoring will be developed, the anti-factor Xa activity is considered the best biological marker to aid with LMWH dosing and is used in practice in the specific scenarios highlighted above.

nant, and separately, the approaches to hemodialysis can influence outcomes independent from the measured anti-Xa activity. Given the limited evidence correlating outcomes with dosing adjustments based on anti-Xa activity, its use as a sole factor for adjusting therapy should be cautioned.

When measuring anti-Xa activity, the sample should be obtained after steady-state concentrations of the LMWH are attained, after the 2nd to 3rd dose. Most available data in the literature support the measurement of peak concentrations, which occur approximately 4 hours after a subcutaneous dose.[47, 55] Trough concentrations can be

> **Clinical Pearl**
>
> Dosing of various LMWHs can be at times confusing as some agents are dosed in milligrams/weight and others as units of antifactor Xa activity/weight. As a practical conversion tool, 1 mg of LMWH-enoxaparin is equivalent to 100 international units antifactor Xa activity.

more useful to rule out drug accumulation, such as in patients with renal failure, and are typically measured just prior to the next dose of the LMWH. While there is some variation in the target concentrations reported in the literature, peak anti-Xa concentrations of 0.1–0.4 units/mL with twice daily dosing are recommended for prevention of VTE, but a more conservative range is 0.2 to 0.4 units/mL. For the treatment of VTE, peak concentrations of 0.4–1.1 units/mL with twice daily dosing have been suggested, but a more conservative therapeutic range is 0.5–1.0 units/mL. With once daily dosing, as higher doses of drug are given per dose, peak concentrations of 1.0–2.0 units/mL have been suggested, but supporting data is even more limited. Although no clear correlation of anti-Xa activity with efficacy and safety outcomes exists, some data suggests that anti-Xa concentrations of greater than 1.0 units/mL in venous indications and greater than 1.5 units/mL in arterial indications have been associated with an increased risk of bleeding.[1, 54-56] Specific algorithms for dosing adjustments based on antifactor Xa activity have not been widely evaluated and are limited at the present time. One dosing approach has been suggested in pediatric patients that can also be potentially applied in adult populations (see Table 11-7).[57]

Side Effects, Precautions, and Contraindications

Similar to UFH, bleeding is the most common complication associated with LMWHs.[1, 37] The frequency of major or life threatening bleeding appears to be similar or in some reports lower with LMWHs than with UFH,[58] although this has not been consistently demonstrated in individual clinical trials. In patients at a high acute risk for bleeding, an UFH infusion for ease of adjusting and reversing anticoagulant effects may be desired. Bruising at the injection site is frequently reported with the use of LMWHs. The incidence of bleeding varies with the patient population treated, the indication, dose, and specific LMWH administered.[1, 37, 46]

Spinal and epidural hematomas have been linked to the use of LMWHs in patients undergoing spinal and epidural anesthesia or spinal puncture.[1, 10, 59] Concurrent use of LMWH and all other agents that impact hemostasis in patients with in-dwelling epidural catheters should be strictly avoided as they further enhance the risk of spinal hematoma formation.[10, 59] When inserting and removing the in-dwelling epidural catheters, great care should be used in appropriately coordinating the timing of the dosing of LMWH (see Table 11-8).

> **Clinical Pearl**
>
> When monitoring anti-Xa activity, verify that the level was drawn at the pre-selected time post dose (i.e., 4 hours post dose for peak levels), and is consistently done this way for subsequent measurements.

Table 11-7.
Sample LMWH Dosing Nomogram for Pediatric Patients

AntiXa Level	Hold Next Dose	Dosage Change	Next AntiXa Level
<0.35 units/mL	No	↑ 25%	4 h after next dose
0.35–0.49	No	↑ 10%	4 h after next dose
0.5–1.0	No	No	Next day, then in 1 week, then monthly
1.1–1.5	No	↓ 20%	Before next dose
1.6–2.0	3 h	↓ 30%	Before next dose and 4 h after next dose
>2.0 units/mL	Until antiXa < 0.5 units/mL	↓ 40%	Before next dose and q12h until antiXa <0.5 units/mL

Source: Adapted from: Monagle P, et al. *Chest.* 2001;119 (suppl 1):344–70.

> **Clinical Pearl**
>
> In patients with planned invasive or surgical procedures associated with increased risk of bleeding, the presence of an LMWH should be recognized and the dose held in a sufficient amount of time to allow for drug elimination in order to reduce potential bleeding complications but at the same time minimizing the risk for thrombosis. This step should be repeated post procedure in determining the appropriate time of restarting anticoagulation.

The incidence if HIT is lower with LMWH compared to UFH.[60] However, low molecular weight heparins cross-react with heparin antibodies *in vitro* and should not be given as an alternative anticoagulant in patients with a diagnosis of HIT. Similarly to UFH, platelet counts should be monitored in all patients receiving an LMWH preparation and any signs of thrombocytopenia should be thoroughly evaluated.[1, 40, 42] The risk of osteoporosis appears to be lower with the long-term use of LMWHs when compared to UFH.[1, 46, 61, 62]

Fondaparinux

Pharmacology

Fondaparinux is the first agent in a class of synthetic anticoagulants that selectively inhibit factor Xa activity. Also known as "pentasaccharide," its molecule is composed of the five specific saccharide units that bind to antithrombin (see Figure 11-1).[2, 6] Similar to UFH and LMWH, fondaparinux, by modifying antithrombin activity, is an indirect inhibitor of factor Xa. Through its interaction with antithrombin, fondaparinux inhibits factor-Xa, which in turn mediates the ultimate steps in the coagulation cascade of inhibiting thrombin generation and thrombus formation. The binding of fondaparinux to antithrombin causes a conformational change in the antithrombin's active site which in turn enhances anti-factor Xa activity by approximately 300-fold. The fondaparinux-antithrombin bond is reversible in nature, and the fondaparinux molecule is released to bind several other antithrombin molecules.[2, 7, 63]

In contrast to UFH and LMWH, at therapeutic plasma concentrations, fondaparinux has no direct effect on thrombin (factor IIa) activity. The selective inhibition of factor Xa without a direct effect on thrombin preserves its regulatory functions in the control of hemostasis, which may confer some beneficial characteristics to fondaparinux in wound healing. Unlike UFH or LMWH, fondaparinux does not affect platelet function. As synthetic drugs, factor-Xa inhibitors like fondaparinux cannot transmit animal pathogens, are consistent from batch-to-batch, and can be available in an unlimited supply.[3, 29, 64] This may also be a factor to consider if a non-porcine derived product is requested by a patient for religious concerns.

> **Clinical Pearl**
>
> To date, no cases of HIT have been reported with the use of fondaparinux. Although published data is very limited, the use of SC fondaparinux in cases of sub-acute HIT (platelets are recovered) as a bridge to warfarin therapy can be an attractive alternative to agents like argatroban or lepirudin. The dose in this setting has not been established and may depend on the specific indication for use.

> **Clinical Pearl**
>
> Removal of epidural catheters should be timed and performed at trough LMWH concentrations, i.e., after a minimum of 12 hours has elapsed after the last dose of the LMWH in patients with normal renal function. The next LMWH dose should not be given sooner then 2 hours after removing the catheter (also see Table 11-8).

Pharmacokinetics/Pharmacodynamics

After subcutaneous administration, fondaparinux is completely (100%) absorbed and peak plasma concentrations are reached within 2 to 3 hours.[2, 63] A long elimination half-life of 17 to 21 hours allows once daily administration, however the anticoagulant effect of fondaparinux will persist for 2 to 4 days after stopping the drug. In patients with renal impairment the anticoagulant effect persists even longer.[2, 6, 65]

Table 11-8.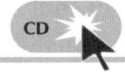

Recommendations for Timing of Anticoagulant Agents in Patients Undergoing Neuraxial Procedures

Anticoagulant Agent	Minimum Time Between Anticoagulant Dose and Insertion of Spinal Needle or Placement of Epidural Catheter	Minimum Time Between Insertion of Spinal Needle or Placement of Epidural Catheter and Anticoagulant Dose	Minimum Time Between Anticoagulant Dose and Removal of the Epidural Catheter	Minimum Time Between Removal of the Epidural Catheter and Anticoagulant Dose
Therapeutic dose UFH (IV or SC)	aPTT < 40 seconds and > 4 h post IV infusion or > 12 h post SC dose	Avoid while catheter is in place	Avoid while catheter is in place; aPTT < 40 seconds and > 4 h post IV infusion or > 12 h post SC dose when anticoagulant effect is at minimum	2 h
Prophylactic dose SC UFH (5,000 units q12h or q8h)	No Time Restrictions Apply			
Fondaparinux: therapeutic or prophylactic doses	36 to 48 h*	Avoid while catheter is in place	Ideally avoid while catheter is in place; Just before the next dose and when anticoagulant effect is at minimum	2 h
Therapeutic dose LMWH (enoxaparin 1mg/kg SC q12h or enoxaparin 1.5 mg/kg SC q24h or dalteparin 100 units/kg SC q12h or dalteparin 200 units/kg SC q24h or tinzaparin 175 units/kg SC q24h)	24 h*	Avoid while catheter is in place	Ideally avoid while catheter is in place; Just before the next dose and when anticoagulant effect is at minimum	2 h
Prophylactic dose LMWH (enoxaparin 30mg SC q12h or enoxaparin 40mg SC q24h or dalteparin 5,000 units SC q24h)	10 to 12 h*	Avoid while catheter is in place	Ideally avoid while catheter is in place; Just before the next dose and when anticoagulant effect is at minimum	2 h

* Longer elimination times will be required in patients with impaired renal function. h = hours.
Source: Horlocker 2003.[59]

> **Clinical Pearl**
>
> To minimize bleeding in patients receiving fondaparinux and who are scheduled for surgical intervention, careful timing of the procedure should be considered as the effect of fondaparinux can persist even as long as 2–4 days after the last dose.

Fondaparinux binds specifically to antithrombin and unlike heparin it does not bind to other cellular proteins such as albumin, glycoprotein, platelets, or platelet factor 4.[2, 3, 63] Due to a predictable and linear dose-response relationship, fondaparinux does not require routine coagulation monitoring or dose adjustments. It is distributed in the blood and elimination is mainly renal as unchanged drug. In patients with renal impairment drug accumulation has been reported.[2, 6, 29, 64] Due to an increased risk of bleeding, fondaparinux is contraindicated in patients with severe renal dysfunction (creatinine clearance < 30 mL/min). As fondaparinux is not metabolized in the liver, it has no major pharmacokinetic drug interactions. However, care should be used when fondaparinux is used concurrently with other antithrombotic agents due to an increased risk of bleeding complications.[65]

Indications

Fondaparinux has been evaluated and has demonstrated efficacy in the prevention and treatment of both venous and arterial thrombosis.[66-68] Fondaparinux is FDA-approved for the prevention of VTE following orthopedic (hip fracture, hip replacement, and knee replacement) surgery, prevention of VTE following abdominal surgery, and for the treatment of acute DVT and PE.[65] Fondaparinux has also been evaluated for the prevention of VTE in medical patients and in the treatment of patients with ACS, however these indications are not currently approved by the FDA.[69-71]

Dosing and Administration

When used for VTE prevention after abdominal surgery, orthopedic surgery, and in medically ill patients, the dose of fondaparinux is 2.5 mg injected subcutaneously once daily (Table 11-6). In surgical patients, the first dose is typically initiated 6 to 8 hours following surgery. Initiating fondaparinux too soon (i.e., < 6 hours) after surgery should be avoided as there is a direct relationship between the timing of the first dose and the risk of major bleeding complications.[65, 66] In cases where immediate post-operative bleeding is a concern, delaying the initiation of the first dose of fondaparinux until the morning after the orthopedic surgery has also been demonstrated to be effective.[72] For VTE prevention, the usual duration of therapy ranges from 5 to 14 days, depending on the patient population and the specific indication. After hip fracture or hip replacement surgery, fondaparinux can also be given as extended VTE prophylaxis for up to 30 days.[10]

> **Clinical Pearl**
>
> The dose of fondaparinux for obese patients (> 100 kg) with VTE is 10 mg SC every 24 hours, and it is not necessary to adjust upwards to total body weight as is the case for the LMWHs.

Interestingly, in the treatment of patients with ACS, the same dosing regimen of 2.5 mg given subcutaneously once daily has been demonstrated to be effective, similar for its use in VTE prevention.[69, 70] The lower dosing regimen of 2.5 mg once daily was selected for the ACS indications due to a lack of dose-efficacy response of fondaparinux at higher doses in the initial Phase II dose ranging studies.[73] Similarly, no dose response for recurrent thrombosis or bleeding with doses up to 10 mg were observed for use in the initial treatment of DVT or PE. Since the higher doses demonstrated to be effective, the phase III trials for DVT and separately PE used dosing based on the patient's actual body weight.[67, 68] For patients who weigh between 50 kg to 100 kg, the dose of fondaparinux is 7.5 mg given SC once daily. Patients who weigh more than 100 kg should be given 10 mg once daily and those who weigh less than 50 kg should receive only 5

> **Clinical Pearl**
>
> Care should be used when fondaparinux is used for an extended time (> 7–10 days) in patients with moderate renal impairment (CrCl 30–50 mL/min), as accumulation of the drug has also been reported in these patients at a rate of approximately 40%.[65]

mg daily. Similar to the LMWHs, fondaparinux is administered via the SC route as a once-daily injection. Injection sites include the abdominal wall and the upper, outer parts of the thighs, and the site should be alternated with each injection.[65]

Monitoring

In patients treated with fondaparinux, due to its predictable dose-response, routine monitoring of coagulation parameters is not required.[2, 63] Fondaparinux has no clinically relevant effect on coagulation tests such as the thrombin time, aPTT and PT. In certain high-risk circumstances (suspected over- or under-dosing, renal insufficiency or severe bleeding complications) anti-factor Xa measurement may be considered in order to examine the biologic activity of fondaparinux in comparison to its plasma concentration and for dose guiding. However, caution must be used as the specific parameters for testing and monitoring are not as well defined for this agent as for the heparins, and as mentioned for phase II trials in ACS and VTE, no dose-related response between bleeding and recurrent thrombotic complications were noted up to 10 mg.[6, 50, 74, 75] When measuring the biologic activity of fondaparinux, the use of a chromogenic anti-factor Xa assay and a fondaparinux standard curve should be used. Chromogenic anti-factor Xa assays calibrated with fondaparinux have been shown to reach the equivalence criteria for plasma samples and provide fairly reliable results.[74-76] Prophylactic treatment with 2.5 mg of fondaparinux in orthopedic surgery patients resulted in concentrations between 0.2 and 0.7 mcg/mL at 3 hours after the subcutaneous injection.[77]

Renal function should be documented at baseline and then closely monitored during the course of therapy. If the creatinine clearance drops below 30 mL/min, fondaparinux therapy should be held. Patients receiving treatment with fondaparinux should be closely monitored for signs and symptoms of bleeding complications. Care should be used especially in patients with a creatinine clearance between 30 and 50 mL/min as drug accumulation can occur. As with other anticoagulants, a CBC should be monitored periodically to screen for possible occult bleeding. In patients who received spinal anesthesia, close monitoring for any signs and symptoms of neurological impairment should be performed.[2, 6, 29, 63]

Side Effects, Precautions, and Contraindications

Similar to the heparins, bleeding is the major side effect associated with fondaparinux therapy. An inverse correlation between patient weight and major bleeding complications has been reported with the VTE prophylaxis dose (2.5 mg) of fondaparinux.[63, 65, 66] Fondaparinux is contraindicated for VTE prophylaxis in patients who weigh less than 50 kg. The VTE treatment dose is reduced to 5 mg given every 24 hours in patients who weigh less than 50 kg.[65] Due to its long half-life and the risk of spinal hematoma, great caution should be used if fondaparinux is administered in patients receiving neuraxial or spinal anesthesia. Appropriate timing of the fondaparinux dosing and also the timing of the placement and pulling of the epidural catheter is extremely critical (Table 11-8).[59, 78] Thrombocytopenia has been reported to a similar extent as with the LMWHs, however no cases of heparin-induced thrombocytopenia have been reported to date with fondaparinux.[2, 63, 64]

Reversal of Anticoagulant Effect

Unfractionated Heparin

Protamine sulfate is the antidote used to reverse the anticoagulant effect of UFH.[1, 79, 80] To minimize the risk of severe adverse reactions such as hypotension and bradycardia linked to its administration, protamine should be given as a slow IV infusion over 3 to 5 minutes. Once administered, protamine neutralizes the effect of UFH in approximately 5 minutes and its activity will last for approximately 2 hours. One mg of protamine sulfate neutralizes approximately 100 units of UFH. The maximum recommended single dose of protamine is 50 mg, however multiple repeated doses may be necessary if hemorrhage persists. Due to the short half-life of UFH ($\sim$ 60 min) when given as an IV infusion, only the dose given over the last 3–4 hours needs to be included in the protamine dose calculation. When given via the SC route, a longer protamine infusion time or repeated administration may be necessary. The patient's coagulation status should be closely monitored using the aPTT test in order to assess response to protamine therapy.[1, 80, 81]

Clinical Pearl

If measurement of anti-factor Xa activity is necessary while a patient is treated with fondaparinux therapy, expect 4-hours peak levels to be higher then those we see typically with the LMWHs as fondaparinux is a pure factor-Xa inhibitor.

LMWH

While there is no complete antidote for LMWHs, protamine can be used as a partial reversal agent for the effects of LMWH.[1, 79] Although protamine neutralizes the antithrombin activity of LMWH, it only neutralizes approximately 60% of their anti-factor Xa activity.[1, 82, 83] If LMWH was given in the previous 8 hours, then 1 mg of protamine should be administered for every 100 units (or 1 mg) of the LMWH. If the LMWH dose was given in the previous 8 to 12 hours, a 0.5-mg dose of protamine should be given for every 100 anti-factor Xa units. The use of protamine sulfate is not recommended if the LMWH was administered more than 12 hours earlier.[1, 79, 81]

Fondaparinux

Fondaparinux is not reversed by protamine, and at this time no specific antidote is available to reverse

> **Clinical Pearl**
>
> Patients with fish allergies are at risk for developing anti-protamine antibodies and allergic reactions to protamine. These patients can be pretreated with steroids and antihistamines.

its antithrombotic activity.[79] In the event of major bleeding, fresh frozen plasma and factor concentrates should be given. In the case of a life-threatening bleed, recombinant factor VIIa has been shown to reverse effects in vitro for 2–4 hours, but is a very costly option and can also promote thrombosis formation.[84, 85]

Special Patient Populations

In selected high-risk populations, such as patients at high risk of bleeding, need for emergent invasive procedures, and presence of renal insufficiency, UFH often is the preferred anticoagulant agent because of its relatively short half-life and its potential for rapid reversal. Acute traumatic injury or extra-corporeal membranous oxygenation (ECMO) are frequently associated with reduced levels of AT and an increased risk for thromboembolic complications. In such situations, a heparin infusion may be desired over other anticoagulants due to the ease of frequently measuring and evaluating the anticoagulant effect.

> **Clinical Pearl**
>
> In patients with anasarca, reduced bioavailability of SC injections may preclude the potential for achieving adequate anticoagulation for either UFH or LMWH. In such situations, UFH infusion targeting a low-intensity increase in the aPTT may be used for VTE prophylaxis.

Renal Impairment

The elimination of UFH is dose-dependent and due to its ability to be monitored and dose adjusted, its use in patients with renal impairment has not been historically considered a major clinical challenge. Irrespective of the anticoagulant used, a higher incidence of major bleeding exists as renal function declines. Thus, UFH may be the preferred agent for patients with notable renal dysfunction, or those requiring hemodialysis.[1, 86] In the setting of intermittent hemodialysis, minimal amounts of systemic heparin may be used, and the dialyzer may be pre-bathed in heparin. In extended duration therapies, and more so in continuous renal replacement therapies, a greater intensity of anticoagulation (typically using heparin) is necessary. Rates can depend on the type on hemodialysis involved. In contrast, the LMWHs and fondaparinux are primarily cleared via renal excretion and pharmacokinetic data suggests that as renal function decreases, the half-life of LMWHs and fondaparinux increases, and their clearance decreases.[87, 88] Reduced elimination can result in increased drug concentrations and an increased bleeding risk. The actual degree of accumulation is different for the various LMWHs and fondaparinux, as there are differences in their pharmacologic profiles (Table 11-9).

Because the large clinical trials have generally excluded patients with renal impairment, efficacy and safety outcomes in these patients are not well-documented, and clear dosing and monitoring guidelines are lacking for most of the agents.[47, 88] Dosing estimates can be however inferred from our understanding of kinetic studies with the various agents. The 7th ACCP panel and many other experts still recommend the use of UFH to provide full therapeutic anticoagulation in patients with severe renal impairment (CrCl less than 30 mL/min).[1, 88] If LMWH is used, then monitoring of anti-Xa activity should be considered in patients with a CrCl less than 30 mL/min, or in patients with mod-

Table 11-9.
Dosing and Monitoring Considerations for LMWH and Fondaparinux in Patients with Renal Impairment

Anticoagulant	Pharmacokinetic Considerations	Dosing and Monitoring Recommendations	Package Insert Recommendations
Dalteparin	CrCl < 30* mL/min: no accumulation noted up to 1 week of therapy CrCl 30 to 50 mL/min: no accumulation noted	CrCl < 30* mL/min: no dose adjustment needed up to 1 week For use > 1 week, consider monitoring of anti-Xa activity and adjust dose if accumulation is noted CrCl 30 to 50 mL/min: no dose adjustment needed	CrCl < 30* mL/min: use with caution
Enoxaparin	CrCl < 30* mL/min: 40% to 50% accumulation noted CrCl 30 to 50 mL/min: 15 to 20% accumulation noted	CrCl < 30* mL/min: Consider a 40% to 50% dose decrease and subsequent monitoring of anti-Xa activity CrCl 30 to 50 mL/min: Consider a 15% to 20% dose decrease with prolonged use (> 10–14 days) and subsequent monitoring of anti-Xa activity	CrCl < 30* mL/min: Prophylaxis–30mg SC daily Treatment–1mg/kg SC daily
Tinzaparin	CrCl < 30* mL/min: 20% accumulation noted CrCl 30 to 50 mL/min: no accumulation noted	CrCl < 30* mL/min: consider a dose decrease of 20% and subsequent monitoring of anti-Xa activity CrCl 30 to 50 mL/min: no dose adjustment needed	CrCl < 30* mL/min: use with caution
Fondaparinux	CrCl < 30* mL/min: 55% accumulation noted CrCl 30 to 50 mL/min: 40% accumulation noted	CrCl < 30 mL/min: only use if able to measure anti-Xa activity to guide with dose adjustment CrCl 30 to 50 mL/min: if prolonged use (> 10–14 days) consider measurement of anti-Xa activity to guide with dose adjustment	CrCl < 30 mL/min: contraindicated CrCl 30 to 50 mL/min: use with caution

* Data is very limited in patients with a CrCl < 20 mL/min; in patients on hemodialysis, limited data is only available for thrombosis prevention in the dialysis circuit but NOT for the prevention and/or treatment of venous or arterial thrombosis. Thus, until further data is available UFH is the agent of choice in patients on hemodialysis or with a CrCl < 20 mL/min.

erate renal impairment with a CrCl 30–50 mL/min and if the LMWHs are used for extended periods of time (greater than 10–14 days).[1,55,56] Fondaparinux is contraindicated in patients with CrCl < 30 mL/min, and care should be used when administered in patients with CrCl of 30 to 50 mL/min as drug accumulation can occur, especially with prolonged used (see Table 11-9).[29,65] Elderly patients are also more likely to have decreased renal function and careful assessment of renal status should be conducted prior to initiating therapy with any of these agents.

Extremes of Body Weight

Total body weight appears to be a good predictor for dosing of LMWHs in obese patients. Setting a maximum dose (or dose capping) is not recommended, and in fact it may result in under-dosing of these patients with a potential increase in thrombotic complications.[48,55,56] Monitoring of anti-Xa activity is generally not recommended; however, as only a very limited number of patients with total body weight greater than 150 kg have been included in the large LMWH treatment clinical trials, it may be reasonable to consider anti-factor Xa measurement in these patients for the purposes of dose guiding.[1, 54, 56] For prophylaxis indications, available data suggest that fixed LMWH doses may not be sufficient in morbidly obese patients.[55, 56] In the absence of clear dosing guidelines of LMWHs for prophylaxis in obese patients, a 25%–30% dose increase or weight based dosing of 50 units/kg/day may be considered.[1, 47, 56]

In contrast, low weight patients (i.e., < 50 kg) may be at risk for drug accumulation and bleeding complications when fixed prophylactic doses of LMWH or fondaparinux are administered. Due to a concern of increased bleeding complications, when used for VTE prophylaxis in surgical patients, fondaparinux is contraindicated in patients who weigh less than 50 kg. When used for VTE treatment, the dose of fondaparinux is lowered to 5 mg daily in patients who weigh less than 50 kg.[1, 56, 65]

Pregnancy

The heparins, UFH or LMWH, are the anticoagulants of choice during pregnancy.[62] UFH is FDA pregnancy category C, and as it does not cross the placenta it has not been associated with teratogenicity.[89] During the last trimester and in the peripartum period, UFH should be used with caution in order to minimize the risk of potential maternal hemorrhage. UFH is not excreted in breast milk and can be used safely by women who are breastfeeding. The LMWHs (dalteparin, enoxaparin, and tinzaparin) are classified as FDA pregnancy category B, they do not cross the placenta, and are not excreted in breast milk.[61, 62] The LMWHs appear to be relatively safe to use during pregnancy and are an attractive alternative to UFH when long-term anticoagulation therapy is required. In contrast to UFH, the LMWHs do not appear to affect bone formation with long-term administration. Because the pharmacokinetics of low-molecular-weight heparins may change during pregnancy, monitoring anti-Xa activity every 3 to 4 weeks for dose guiding should be considered.[61, 62] Induction of labor is advisable so that UFH and LMWH can be discontinued prior to delivery to minimize the risk for excessive bleeding during delivery.[62]

Fondaparinux is categorized as FDA pregnancy category B as it does not appear to cross the placental barrier.[65, 90] There is limited information regarding the use of fondaparinux during pregnancy.[91] Fondaparinux is excreted in the milk of lactating rats, but excretion in human milk is unknown. Until more data becomes available, UFH and LMWH should remain the agents of choice in pregnant patients.[65]

> **Clinical Pearl**
>
> Women who develop HIT during pregnancy or have a recent history of HIT (e.g., less than 3 months) cannot use UFH or LMWH safely. Potential treatment alternatives with a DTI should be considered. Lepirudin is known to cross the placenta, however case reports suggest it may be safe for the management of HIT with thrombosis in pregnancy. Limited case reports suggest that fondaparinux may also be a future potential alternative in pregnant patients, however, a dose has not been established.

Pediatric Patients

UFH and LMWH are commonly used anticoagulants in children requiring antithrombotic therapy. The most common form of thrombosis in children is usually seen in the upper extremity where vascular access lines have been placed. For the treatment of acute thrombosis, the dosage of UFH will vary with age. An initial loading dose of 75 to 100 units/kg over 10 minutes followed by a maintenance dose of 28 units/kg/hour for infants up to 12 months and 20 units/kg/hour for children 1 year old or greater has been suggested.[92, 93] Unfortunately, heparin adjustment protocols and algorithms are not readily available in the pediatric population. Some algorithms have proposed adjustments based on a percentage of the dose. In patients requiring very small amounts of UFH, the required changes in infusion rate may be very small, thus requiring a considerable amount of time to achieve desired target values. In contrast, high infusion rates may lead to overshooting the target values secondary to more notable changes required in the infusion rate. It should also be noted that most of the laboratory target values are based on data from adults, and have not been necessarily validated in the pediatric population.[92]

Due to their convenience of use, the LMWHs are becoming the preferred agents in pediatric populations despite limited data to test their safety and effectiveness in this setting. Weight-based LMWH doses provide a less predictable anticoagulant response in children compared to adults, thus periodic monitoring of anti-Xa activity for dose guiding should be considered (Table 11-7).[92, 94] Neonates or infants are at increased risk for having antithrombin deficiency. Various anti-Xa activity assays are currently available that may or may not include a step to spike the sample with antithrombin prior to measuring. If such a step is present, the presence of subtherapeutic anticoagulation may be missed. Because of the challenges in monitoring UFH or using warfarin in pediatric patients, the use of LMWHs has been explored. Although the incidence of HIT in pediatric patients is most likely lower then in adults, HIT has also been reported in these patients and it should be considered when monitoring therapy.[95]

For enoxaparin, suggested therapeutic doses are 1.5 mg/kg every 12 hours for infants younger then 2 months and 1.0 mg/kg every 12 hours for those older then 2 months. The suggested dose for dalteparin is 86 to 172 units/kg every 24 hours keeping in mind that neonates appear to require higher doses/kg than older children or adults.[92,94,96] Fondaparinux use in pediatric populations has not been studied. When used in smaller doses, enoxaparin may have to be diluted to accurately allow for measurement of the dose. This dilution has been shown to maintain appropriate anti-Xa activity for up to 2 weeks.[97]

Conclusion

A complexity of factors can affect the appropriate and safe use of UFH, LMWH and fondaparinux in daily clinical practice. Clinicians involved in managing and monitoring various antithrombotic therapies need to carefully consider all the clinical nuances in selecting, dosing, and monitoring UFH, LMWH, and fondaparinux to allow for their effective use and minimize related complications.

Clinical Pearl

Monitoring of anti-Xa activity for LMWH has been suggested in multiple populations where unique dosing approaches may be present. Unfortunately, specifics and outcomes with this approach are limited at best. When using an anti-Xa activity level, consider how you will respond when the value is reported. Use caution if consistently low values lead to notably high dosing regimens and potentially increasing the risk for bleeding. In contrast, consistently high values may drive the dosing regimen down and increase risk for thromboembolism.

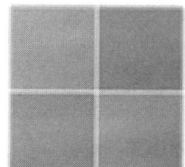

Patient Case

KE is a 29-year-old female who presents to the ER with complaints of LLE pain, erythema, and swelling. Her symptoms started 4 days ago and have gotten progressively worse. Of note is that she is 3 months pregnant, with no previous pregnancies reported. An ultrasound was ordered and she was diagnosed with a DVT involving her L iliac and femoral veins. She is admitted for treatment.

Past Medical History:
Pregnancy loss x 2
Family History:
Mother died of a PE
Maternal grandmother died of a stroke
Social History:
Non significant
Current Medications:
Pre-natal vitamin 1 tablet by mouth daily
Folic acid 1 mg daily
Allergies:
No known drug allergies
Physical Examination:
Vital signs: blood pressure = 125/65, heart rate = 92, respiratory rate = 20, temperature = 38 °C
Weight: 69 kg; height: 65 inches
Labs:
Within normal limits
Estimate GFR = 101 mL/min
Tests:
Doppler US: (+) for ileo-femoral DVT

1. **What are appropriate acute-phase treatment options in this patient?**

   Anticoagulation therapy needs to be initiated promptly in order to minimize clot extension and PE. For the initial acute phase therapy, full therapeutic doses of IV UFH or SC LMWH are both appropriate treatment options. As the patient is hospitalized, UFH is selected as initial therapy.

2. **Discuss dosing and monitoring of UFH in this patient.**

   A weight-based UFH dosing regimen should be considered, as these regimens are more likely to reach the therapeutic aPTT threshold in the first 24 hours after initiating treatment as compared to more traditional dosing regimens. UFH can be safely used in pregnancy. An IV bolus dose of UFH of 80 units/kg (5,500 units) should be given, followed by an infusion at a rate of 18 units/kg/hour (1,200 units/hour). The patient's actual body weight should be used for dose calculation. Loading doses are usually rounded to the nearest 500 units and infusion rates are rounded to the nearest 100 units for ease of administration. The aPTT should be obtained at baseline, and then at 6 hours after initiating the UFH infusion. Subsequent aPTTs should be obtained at 6 hours after each dose change. Once the patient is stabilized and the aPTT is within therapeutic range, monitoring can be extended to every 24 hours as long as the patient is on therapy. The goal aPTT will be institution specific, to correspond to a plasma heparin concentration by anti-factor Xa activity of 0.3–0.7 units/mL. At this institution, the target aPTT range has been determined by the laboratory to be 60 to 90 seconds.

3. The first aPTT, drawn 6 hours after initiating the UFH infusion, comes back at 102 seconds. The UFH infusion rate needs to be decreased according to the nomogram highlighted in Table 11-5 (or a similar institution based nomogram). A dose decrease by 1 unit/kg/hour ($\sim$ 70 units/hour down from 1,200 units/hour to 1,100 units/hour) is suggested in this patient. The aPTT should be checked again at 6 hours after the new infusion rate has been initiated, and further dosing adjustments should be made as necessary.

4. **After additional dose adjustments, the patient's UFH infusion has been maintained at 1,000 units/hour. After completing 5 days of IV UFH therapy, the decision was made to send the patient home. Discuss anticoagulant agent selection, dosing, and monitoring considerations.**

As this patient is not a candidate for warfarin, due to its teratogenic potential in pregnancy, she will need to be treated with a SC anticoagulant (SC adjusted dose UFH or SC therapeutic LMWH) for the remainder of her pregnancy. Adjusted-dose SC UFH is selected as she cannot afford to pay the cost of an LMWH, due to lack of insurance coverage for medications. The patient's 24-hour UFH dose requirement is calculated at 24,000 units. This dose is then increased (usually by 10%–20%) to account for the more limited bioavailability of the SC route of administration. In our patient, a reasonable dose adjustment would be to increase the dose to 27,000 units or approximately a 12.5% increase in dose. This dose is then divided in two, and the patient's initial SC UFH will be 13,500 units SC given every 12 hours. The IV UFH infusion is discontinued and within 1 hour of stopping the infusion, the first SC UFH dose should be administered to ensure that the peak anticoagulant levels are reached in a timely fashion. The aPTT should be checked at 6 hours after the SC dose and monitored frequently until the patient's dose is stabilized. Once the dose is stabilized, monitoring of aPTT should be performed at least weekly throughout her pregnancy as dose requirements may change due to progressive weight gain and changes in glomerular filtration rate.

References

1. Hirsh J, Raschke R. Heparin and low-molecular-weight heparin: the Seventh ACCP Conference on Antithrombotic and Thrombolytic Therapy. *Chest.* 2004;126(3 Suppl):188S-203S.
2. Weitz JI, Hirsh J, Samama MM. New anticoagulant drugs: the Seventh ACCP Conference on Antithrombotic and Thrombolytic Therapy. *Chest.* 2004;126(3 Suppl):265S-286S.
3. Hoppensteadt D, Walenga JM, Fareed J, Bick RL. Heparin, low-molecular-weight heparins, and heparin pentasaccharide: basic and clinical differentiation. *Hematol Oncol Clin North Am.* 2003;17(1):313-41.
4. Heparin Sodium Prescribing Information. Accessed January 2007.
5. Hirsh J, Anand SS, Halperin JL, Fuster V. Guide to anticoagulant therapy: heparin. *Circulation.* 2001;103:2994-3018.
6. Nutescu EA, Shapiro NL, Chevalier A, Amin AN. A pharmacologic overview of current and emerging anticoagulants. *Cleve Clin J Med.* 2005;72 Suppl 1:S2-6.
7. Alban S. From heparins to factor Xa inhibitors and beyond. *Eur J Clin Invest.* 2005;35(Suppl 1):12-20.
8. Bussey H. Traditional anticoagulant therapy: why abandon half a century of success? *Am J Health-Syst Pharm.* 2002;59(20 Suppl 6):S3-6.
9. Hirsh J, Raschke R. Heparin and low-molecular-weight heparin. *Chest.* 2004;126:188S-203S.
10. Geerts WH, Pineo GF, Heit JA, et al. Prevention of venous thromboembolism: the Seventh ACCP Conference on Antithrombotic and Thrombolytic Therapy. *Chest.* 2004;126(3 Suppl):338S-400S.
11. Raschke RA, Reilly BM, Guidry JR, et al. The weight-based heparin dosing nomogram compared with a "standard care" nomogram. *Ann Intern Med.* 1993;119:874-881.
12. Reilly BM, Raschke RA. New method to predict patients' intravenous heparin dose requirements. *J Gen Intern Med.* 1996;11(3):168-173.
13. Raschke RA, Gollihare B, Peirce JC. The effectiveness of implementing the weight-based heparin nomogram as a practice guideline. *Arch Intern Med.* 1996;156(15):1645-9.
14. Rosborough TK, Shepherd MF. Achieving target antifactor Xa activity with a heparin protocol based on sex, age, height, and weight. *Pharmacotherapy.*

2004;24(6):713-9.
15. Rosborough TK. In unfractionated heparin dosing, the combination of patient age and estimated plasma volume predicts initial antifactor Xa activity better than patient weight alone. *Pharmacotherapy.* 1998;18(6):1217-23.
16. Braunwald E, Antman EM, Beasley JW, et al. ACC/AHA guidelines for the management of patients with unstable angina and non-ST-segment elevation myocardial infarction: executive summary and recommendations. A report of the American College of Cardiology/American Heart Association task force on practice guidelines (committee on the management of patients with unstable angina). *Circulation.* 2000;102(10):1193-1209.
17. Braunwald E, Antman EM, Beasley JW, et al. ACC/AHA guideline update for the management of patients with unstable angina and non-ST-segment elevation myocardial infarction—2002: summary article: a report of the American College of Cardiology/American Heart Association Task Force on Practice Guidelines (Committee on the Management of Patients With Unstable Angina). *Circulation.* 2002;106(14):1893-1900.
18. Antman EM, Anbe DT, Armstrong PW, et al. ACC/AHA guidelines for the management of patients with ST-elevation myocardial infarction: a report of the American College of Cardiology/American Heart Association Task Force on Practice Guidelines (Committee to Revise the 1999 Guidelines for the Management of Patients with Acute Myocardial Infarction). *Circulation.* 2004;110(9):e82-292.
19. Smith SC, Jr., Feldman TE, Hirshfeld JW, Jr., et al. ACC/AHA/SCAI 2005 guideline update for percutaneous coronary intervention: a report of the American College of Cardiology/American Heart Association Task Force on Practice Guidelines (ACC/AHA/SCAI Writing Committee to Update 2001 Guidelines for Percutaneous Coronary Intervention). *Circulation.* 2006;113(7):e166-286.
20. Hull RD, Raskob GE, Brant RF, Pineo GF, Valentine KA. The importance of initial heparin treatment on long-term clinical outcomes of antithrombotic therapy. The emerging theme of delayed recurrence. *Arch Intern Med.* 1997;157(20):2317-21.
21. Anand SS, Bates S, Ginsberg JS, et al. Recurrent venous thrombosis and heparin therapy: an evaluation of the importance of early activated partial thromboplastin times. *Arch Intern Med.* 1999;159(17):2029-32.
22. Prandoni P, Carnovali M, Marchiori A. Subcutaneous adjusted-dose unfractionated heparin vs. fixed-dose low-molecular-weight heparin in the initial treatment of venous thromboembolism. *Arch Intern Med.* 2004;164(10):1077-83.
23. Buller HR, Agnelli G, Hull RD, Hyers TM, Prins MH, Raskob GE. Antithrombotic therapy for venous thromboembolic disease: the Seventh ACCP Conference on Antithrombotic and Thrombolytic Therapy. *Chest.* 2004;126(3 Suppl):401S-28S.
24. Kearon C, Ginsberg JS, Julian JA, et al. Comparison of fixed-dose weight-adjusted unfractionated heparin and low-molecular-weight heparin for acute treatment of venous thromboembolism. *JAMA.* 2006;296:935-942.
25. Dobesh PP. Unfractionated heparin dosing nomograms: road maps to where? *Pharmacotherapy.* 2004;24(8 Pt 2):142S-5S.
26. Schwiesow SJ, Wessell AM, Steyer TE. Use of a modified dosing weight for heparin therapy in a morbidly obese patient. *Ann Pharmacother.* 2005;39(4):753-6.
27. Levine MN, Hirsh J, Gent M, et al. A randomized trial comparing activated thromboplastin time with heparin assay in patients with acute venous thromboembolism requiring large daily doses of heparin. *Arch Intern Med.* 1994;154(1):49-56.
28. Hull RD, Pineo GF. Heparin and low-molecular-weight heparin therapy for venous thromboembolism: will unfractionated heparin survive? *Semin Thromb Hemost.* 2004;30 Suppl 1:11-23.
29. Dinwoodey DL, Ansell JE. Heparins, low-molecular-weight heparins, and pentasaccharides. *Clin Geriatr Med.* 2006;22(1):1-15, vii.
30. Raschke R, Reilly B. Monitoring heparin therapy. *Ann Intern Med.* 1994;120(2):169-70.
31. Olson JD, Arkin CF, Brandt JT, et al. College of American Pathologists Conference XXXI on laboratory monitoring of anticoagulation therapy. Laboratory monitoring of unfractionated heparin therapy. *Arch Pathol Lab Med.* 1998;122(9):782-788.
32. Kitchen S, Preston FE. The therapeutic range for heparin therapy: relationship between six activated partial thromboplastin time reagents and two heparin assays. *Thromb Haemost.* 1996;75(5):734-9.
33. Kitchen S, Theaker J, Preston FE. Monitoring unfractionated heparin therapy: relationship between eight anti-Xa assays and a protamine titration assay. *Blood Coagul Fibrinolysis.* 2000;11(2):137-44.
34. Taylor CT, Petros WP, Ortel TL. Two instruments to determine activated partial thromboplastin time: implications for heparin monitoring. *Pharmacotherapy.* 1999;19(4):383-7.
35. Kovacs MJ, Keeney M, MacKinnon K, Boyle E. Three different chromogenic methods do not give equivalent anti-Xa levels for patients on therapeutic low molecular weight heparin (dalteparin) or unfractionated heparin. *Clin Lab Haematol.* 1999;21(1):55-60.
36. Zidane M, Schram MT, Planken EW, et al. Frequency of major hemorrhage in patients treated with unfractionated intravenous heparin for deep venous thrombosis or pulmonary embolism: a study in routine clinical practice. *Arch Intern Med.* 2000;160(15):2369-73.
37. Levine MN, Raskob G, Beyth RJ, Kearon C, Schulman S. Hemorrhagic complications of anticoagulant treatment: the Seventh ACCP Conference on Antithrombotic and Thrombolytic Therapy. *Chest.* 2004;126(3 Suppl):287S-310S.
38. Hyers TM. Heparin and other rapidly acting anticoagulants. *Semin Vasc Surg.* 2005;18(3):130-3.
39. Warkentin TE. Heparin-induced thrombocytopenia: pathogenesis and management. *Br J Haematol.* 2003;121(4):535-555.
40. Warkentin TE, Greinacher A. Heparin-induced thrombocytopenia: recognition, treatment, and prevention: the Seventh ACCP Conference on Antithrombotic and Thrombolytic Therapy. *Chest.* 2004;126(3 Suppl):311S-37S.
41. Warkentin TE. New approaches to the diagno-

sis of heparin-induced thrombocytopenia. *Chest.* 2005;127(2 Suppl):35S-45S.
42. Warkentin TE. Heparin-induced thrombocytopenia: diagnosis and management. *Circulation.* 2004;110(18):e454-8.
43. Arepally GM, Ortel TL. Clinical practice. Heparin-induced thrombocytopenia. *N Engl J Med.* 2006;355(8):809-17.
44. Warkentin TE, Kelton JG. Temporal aspects of heparin-induced thrombocytopenia. *N Engl J Med.* 2001 2001;344(17):1286-92.
45. Brewer D. Low-molecular-weight heparin for initial treatment of venous thromboembolism. *Am Fam Physician.* 2005;72(1):75-76.
46. Bick RL, Frenkel EP, Walenga J, Fareed J, Hoppensteadt DA. Unfractionated heparin, low molecular weight heparins, and pentasaccharide: basic mechanism of actions, pharmacology, and clinical use. *Hematol Oncol Clin North Am.* 2005;19(1):1-51.
47. Duplaga BA, Rivers CW, Nutescu E. Dosing and monitoring of low-molecular-weight heparins in special populations. *Pharmacotherapy.* 2001;21(2):218-34.
48. Spinler SA. The skinny on treatment of venous thromboembolism in obesity. *J Thromb Haemost.* 2005;3(5):854-5.
49. Spinler SA, Dobesh P. Dose capping enoxaparin is unjustified and denies patients with acute coronary syndromes a potentially effective treatment. *Chest.* 2005;127(6):2288-9; author reply 2289-90.
50. Michota F, Merli G. Anticoagulation in special patient populations: are special dosing considerations required? *Cleve Clin J Med.* 2005;72 Suppl 1:S37-42.
51. Sanderink GJ, Le Liboux A, Jariwala N, et al. The pharmacokinetics and pharmacodynamics of enoxaparin in obese volunteers. *Clin Pharmacol Ther.* 2002;72(3):308-18.
52. Hainer JW, Barrett JS, Assaid CA, et al. Dosing in heavy-weight/obese patients with the LMWH, tinzaparin: a pharmacodynamic study. *Thromb Haemost.* 2002;87(5):817-23.
53. Lovenox Prescribing Information. Accessed January 2007.
54. Laposata M, Green D, Van Cott EM, Barrowcliffe TW, Goodnight SH, Sosolik RC. College of American Pathologists Conference XXXI on laboratory monitoring of anticoagulant therapy: the clinical use and laboratory monitoring of low-molecular-weight heparin, danaparoid, hirudin and related compounds, and argatroban. *Arch Pathol Lab Med.* 1998;122(9):799-807.
55. Howard PA. Low molecular weight heparins in special populations. *J Infus Nurs.* 2003;26(5):304-10.
56. Wittkowsky AK, Nutescu EA. Thrombosis: Treatment and prevention in patients with chronic illness. In: Schumock G, Brundage D, Chapman M, et al, eds. *Pharmacotherapy Self-Assessment Program.* 5th ed. Lexena, KS: American College of Clinical Pharmacy; 2005;169-191.
57. Monagle P, Michelson AD, Bovill E, Andrew M. Antithrombotic therapy in children. *Chest.* 2001 2001;119(1 Suppl):344S-70S.
58. Dolovich L, Ginsberg JS, Douketis J, et al. A meta-analysis comparing low-molecular-weight heparins with unfractionated heparin in the treatment of venous thromboembolism. *Arch Intern Med.* 2000;160:181-8.
59. Horlocker TT, Wedel DJ, Benzon H, et al. Regional anesthesia in the anticoagulated patient: defining the risks (the second ASRA Consensus Conference on Neuraxial Anesthesia and Anticoagulation). *Reg Anesth Pain Med.* 2003;28(3):172-97.
60. Martel N, Lee J, Wells PS. Risk for heparin-induced thrombocytopenia with unfractionated and low-molecular-weight heparin thromboprophylaxis: a meta-analysis. *Blood.* 2005;106(8):2710-15.
61. Greer IA. Anticoagulants in pregnancy. *J Thromb Thrombolysis.* 2006;21(1):57-65.
62. Bates SM, Greer IA, Hirsh J, Ginsberg JS. Use of antithrombotic agents during pregnancy: the Seventh ACCP Conference on Antithrombotic and Thrombolytic Therapy. *Chest.* 2004;126(3 Suppl):627S-44S.
63. Turpie AG. Fondaparinux: a Factor Xa inhibitor for antithrombotic therapy. *Expert Opin Pharmacother.* 2004;5(6):1373-84.
64. Dager WE, Andersen J, Nutescu E. Special considerations with fondaparinux therapy: heparin-induced thrombocytopenia and wound healing. *Pharmacotherapy.* 2004;24(7 Pt 2):88S-94S.
65. Arixtra Prescribing Information. Accessed January 2007.
66. Turpie AG, Bauer KA, Eriksson BI, Lassen MR. Fondaparinux vs enoxaparin for the prevention of venous thromboembolism in major orthopedic surgery: a meta-analysis of 4 randomized double-blind studies. *Arch Intern Med.* 2002;162(16):1833-40.
67. Buller HR, Davidson BL, Decousus H, et al. Subcutaneous fondaparinux versus intravenous unfractionated heparin in the initial treatment of pulmonary embolism. *N Engl J Med.* 2003;349(18):1695-1702.
68. Buller HR, Davidson BL, Decousus H, et al. Fondaparinux or enoxaparin for the initial treatment of symptomatic deep venous thrombosis: a randomized trial. *Ann Intern Med.* 2004;140(11):867-73.
69. Yusuf S, Mehta SR, Chrolavicius S, et al. Effects of fondaparinux on mortality and reinfarction in patients with acute ST-segment elevation myocardial infarction: the OASIS-6 randomized trial. *JAMA.* 2006;295(13):1519-30.
70. Yusuf S, Mehta SR, Chrolavicius S, et al. Comparison of fondaparinux and enoxaparin in acute coronary syndromes. *N Engl J Med.* 2006;354(14):1464-76.
71. Cohen AT, Davidson BL, Gallus AS, et al. Efficacy and safety of fondaparinux for the prevention of venous thromboembolism in older acute medical patients: randomized placebo controlled trial. *BMJ.* 2006;332(7537):325-9.
72. Colwell CW, Jr., Kwong LM, Turpie AG, Davidson BL. Flexibility in administration of fondaparinux for prevention of symptomatic venous thromboembolism in orthopaedic surgery. *J Arthroplasty.* 2006;21(1):36-45.
73. Simoons ML, Bobbink IW, Boland J, et al. A dose-finding study of fondaparinux in patients with non-ST-segment elevation acute coronary syndromes: the Pentasaccharide in Unstable Angina (PENTUA) Study. *J Am Coll Cardiol.* 2004;43(12):2183-90.
74. Smogorzewska A, Brandt JT, Chandler WL, et al. Effect of fondaparinux on coagulation assays: results

74. ...of College of American Pathologists proficiency testing. *Arch Pathol Lab Med.* 2006;130(11):1605-11.
75. Damgen-von Brevern G, Klaffling C, Lindhoff-Last E. [Monitoring anticoagulation by fondaparinux: determination of anti factor Xa-level]. *Hamostaseologie.* 2005;25(3):281-5.
76. Paolucci F, Frasa H, Van Aarle F, et al. Two sensitive and rapid chromogenic assays of fondaparinux sodium (Arixtra) in human plasma and other biological matrices. *Clin Lab.* 2003;49(9-10):451-460.
77. Klaeffling C, Piechottka G, Daemgen-von Brevern G, et al. Development and clinical evaluation of two chromogenic substrate methods for monitoring fondaparinux sodium. *Ther Drug Monit.* 2006;28(3):375-81.
78. Gogarten W. The influence of new antithrombotic drugs on regional anesthesia. *Curr Opin Anaesthesiol.* 2006;19(5):545-50.
79. Warkentin TE, Crowther MA. Reversing anticoagulants both old and new. *Can J Anaesth.* 2002;49(6):S11-25.
80. Haverkamp D, Hutten BA, Buller HR, Gallus AS, Lensing AW, Prins MH. The use of specific antidotes as a response to bleeding complications during anticoagulant therapy for venous thromboembolism. *J Thromb Haemost.* 2003;1(1):69-73.
81. Schulman S, Bijsterveld NR. Anticoagulants and their reversal. *Transfus Med Rev.* 2007;21(1):37-48.
82. Makris M, Hough RE, Kitchen S. Poor reversal of low molecular weight heparin by protamine. *Br J Haematol.* 2000;108(4):884-885.
83. Chawla LS, Moore G, Seneff MG. Incomplete reversal of enoxaparin toxicity by protamine: implications of renal insufficiency, obesity, and low molecular weight heparin sulfate content. *Obes Surg.* May 2004;14(5):695-698.
84. Kessler CM. Antidotes to haemorrhage: recombinant factor VIIa. *Best Pract Res Clin Haematol.* 2004;17(1):183-97.
85. Levi M, Peters M, Buller HR. Efficacy and safety of recombinant factor VIIa for treatment of severe bleeding: a systematic review. *Crit Care Med.* 2005;33(4):883-90.
86. Sonawane S, Kasbekar N, Berns JS. The safety of heparins in end-stage renal disease. *Semin Dial.* 2006;19(4):305-10.
87. Grand'Maison A, Charest AF, Geerts WH. Anticoagulant use in patients with chronic renal impairment. *Am J Cardiovasc Drugs.* 2005;5(5):291-305.
88. Lim W, Dentali F, Eikelboom JW, Crowther MA. Meta-analysis: low-molecular-weight heparin and bleeding in patients with severe renal insufficiency. *Ann Intern Med.* 2006;144(9):673-684.
89. Bates SM, Greer IA, Hirsh J, Ginsberg JS. Use of antithrombotic agents during pregnancy. *Chest.* 2004;126:627S-644S.
90. Lagrange F, Brun JL, Vergnes MC, et al. Fondaparinux sodium does not cross the placental barrier: study using the in-vitro human dually perfused cotyledon model. *Clin Pharmacokinet.* 2002;41 Suppl 2:47-9.
91. Mazzolai L, Hohlfeld P, Spertini F, Hayoz D, Schapira M, Duchosal MA. Fondaparinux is a safe alternative in case of heparin intolerance during pregnancy. *Blood.* 2006;108(5):1569-70.
92. Monagle P, Chan A, Massicotte P, Chalmers E, Michelson AD. Antithrombotic therapy in children. *Chest.* 2004;126:645S-87S.
93. Streif W, Mitchell LG, Andrew M. Antithrombotic therapy in children. *Curr Opin Pediatr.* 1999;11(1):56-64.
94. Sutor AH, Chan AK, Massicotte P. Low-molecular-weight heparin in pediatric patients. *Semin Thromb Hemost.* 2004;30 Suppl 1:31-9.
95. Dager WE, White RH. Low-molecular-weight heparin-induced thrombocytopenia in a child. *Ann Pharmacother.* 2004;38(2):247-50.
96. Punzalan RC, Hillery CA, Montgomery RR, Scott CA, Gill JC. Low-molecular-weight heparin in thrombotic disease in children and adolescents. *J Pediatr Hematol Oncol.* 2000;22(2):137-142.
97. Dager WE, Gosselin RC, King JH, Christensen CL, Owings JT, Larkin EC. Anti-Xa stability of diluted enoxaparin for use in pediatrics. *Ann Pharmacother.* 2004;38(4):569-73.

Chapter 12

Essential Direct Thrombin Inhibitor Knowledge

William Dager

Chapter Outline

- Introduction
- Pharmacology
- Pharmacokinetics/pharmacodynamics
  - Lepirudin
  - Bivalirudin
  - Argatroban
- Indications
  - DTIs in HIT
- Initializing a DTI infusion
- Contraindications/precautions
  - Hypersensitivity
- Monitoring
- Transitioning to warfarin
- Reversal
- Conclusion
- Patient case
- References

Introduction

When vascular injury occurs, proenzymes and procofactors are converted into active substances that work in concert to generate thrombin as part of the hemostatic repair process. Thrombin has a central role in this process as both a procoagulant and anticoagulant. Thrombin regulated procoagulation includes conversion of soluble fibrinogen to fibrin, activation of factors V, VIII and XIII; increasing formation of fibrin cross linking and clot stabilization.[1-3] Process that causes activation of thrombin can lead to undesirable arterial or venous thromboembolism. Inactivation of thrombin may eliminate its ability mediate additional thrombus formation.

Pharmacology

The activity of thrombin can be inhibited by currently available agents that bind directly to either the catalytic or active site, substrate recognition site (exocite 1), or heparin-binding site (exocite 2). Unfractionated heparin (UFH), low molecular weight heparin (LMWH) and fondaparinux are considered to be indirect anticoagulants because of their ability to catalyze the inhibitory effects of antithrombin (AT) against thrombin. When heparin binds simultaneously to exocite 2 and AT, a heparin-thrombin-antithrombin complex is formed. Heparin can also act as a bridge between fibrin and thrombin via exocite 2. The occupation of both sites on thrombin protects the enzymatic activity from inactivation but reduces its ability to inhibit thrombin already bound to fibrin and thrombus growth.[1]

In contrast, direct thrombin inhibitors (DTI) bind directly to the catalytic region on thrombin responsible for enzymatic activity. Binding to the catalytic region or active site on thrombin inhibits several of the actions of thrombin including platelet activation and cleavage of fibrinogen involved in thrombus formation. The bivalent DTIs (lepirudin and bivalirudin) also bind to the substrate recognition (exocite 1) on thrombin where fibrinogen can bind. Since the DTIs do not bind to exocite 2, they are capable of inhibiting the effects of thrombin already bound to fibrin (clot bound thrombin). Direct thrombin inhibitors can also block thrombins ability to activate platelets, stimulate granule release, surface receptor expression and aggregation in addition to a plethora of other factors that mediate vascular integrity.[2]

Pharmacokinetics/Pharmacodynamics

Currently, three parenteral DTIs are available in U.S.: bivalirudin, lepirudin, and argatroban. Notable pharmacokinetic and pharmacodynamic differences between the three agents result in agent specific dosing regimens and effects on clot based laboratory assays (Table 12-1).

Lepirudin

The first DTI to become available in the U.S. was lepirudin, a recombinant product derived from leech (Hirudo Medicinalis) saliva, which has been observed to have anticoagulant properties since 1884. Of the three DTIs, lepirudin has the tightest binding to thrombin, with a dissociation constant around 2×10^{-14} M. Because of the low dissociation constant, lepirudin can inhibit thrombin at a very low concentration compared to the other DTIs.[3] The inhibition of thrombin can also continue for up to 18 hours after administration. The kidney is the primary site for removal of lepirudin, accounting for 50%–60% of clearance with additional elimination via the bile and liver. Pharmacokinetic studies have observed an elimination half-life of approximately 1.3 hours in healthy subjects with normal renal function, which can be prolonged as creatinine clearance (CrCl) decreases.[2]

Bivalirudin

Bivalirudin is a recombinant analog of hirudin that has the most rapid elimination rate of the three DTIs, having a half-life of approximately 30 minutes with 20% eliminated unchanged in the urine in healthy controls.[2] The dissociation constant of bivalirudin is approximately 1.9 nM. In patients receiving bivalirudin for PTCA, serum concentrations correlated with measured aPTT values.[2] Bivalirudin is inactivated by enzymatic cleavage of the Arg–Pro bond in the amino-terminal domain by thrombin itself in addition to dissociating from the thrombin complex, allowing thrombin to recover its activity.[2] Because of the enzymatic cleavage by thrombin, the reduction in dosing of bivalirudin may not be as notable as lepirudin or argatroban in patients with reduced renal or hepatic function, respectively.[4] Because of thrombins ability to enzymatically inactivate bivalirudin, pooled blood in the field outside the circulation (during surgery), or in a cell-saver reservoir may be prone to clotting.[5] Reduced dosing has been suggested when renal insufficiency is present; however, the dose may need to be subsequently increased during hemodialysis, as hemofiltration has been shown to remove bivalirudin.[6-8]

Argatroban

Argatroban is a synthetic derivative of arginine that selectively inhibits only the active site on thrombin, with a dissociation constant of 3.9×10^{-8} mol/L.[2] Argatroban can effectively inhibit the activity of circulating and bound thrombin.[2,9] It is primarily eliminated hepatically, with an elimination half-life in healthy control subjects of 31–51 seconds. A notable increases in the elimination half-life was observed in the presence of mild to moderate hepatic insufficiency.[10]

Concurrent agents such as aspirin have not been observed to alter the elimination of DTIs. It should be noted that clinical trials have typically excluded patients with liver or renal impairment, and thus the true pharmacokinetic to pharmaco-

Table 12-1.
Pharmacokinetics of Available Antithrombin Agents[11-13]

Agent	Argatroban	Bivalirudin	Lepirudin
Route of administration	IV	IV	IV/SC
Plasma half-life normal subjects	39–51 min	10–24 min	1.3 hours
Primary elimination route	Hepatic	Enzymatic	Renal
Fraction excreted unchanged in the urine (Fe)	16%	20%	35%

dynamic responses in these patients as not been established.

Indications

Lepirudin and argatroban are indicated for anticoagulation therapy in the setting of prophylaxis or treatment of thrombosis in heparin induced thrombocytopenia (HIT). Argatroban and bivalirudin are indicated for patients with HIT requiring percutaneous coronary intervention (PCI). Bivalirudin is also indicated in the setting of unstable angina undergoing percutaneous transluminal coronary angioplasty (PTCA) or PCI in non-HIT patients.[11-13]

DTIs in HIT

Because HIT was a catastrophic disease without an approach for management, the parenteral DTIs were not extensively studied in dose ranging phase II trials. Instead, clinical trials comparing argatroban or lepirudin to a historical were undertaken simultaneously as it was determined that a blinded randomized control trial would be unethical. The argatroban trial was predominantly done in North America, selecting an aPTT target range of 1.5 to 3 times control. In contrast, lepirudin was investigated in Germany with an aPTT target of 1.5 to 2.5 times control. Because of the numerous differences in the populations studied including the duration of DTI therapy, degree of thrombocytopenia, or confirmation of antibody test, it would be difficult to directly compare observed results between the two agents for differences in efficacy or complication rates. Some notable observations from the trials however continue to influence how clinicians use these agents in the management of HIT.

Of the three parenteral DTIs, lepirudin has an elimination half-life long enough to facilitate administration by the subcutaneous route. A linear dose response in the aPTT was observed with SC lepirudin, 0.75 mg, 1.25mg and 2 mg SC every 12 hours over a 5 day period in initial management of DVT.[14] In the setting of HIT, case studies have suggested 25-50mg SQ ever 12 hours can prevent thrombosis complications after initial management with a DTI infusion.[15-17] Outside HIT, DTIs may offer an alternative approach to anticoagulation when antithrombin deficiency or concerns for hypersensitivity to heparin are present.

Initiating a DTI Infusion

The initial dosing regimen for a DTI will depend on the indication for anticoagulation, clinical presentation of the patient, and the desired intensity of parenteral anticoagulation, as is also the case with the use of heparin. In the setting of HIT, antithrombin deficiency or treatment of thromboembolic complications, a lower intensity of anticoagulation is targeted compared to treatment of acute coronary syndrome. The initial dose may depend on the presence of thrombosis, impaired organ function and presence of active bleeding or risk factors for bleeding (Table 12-2).[8] When concerns for bleeding are present in the absence of thrombosis, the lower end of the reduced intensity target range may be considered. In the presence of acute thrombosis and limited risk for bleeding, the higher end of the target range may be considered.

Table 12-2.
Steps in the Initiation, Monitoring, and Transition Off DTI Therapy

Initiating DTI therapy
1. Draw baseline aPTT and INR if not previously done.
2. Evaluate renal, liver and cardiac function for potential reasons to reduce the dose.
3. Initiate DTI depending on target goals and indication for use.
   a. Consider a regimen with a sliding scale in mg/h for simplicity
   b. Consider a simple standard dilution (1 mg/mL) and rates in "mg/h" if possible to decrease confusion in administration rates and charting.

Monitoring the DTI infusion
1. Draw aPTT at a predetermined time within 2–6 hours to reduce the risk of over-targeting or under-targeting the selected aPTT goal.
   a. Adjust upwards any value notably below a ratio of 1.5 × baseline.
   b. Consider adjusting downward if the upper end of the target range, or above prior to achieving steady state.
   c. Follow platelet count, patient and HCT (or hemoglobin) for any evidence of bleeding.
2. If an INR is requested, consider including an aPTT to determine amount of DTI effect on the INR value.

For lepirudin, the initial starting dose in isolated HIT (thrombocytopenia without acute thrombosis) is 0.1 mg/kg/h with no bolus.[18-19] In a meta analysis of the three primary lepirudin trials, the mean dose in this setting was 0.06 mg/kg/h.[20] If acute thrombosis is present, than a bolus of 0.4 mg/kg followed by a infusion of 0.15 mg/kg/h is suggested. Since lepirudin is primarily eliminated via the kidney, a dose reduction is suggested as renal function declines based on reliable methods for estimating function.[12,21-22] Subsequent analysis of dosing in the clinical trial in addition to independent observations suggest that a trend towards doses lower then provided in the prescribing information are fairly common.[23-24] This might be attributed to the identified target range, sensitivity in the aPTT assay, use in sicker patients and influence of reduced cardiac, hepatic or renal function.

In patients requiring hemodialysis, the half-life of lepirudin was observed to be 30 times longer (51.8 ± 15.6 hours) than observed in a normal renal function control comparator (1.7 ± 1.5 hours).[25] In patients with severe renal dysfunction, removal and dosing adjustment may depend on the degree of residual renal function observed by current urine output.[26] Lepirudin can be removed to some extent during hemodialysis, with potentially greater elimination observed when dialyzers with a greater negative charge on the membrane surfaces are used.[22, 27] Antibodies to lepirudin that can reduce clearance have been observed with prolonged use.[28]

The elimination half-life of lepirudin administered subcutaneous is approximately 4 to 8 hours with peak observed 1.3–2.5 hours post the dose, allowing effective anticoagulation using twice daily dosing.[29] In a dose-ranging analysis comparing twice daily SC lepirudin to heparin in the treatment of proximal DVT, a linear response in aPTT was observed between 0.75 to 2 mg/kg.[14] The 1.25 mg/kg lepirudin dose was just as effective as heparin, with fewer adverse effects compared to the higher 2 mg/kg dose. Measured aPTT ratio values prior to a dose were between 1.5 and 2.0, and peak (3 hours post injection) approximately 2.2 and 2.7 times control. Peak levels 2 hours post administration targeting an aPTT ratio of approximately 2–2.5 times control showed no evidence of accumulation over the 2–3 weeks.[15]

For argatroban, the initial starting dose for treatment of HIT was 2 mcg/kg/min, with a mean dose maintenance infusion of 1.6 to 1.7 mcg/kg/min observed in the clinical trials.[30-32] Lower mean doses than observed in clinical trials have been described in reports from individual institutions.[23-24] Since argatroban is hepatically eliminated, the dose should be reduced to 0.25 mcg/kg/min in patients with mild to moderate liver failure.[10] In patients with major hepatic failure, lower doses and very prolonged effects have been observed.[33-34] Argatroban is eliminated to a limited extent renally. Initially, this was considered to be insignificant, and no alteration in dosing was recommended based on observations in the clinical trials.[11,35] Subsequent reports describe requirements for lower infusion rates depending on the degree of renal insufficiency.[36-38] In one report, the mean argatroban maintenance dose to maintain an aPTT value of 60 seconds was 2.2 ± 0.34 mcg/kg/min for creatinine clearances over 60 ml/min, 1.2 ± 0.15 mcg/kg/min for creatinine clearance of 31–60 mL/min and 0.8 ± 0.4 mcg/kg/min for creatinine clearance below 31 mL/min were observed.[38] Unlike lepirudin or bivalirudin, argatroban is not eliminated during hemodialysis, making it unnecessary for any dosing adjustments.[33,39]

As with heparin, a higher degree of anticoagulation may be necessary in selected situations such as bypass surgery or coronary intervention. The DTI dose may depend on use of other concurrent medications such as a glycoprotein IIb/IIIa inhibitor in PCI, or if on pump or off pump coronary bypass surgery is undertaken. For cardiac bypass surgery, dosing approaches may include a selected bolus dose, infusion rate of the subsequent DTI, preservation of the cell saver; and timing of infusion discontinuation. In these settings, a planned dosing approach should consider available trials and the perspective agent chosen. As the result of reduced cardiac output of transient hypoperfusion to the kidney or liver during surgery, a reduced DTI dose may achieve target goals postoperatively. As cardiac function and perfusion increases in subsequent days, the infusion rate may need to be increased.

Contraindications/Precautions

In clinical trials for any anticoagulant, the efficacy of primary and secondary outcomes is typically influenced by the incidence of minor, major and life-threatening bleeding. Unfortunately, no standardized definition of bleeding in either category exists, and there are no well-controlled direct comparisons between the different DTIs. Current dosing strategies have evolved as appreciation for renal function or hepatic function in post marketing analysis or reports from individual centers recognized a need to adjust the dose downward, potentially reducing in the risk for bleeding. Since the DTIs are dosed differently in both HIT and ACS, the incidence of bleeding may depend on which setting they are being used.

In the initial lepirudin trials for treatment of HIT, major bleeding was associated with higher aPTT values (67 to 79 seconds) compared to 47 to

Chapter 12 ■ Essential Direct Thrombin Inhibitor Knowledge

> **Clinical Pearl**
>
> In severe renal impairment, argatroban may be preferred secondary to its hepatic elimination and pharmacokinetic and pharmacodynamic evidence suggesting no alteration of elimination in hemodialysis.[40]

60 seconds without any difference in the rate of thrombotic complications.[40-43] As the relationship between renal function and initial lepirudin dosing became apparent, the incidence of excessive values and bleeding declined. In a post marketing analysis of the use of lepirudin, not only was a lower incidence of both limb amputations and new thrombotic complications observed, but also a 3-fold reduction in major bleeding from the original trials.[44] Recent analysis of the original argatroban trial and two subsequent trials demonstrated a similar rate of major bleeding between argatroban and control patients.[45]

Overall, the reductions in both thromboembolic and major bleeding can be attributed in part to increased familiarity with the use of these agents; however, voluntary reporting may have reduced the proportion of negative results. Prior to starting a DTI, the benefits of thrombosis management should be balanced with the risk for bleeding when developing a management plan. Considerations may include the desired intensity of anticoagulation.

An important challenge with the DTIs is the lack of a reversal agent. The relatively short half-life in the absence of organ dysfunction may reduce their potential ability to inhibit formation of a fibrin plug for prolonged periods of time. In patients at risk for bleeding, selecting the DTI with the shortest half-life after assessing renal and hepatic function may reduce challenges in controlling any bleeding events. Such may be the case when patients require invasive procedure, are intubated with risk for tracheal trauma, or have open wounds where excessive bleeding is not desired.

Hypersensitivity

Antibodies to lepirudin have been reported to form during prolonged infusions resulting in a greater aPTT response, leading to lower infusion rates.[46] There was no correlation with the presence of antibodies and incidence of amputations, thrombotic complications and major bleeding. Separately, anaphylactic reactions (0.015%) are reported, with a higher yet still rare occurrence (0.16%) for a severe reaction if there has been a previous exposure to lepirudin in recent months.[47-48] Epitopes on bivalirudin may recognize antibodies to lepirudin, however, any clinical significance for this is unclear.[49] Any previous exposure to either lepirudin or bivalirudin should be incorporated in the process of agent selection. Patients with a history of exposure to lepirudin should be monitored for potential, albeit rare, symptoms of a hypersensitivity response, which may include an unexplained need to alter the infusion rate to maintain the targeted degree of anticoagulation. All three DTI are contraindicated in patients with known hypersensitivity to the DTI involved.

> **Clinical Pearl**
>
> Differences in sensitivities for aPTT reagents between heparin or DTI can occur, and thus the target aPTT range for a DTI may not be the same as heparin for a particular reagent and may very between institutions with different aPTT assay.

> **Clinical Pearl**
>
> Acutely ill patients such as those with renal, hepatic or cardiac dysfunction may reach target aPTT values at doses notably lower than observed in the clinical trials. Alterations in dosing requirements may be necessary as the dynamic clinical presentation of the patient changes. Measured aPTT values should take this under consideration to adapt infusion rates, and prevent under or overshooting target goals.

Monitoring

The laboratory parameters to measure the degree of anticoagulation may depend on the situation and desired intensity of anticoagulation. Generally, the aPTT is used for management of HIT or treatment of a venous or peripheral arterial thromboembolism. The intensity of anticoagulation with a DTI in the setting of HIT is an aPTT ratio for bivalirudin or lepirudin of 1.5 to 2.5 times the

Managing Anticoagulation Patients in the Hospital: The Inpatient Anticoagulation Service

> **Clinical Pearl**
>
> The choice for an initial DTI dose may depend on the setting, risk or presence of acute thrombosis, and, separately, bleeding. During use in coronary interventional therapy, this may be confounded by the addition of parenteral antiplatelet agents, or when using the activated clotting time (ACT) used for any adjustment in the infusion rate. In the setting of HIT, the aPTT is typically used, targeting the lower end of the aPTT range if bleeding risk is high and risk for thromboembolism low. The higher end of the range is targeted if bleeding risk is low and acute thromboembolism (or high risk for one) is present.[2]

as examples are present. However, the importance of maintaining an aPTT ratio above 1.5 should be noted, as frequent values below has been associated with increased risk for thrombosis.[20] To avoid aPTT values below the target range, a slightly higher low end ratio goal above 1.5, such as 1.6 to 1.8, may be a consideration.

Since the mechanism of DTIs and sensitivity of the aPTT assays are different than UFH, the intensity of anticoagulation and target range for a given aPTT value may be different. Thus, target aPTT ranges for either agent (heparin and separately a DTI) to a given assay should be independent of each other.[50] The sensitivity of the aPTT to a given DTI concentration may also vary between reagents.[51] An additional note is that a flattening of the aPTT dose response curve has been observed at higher degrees of anticoagulation intensity with minimal change in the aPTT as the DTI concentration increases.[19] The activated clotting time (ACT) may be used in situations where a higher degree of anticoagulation may be required, such as invasive cardiac or selected surgical procedures (i.e., coronary intervention, coronary bypass or ECMO). Given that higher DTI doses are used, excessive INR result may be observed in these settings if measured.

Once the DTI infusion is started in the setting of HIT, an aPTT should be drawn within 2-6 hours depending on the need for aggressive anticoagulation or concerns for bleeding to determine if an adjustment in dosing is needed to achieve target goals (Table 12-2). Frequently, patients requiring

patient's baseline value (lepirudin, maximum of 100 seconds), or 1.5 to 3 times baseline with argatroban based on the endpoints set in the original trials. In the absence of a baseline aPTT value, then the laboratory median normal aPTT value can be considered. The upper end of the targeted range may be considered when the risk of thrombosis far exceeds concerns for bleeding. In contrast, the lower end of the target range may be desired when notable bleeding concerns such as recent surgery, intubation, open wounds, or recent major bleeding

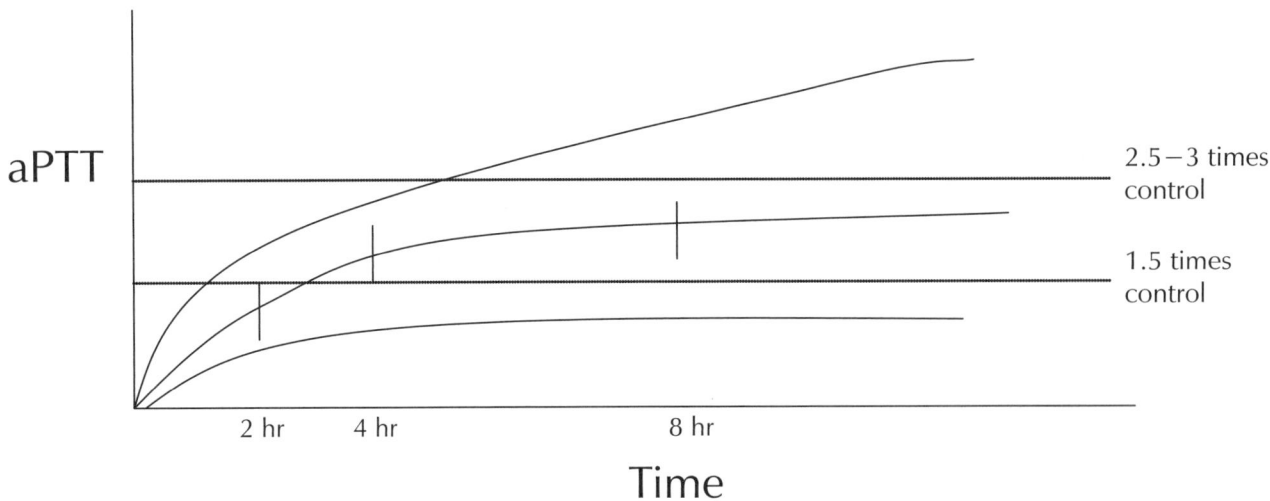

Figure 12-1. If clearance of the DTI is reduced, steady state may not occur for an extended period of time. Measuring the aPTT prior to steady state may assist in determining if the rise is too rapid, even if it is within the target range, or so small that an increase in the infusion rate may be necessary. Waiting to draw the aPTT at steady state may create the risk of prolonged periods time above or below the target range.

DTI therapy have longer elimination half-lives than observed in healthy subjects. As such, the time to steady state can be notably longer, especially if hepatic, renal or impaired cardiac function is present.[8,33,52-54] Waiting for steady state prior to checking an aPTT value may also be to late to avoid undesirable low or excessive values. Checking an aPTT earlier may assist in showing the trend of rise, and allow for any necessary rate adjustment (Figure 12-1). Once steady state has been achieved, the infusion rate can also assist in suggesting how long the effects of the DTI will last once the infusion is discontinued. A low dose DTI regimen achieving target aPTT values may suggest reduced clearance and a longer time for the effects of the DTI to dissipate once stopped. All three DTIs can falsely increase measured INR values in the clinical laboratory, with the most notable effects with argatroban followed to a lesser extent by bivalirudin and lepirudin.[55]

Transitioning to Warfarin

In situations where prolonged anticoagulation is needed, therapy may transition to an anticoagulant more suitable for long-term management. In the case of warfarin, this is a unique challenge because of the DTIs ability to independently elevate the INR. The elevated INR is primarily an in-vitro effect that occurs in the laboratory, and does not, at least for argatroban, reflect an elevated degree of anticoagulation in the patient.[56] Clinicians should thus be cautious not to stop a DTI infusion in the absence of warfarin because of a elevated INR value. Both the DTI concentration and higher international sensitivity indexes (ISI) values of the test can also influence the observed rise in the INR.

In the setting of HIT, warfarin therapy should not be initiated until target aPTT values with the DTI are achieved, and the platelet count is under sufficient recovery. A minimum of 5 days overlapping DTI and warfarin therapy and adequate recovery in platelet count in the setting of acute HIT is also recommended.[57] To avoid the potential for warfarin related venous limb gangrene associated with HIT, warfarin should be initiated cautiously (lower dose) to avoid early excessive anticoagulation while DTI therapy is continued until adequate platelet count recovery has occurred. This may be difficult to determine when a mixed source of thrombocytopenia is present (lack of rise in the platelet count), or suspicion that HIT was not present. Since presence of a DTI can increase the INR, and warfarin the aPTT, determining the degree of anticoagulation independently for either agent when both are present can be difficult.[55,58] Selected parameters have been suggested, however, the multiple variables in assays and their sensitivities can make application of these approaches difficult.

One approach to determine if the target INR for warfarin has been reached is to start with a baseline INR on DTI therapy alone once target aPTT values are achieved (Table 12-3). When the aPTT is stable and the INR value after 5 days of therapy has risen 1.5 to 2 times with minimal change in the aPTT, the target intensity of warfarin anticoagulation may have been achieved. The DTI infusion can be held for a period of time to allow sufficient loss of effects. To simplify the process, the infusion may be held over the night, and an INR with an aPTT drawn at a pre-selected time for assessment in the morning to determine if the infusion needs to be restarted, or discontinued if the INR is within target. The INR can be used to assess the degree of warfarin anticoagulation, and the aPTT to determine if any residual DTI effects continue to be present. Chromogenic factor II or Xa have also been used as a means to monitor warfarin response in settings where additional factor are in-

Table 12-3.
Transitioning from a DTI to Warfarin

1. Draw a baseline INR with an aPTT on DTI therapy alone.
2. Initiate warfarin and identify a desired 1.5–2 point increase in the INR, or a pre-selected INR, that considers the DTI-induced INR prolongation (with minimal change in the aPTT).
3. Once the desired number of overlap days and desired platelet recovery has occurred and the desired INR target is reached, hold the DTI for 4–8 hours and recheck the INR and aPTT. If the INR is between 2–3 with an aPTT close to baseline (accounting for warfarin related elevation), then the DTI can be discontinued. It may take longer for the effects of a DTI to diminish if a very low infusion rate with aPTT values in the target range.
4. Another option may be the use of chromogenic factor Xa or factor II to assess if an adequate anticoagulation response with warfarin has occured.[59-60]

Managing Anticoagulation Patients in the Hospital: The Inpatient Anticoagulation Service

> **Clinical Pearl**
>
> The DTI can independently elevate the INR value by interfering with the assay in the laboratory. Absent of warfarin, this should not be interpreted as an elevated degree of anticoagulation. The degree of effect on the INR may correlate with the concentration of the DTI present, which may be represented by the intensity of rise in the aPTT.

fluencing INR values are creating difficulties in determining the degree of warfarin anticoagulation.[59-60]

Reversal

Currently, there is no easy means to expedite reversal of a DTI. The use of activated recombinant factor VIIa has been suggested, but observations have been mixed on its effectiveness.[61] In addition are concerns of increased risk of thromboembolism with it use.[62] Hemodialysis and plasmapheresis can enhance the removal of both lepirudin and bivalirudin. The extent of removal for lepirudin during hemodialysis may depend on charge on the membrane surface of the dialyzer, with greater removal observed when negatively charged membranes are used.[27] The removal of bivalirudin may depend on the duration of dialysis, type of circuit and pore size of the membrane, and, to a limited extent, the electrostatic charge or the membrane.[6,63] In general, argatroban does not appear to be removed to any significant extent during hemodialysis.[33,39]

Conclusion

The DTIs represent a potent class of anticoagulants that can independently inhibit the functions of thrombin. Dosing can vary considerably depending on the indication for use, agent selected and clinical presentation of the patient. Then unique effects on coagulation related assays should be understood and incorporated into management plans. Careful consideration and understanding of these concepts are critical to optimizing the use of DTIs, which frequently occurs during acute, clinically concerning thrombosis related situations.

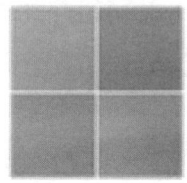

Patient Case

JM is a 67-yo, 85-kg, 5'6" female with hypertension, CHF, and chromic kidney disease (CKD stage III) who was admitted with chest pain and shortness of breath. The EKG was normal, however, there is a suspicion of a urinary tract infection. She was started on a heparin infusion for suspicion of a pulmonary embolism. Two days later the CT scan showed no evidence of a pulmonary embolism, and ultrasound of her legs showed no evidence of thrombus. She also was noted to have exacerbation of her CHF (ejection fraction 25%) and was continued on her heparin infusion for prophylaxis while being treated for the UTI with ceftriaxone. On hospital day 7, she was noted to have a platelet count decline to 75 from her baseline value or 289 on admission. The aPTT prior to starting heparin was 28 seconds.

Question 1: What alterations in the anticoagulation regimen and management plan would you consider?

Answer: The timing of heparin exposure fits the typical onset pattern for HIT along with a 50% drop in platelet count where a clear association with a separate primary cause is not present. Since the suspicion of HIT is not low, changing from heparin to a direct thrombin inhibitor may be considered along with a request for a heparin antibody test. Because the patient has renal insufficiency, argatroban may be the DTI to select. No acute thrombosis is present, so their may be time to initiate therapy at a lower infusion rate to avoid increased risk for bleeding associated with renal insufficiency, and the presence of heart failure with a low ejection fraction potentially reducing elimination.

An initial dose of 1 mcg/kg/min is chosen (approximated to 5 mg/h), with an aPTT requested 4 hours after starting the infusion. A target range of approximately 1.6–2.2 time control, or approximately 45 to 60 seconds was set since no thrombus was present. The aPTT at 4 hours is 59 seconds (INR 3.5). The infusion is continued at the current rate. Another aPTT 6 hours later with a.m. labs is 89 seconds with an INR of 4.5. The infusion is held and fresh frozen plasma (FFP) plus vitamin K 5 mg PO is ordered. The test for HIT antibody was reported as positive, with an optical density of 1.4 (negative cut-off < 0.4).

Question 2: Is discontinuing the Argatroban and administering FFP and Vitamin K clearly indicated?

Answer: Time to steady state is prolonged when clearance is reduced. The 59-second aPTT value at 4 hours, which could be steady state in healthy subjects, may not represent steady state in this patient and might continue to rise. As the aPTT value increased, so did the INR, suggesting an argatroban effect. The INR elevation did not represent a true state of excessive anticoagulation, so the request for vitamin K and FFP was likely not necessary. Holding the DTI for a prolonged period of time may also leave the patient with a very hypercoagulable condition unprotected against thrombosis formation, especially if the platelets have not recovered.

The argatroban is restarted, and, by day three, the argatroban infusion had been adjusted to 3 mg/h (approximately 0.6 mcg/kg/min) with an aPTT of 55 seconds (and INR 3.3), with a platelet count increased to 120 K/mm^3. Warfarin was requested for prophylaxis against HIT related thrombosis for 4 weeks. The initial dose was 10 mg PO times one.

Question 3: Is this an appropriate starting dose of warfarin in an HIT patient?

Answer: Overaggressive warfarin therapy in the setting of HIT is discouraged because of the risk for venous limb gangrene associated with overshooting warfarin related anticoagulation early in therapy. A more conservative regimen (5 mg or less) should be considered.

Question 4: When can a direct thrombin inhibitor be safely discontinued when transitioning to warfarin?

Answer: A measured INR around 5.0 while the aPTT is still within range may reflect a 1.5 to 2 point rise in the INR and a value of around 2.0 off the DTI. At this point, the infusion can be stopped as long as the platelet count has sufficiently recovered (at least to 100,000) with an INR and aPTT checked to verify adequate anticoagulation from warfarin alone. The low argatroban infusion rate may suggest a reduced clearance and that a longer hold (8–12 hours) may be necessary for the DTI effects to dissipate.

References

1. Di Nisio M, Middeldorp S, Buller HR. Direct Thrombin Inhibitors. *N Engl J Med.* 2005;353:1028-40.
2. Kaplan KL. Direct thrombin inhibitors. *Expert Opin Pharmacother.* 2003;4:653-66.
3. Adams TE, Everse SJ, Mann KG. Predicting the pharmacology of thrombin inhibitors. *J Thromb Haemost.* 2003;1:1024-7.
4. Seybert AL, Coons JC, Zerumsky K. Treatment of Heparin-Induced Thrombocytopenia: Is their a role for bivalirudin? *Pharmacotherapy.* 2006;26:229-41.
5. Greinacher A. The use of direct thrombin inhibitors in cardiovascular surgery in patients with heparin-induced thrombocytopenia. *Semin Thromb Hemost.* 2004;30:315-27.
6. Mann MJ, Tseng E, Ratcliffe M, et al. Use of bivalirudin, a direct thrombin inhibitor, and its reversal with modified ultrafiltration during heart transplantation in a patient with heparin-induced thrombocytopenia. *J Heart Lung Transplant.* 2005;24:222-5.
7. Stratmann G, deSilva AM, Tseng EE, et al. Reversal of direct thrombin inhibition after cardiopulmonary bypass in a patient with heparin-induced thrombocytopenia. *Anesth Analg.* 2004;98:1635-9.
8. Dager WE, Dougherty JA, Nguyen PH, et al. Heparin-induced thrombocytopenia: treatment options and special considerations. *Pharmacotherapy.* 2007;27:564-87.
9. Hantgan RR, Jerome WG, Hursting MJ. No effect of clot age or thrombolysis on fibrin- or clot-incorportated thrombin: comparison with heparin and recombinant hirudin. *Thromb Haemost.* 1994;72:381-6.
10. Swan SK, Hursting MJ. The pharmacokinetics and pharmacodynamics of argatroban: effects of age, gender, and hepatic or renal dysfunction. *Pharmacotherapy.* 2000;20:318-29.
11. Prescribing Information. Argatroban. Research Triangle Park, NC; GlaxoSmithKline Pharmaceuticals. February 2005.
12. Prescribing Information. Refludan (lepirudin). Wayne, NJ: Berlex Laboratories. October 2004.
13. Prescribing Information. Angiomax (bivalirudin) Parsippany, NJ; The Medicines Company. February 2005.
14. Schiele F, Lindgaerde F, Eriksson H, et al. Subcutaneous recombinant hirudin (HBW 023) versus intravenous sodium heparin in treatment of established acute deep vein thrombosis of the legs: a multicentre prospective dose-ranging randomized trial. International Multicentre Hirudin Study Group. *Thromb Haemost.* 1997;77:834-48.
15. Huhle G, Hoffmann U, Hoffmann I, et al. A new therapeutic option by subcutaneous recombinant hirudin in patients with heparin-induced thrombocytopenia type II: a pilot study. *Thromb Res.* 2000;99:325-34.
16. Deitcher SR, Ngengwe R, Kaplan R, et al. Subcutaneous lepirudin for heparin-induced thrombocytopenia and when other anticoagulants fail: illustrative cases. *Clin Advance Hem Oncol.* 2004;2:382-4.
17. Andreescu ACM, Cushman M, Hammond JM, et al. Trousseau's Syndrome treated with long term subcutaneous lepirudin (case report and review of the literature). *J Thromb Thrombolysis.* 2001;11:33-7.

18. Greinacher A. Treatment options for heparin-induced thrombocytopenia. *Am J Health-Syst Pharm.* 2003;60 Suppl 5:S12-8.
19. Greinacher A, Warkentin TE. Recognition, treatment, and prevention of heparin-induced thrombocytopenia: Review and update. *Thromb Res.* 2006; 118:165-76.
20. Lubenow N, Eichler P, Leitz T, et al. Lepirudin for prophylaxis of thrombosis in patients with acute isolated heparin-induced thrombocytopenia: an analysis of 3 prospective studies. *Blood.* 2004;104:3072-7.
21. Dager WE, White RH. Low-molecular-weight heparin-induced thrombocytopenia in a child. *Ann Pharmacother.* 2004;38:247-50.
22. Fischer KG. Hirudin in renal insufficiency. *Semin Thromb Hemost.* 2002; 28:467-82.
23. Smythe MA, Stephens JL, Koerber JM, et al. A comparison of lepirudin and argatroban outcomes. *Clin Appl Thromb Hemost.* 2005;11:371-4.
24. Kiser TH, Fish D. Evaluation of bivalirudin treatment for heparin-induced thrombocytopenia in critically ill patients with hepatic and/or renal dysfunction. *Pharmacotherapy.* 2006;26:452-60.
25. Vanholder R, Camez A, Veys N, et al. Pharmacokinetics of recombinant hirudin in hemodialyzed end-stage renal failure patients. *Thromb Haemost.* 1997;77:650-5.
26. Dager WE, White RH. Use of lepirudin in patients with heparin-induced thrombocytopenia and renal failure requiring hemodialysis. *Ann Pharmacother.* 2001;35:885-90.
27. Willey ML, de Denus S, Spinler SA. Removal of lepirudin, a recombinant hirudin, by hemodialysis, hemofiltration, or plasmapheresis. *Pharmacotherapy.* 2002;22:492-9.
28. Eicher P, Friesen HJ, Lubenow N, et al. Antihirudin antibodies in patients with heparin-induced thrombocytopenia treated with lepirudin: incidence, effects on aPTT, and clinical relevance. *Blood.* 2000;96:2373-8.
29. Verstraete M, Nurmohohamed M, Kienast J, et al. Biologic effects of recombinant hirudin (CGP 39393) in human volunteers. *J Am Coll Cardiol.* 1993;22:1080-1088.
30. Verme-Gibboney CN, Hursting MJ. Argatroban dosing in patient with heparin-induced thrombocytopenia. *Ann Pharmacother.* 2003;37:970-5.
31. Lewis BE, Wallis DE, Berkowitz SD, et al. Argatroban anticoagulant therapy in patients with heparin-induced thrombocytopenia. *Circulation.* 2001;103:1838-43.
32. Lewis BE, Wallis DE, Leya F, et al. Argatroban anticoagulation in patients with heparin-induced thrombocytopenia. *Arch Intern Med.* 2003;163:1849-56.
33. Dager WE, White RH. Argatroban for heparin induced thrombocytopenia in hepato-renal failure and CVVHD. *Ann Pharmacother.* 2003;37:1232-6.
34. Williamson DR, Boulanger I, Tardif M, et al. Argatroban dosing in intensive care patients with acute renal failure and liver dysfunction. *Pharmacotherapy.* 2004;24:409-14.
35. Reddy BV, Grossman EJ, Trevino SA, et al. Argatroban anticoagulation in patients with heparin-induced thrombocytopenia requiring renal replacement therapy. *Ann Pharmacother.* 2005;39:1601-5.
36. Yeo EL, Hicks L, Huh J. Experience with argatroban dosing for heparin induced thrombocytopenia at a large, tertiary, teaching hospital [abstract]. *Blood.* 2003;102:128b (abstract 4218).
37. Baghdasarian SB, Singh I, Militello MA, et al. Argatroban dosage in critically ill patients with HIT [abstract]. *Blood.* 2004;104:493a (abstract 1779).
38. Arpino PA, Hallisey RK. Effect of renal function on the pharmacodynamics of argatroban. *Ann Pharmacother.* 2004;38:25-9.
39. Tang IY, Cox DS, Patel K, et al. Argatroban and renal replacement therapy in patients with heparin-induced thrombocytopenia. *Ann Pharmacother.* 2005;39:231-6.
40. Dager WE, White RH. Pharmacotherapy of heparin-induced thrombocytopenia. *Expert Opin on Pharmacother.* 2003:4:919-40.
41. Greinacher A, Volpel H, Janssens U, et al. Recombinant hirudin (lepirudin) provides safe and effective anticoagulation in patients with heparin-induced thrombocytopenia: a prospective study. *Circulation.* 1999;99:73-80.
42. Greinacher A, Janssens U, Berg G, et al. Lepirudin (recombinant hirudin) for parenteral anticoagulation in patients with heparin-induced thrombocytopenia. Heparin-Associated Thrombocytopenia Study (HAT) investigators. *Circulation.* 1999;100:587-93.
43. Lubenow N, Eicher P, Lietz T, Greinacher A, HIT Investigators group. Lepirudin in patients with heparin-induced thrombocytopenia–results of the third prospective study (HAT-3) and a combined analysis of HAT-1, HAT-2, and HAT-3. *J Thromb Haemost.* 2005;3:2428-36.
44. Lubenow N, Eichler P, Greinacher A. Results of a large drug monitoring program confirms the safety and efficacy of Refludan (lepirudin) in patients with immune-mediated heparin-induced thrombocytopenia (HIT) [abstract]. *Blood.* 2002;100:502a.
45. Lewis BE, Wallis DE, Hursting MJ, et al. Effects of argatroban therapy, demographic variables, and platelet count on thrombotic risk in heparin-induced thrombocytopenia. *Chest.* 2006;129:1407-16.
46. Eicher P, Friesen HJ, Lubenow N, et al. Antihirudin antibodies in patients with heparin-induced thrombocytopenia treated with lepirudin: incidence, effects on aPTT, and clinical relevance. *Blood.* 2000;96:2373-8.
47. Greinacher A, Lubenow N, Eicher P. Anaphylactic and anaphylactoid reactions associated with lepirudin in patients with heparin-induced thrombocytopenia. *Circulation.* 2003;108:2062-5.
48. Badger NO, Butler K, Hallman LC. Excessive anticoagulation and anaphylactic reaction after rechallenge with lepirudin in a patient with heparin-induced thrombocytopenia. *Pharmacotherapy.* 2004;24:1800-3.
49. Eicher P, Lubenow N, Strobel U, et al. Antibodies against lepirudin are polyspecific and recognize epitopes on bivalirudin. *Blood.* 2004;103:613-6.
50. Gray E, Harenberg J. Collaborative study on monitoring methods to determine direct thrombin inhibitors lepirudin and argatroban. *J Thromb Haemost.* 2005;3:2096-7.
51. Gosselin RC, King JH, Janatpour KA, et al. Comparing direct thrombin inhibitors using aPTT, ecarin

clotting times, and thrombin inhibitor management testing. *Ann Pharmacother.* 2004;38:1383-8.
52. Jusko WJ. Guidelines for collection and analysis of pharmacokinetic data. (chapter 2). In Burton ME, Shaw LM, Schentag JJ, Evans WE, eds. Applied Pharmacokinetics and Pharmacodynamics. Baltimore, MD: Lippincott Williams & Wilkins; 2005:3-29.
53. van Griensven JM, Koster RW, Burggraaf J, et al. Effects of liver blood flow on the pharmacokinetics of tissue-type plasminogen activator (alteplase) during thrombolysis in patients with acute myocardial infarction. *Clin Pharmacol Ther.* 1998;63:39-47.
54. Reichert MG, MacGregor DA, Kincaid EH, et al. Excessive argatroban anticoagulation for heparin-induced thrombocytopenia. *Ann Pharmacother.* 2003;37:652-4.
55. Gosselin RC, Dager WE, King JH, et al. Effect of direct thrombin-inhibitors: bivalirudin, lepirudin and argatroban, on prothrombin time and INR measurements. *Am J Clin Pathol.* 2004;121:593-9.
56. Brown PM, Hursting MJ. Lack of pharmacokinetic interactions between argatroban and warfarin. *Am J Health-Syst Pharm.* 2002;59:2078-83.
57. Warkentin TE, Greinacher A. Heparin-induced thrombocytopenia: recognition, treatment, and prevention: the Seventh ACCP Conference on Antithrombotic and Thrombolytic Therapy. *Chest.* 2004;126(3 suppl):311S-337S.
58. Olson JD, Arkin CF, Brandt JT, et al. College of American pathologists conference XXXI on laboratory monitoring of anticoagulant therapy. Laboratory monitoring of unfractionated heparin therapy. *Arch Pathol Lab Med.* 1998;122:782-98.
59. Arpino PA, Demirjian Z, Van Cott EM. Use of the chromogenic factor X assay to predict the international normalized ratio in patients transitioning from argatroban to warfarin. *Pharmacotherapy.* 2005;25:157-64.
60. Trask AS, Gosselin RC, Diaz JA, et al. Warfarin initiation and monitoring with clotting factors II, VII, and X. *Ann Pharmacother.* 2004;38:251-6.
61. Wolzt M, Levi M, Sarich TC, et al. Effect of recombinant factor VIIa on melagatran-induced inhibition of thrombin generation and platelet activation in healthy volunteers. *Thromb Haemost.* 2004;91:1090-6.
62. O'Connell KA, Wood JJ, Wise RP, et al. Thromboembolic adverse events after use of recombinant human coagulation factor VIIa. *JAMA.* 2006;295:293-8.
63. Koster A, Chew D, Grundel M, et al. An assessment of different filter systems for extracorporeal elimination of bivalirudin: an in vitro study. *Anesth Analg.* 2003;96:1316-9.

Chapter 13

Helpful References and Preparing for the Future

Michael Gulseth

Chapter Outline

- Introduction
- Helpful resources
  - Journals
  - Textbooks
  - Conferences
  - Credentials
- Preparing for the future
  - New anticoagulants
  - The "antithrombosis service"
- Conclusion
- References

Introduction

Approaches for managing anticoagulation therapy have undergone tremendous change in the past 10–15 years, and show no sign of slowing down. In addition, preventing or treating thromboembolism has become complex enough that focused practices in anticoagulation therapy have become a reality in both the outpatient and inpatient settings. This text is evidence of this by exploring the evolving role of inpatient anticoagulation services to facilitate patient care needs given the ever expanding complexity of the acutely ill inpatient and complexity of anticoagulation therapy. Practitioners desiring to be successful either in establishing or practicing in an inpatient anticoagulation service will be constantly challenged with keeping up with the rapid changes in this area. The purpose of this final chapter is to:

- explore helpful resources (many of which were used heavily in preparing this text) to an inpatient anticoagulation service.
- identify future approaches to anticoagulant therapy on the horizon and how they may alter the anticoagulation treatment landscape.
- briefly discuss the concept of the antithrombosis service.

Helpful Resources

Journals

Perhaps the single most helpful clinical reference for any anticoagulation service is the most recent practice recommendation of American College of Chest Physicians Consensus Conference on Antithrombotic Therapy, commonly referred to as the "Chest" guidelines.[1] The current version of this document is the September 2004 supplement to *Chest* and it is updated every 2–3 years. The document is a comprehensive review of the evidence supporting the use of all antithrombotics. The expert panel uses medical evidence to formulate expert practice recommendations that are graded based on the strength of the evidence. It contains information that focuses both on important disease states (such as atrial fibrillation, deep vein thrombosis, etc.) and different classes of antithrombotics (warfarin, heparins, anti-platelets, etc.). It may be worth while to have hard copies or electronic access to this important document easily accessible for all pharmacists working in an anticoagulation service.

The American Heart Association, in conjunction with the American College of Cardiology, regularly publishes expert recommendations on how to treat different disease states based on the most current evidence. They are also graded, much like the Chest guidelines, based on the strength of the evidence. Examples of diseases covered by these expert recommendations are different types of acute coronary syndromes[2,3] and peripheral arterial disease.[4] They are available for free on-line at http://my.americanheart.org/portal/professional/guidelines. One particular guideline that is medication specific is their "Foundation Guide to Warfarin Therapy."[5] This guideline is a helpful review of warfarin similar to the vitamin K antagonist chapter of the Chest guidelines.[6] It is important to note that all of the guidelines above may contain outdated information by the time they are published, still are prone to opinions of the selected authors, and may be heavily weighted on evidence based on clinical trials that may have excluded many of situations where anticoagulation is utilized in the inpatient setting.

It is quite common to find excellent articles on both the clinical and practice issues relative to anticoagulation therapy in the inpatient setting in different pharmacy journals. *Pharmacotherapy*[7] and *The Annals of Pharmacotherapy*[8,9] often have both primary and tertiary articles on anticoagulation related topics. The *American Journal of Health-System Pharmacy* has also had excellent articles on anticoagulation related topics.[10,11] An anticoagulation pharmacist should regularly review articles in both pharmacy and medical journals to keep current his or her practice.

Textbooks

While textbooks do not have the currency of content provided in more often published journals, they offer solid and comprehensive information that can be referred to and applied to practice on a daily basis. An excellent textbook that deals extensively with warfarin management is *Managing Oral Anticoagulation Therapy: Clinical and Operational Guidelines* available from Facts and Comparisons at http://www.factsandcomparisons.com/Products/index.aspx?cat=6&id=1077. This text covers both the operational and clinical components of setting up and running an outpatient anticoagulation clinic. Although the text focuses on the outpatient setting, many concepts presented can be applied to the inpatient setting. Much of this information, particularly the clinical information, will also be helpful for an inpatient anticoagulation pharmacist.

Another extremely helpful textbook is *Staff Development for Pharmacy Practice*, written by Christine M. Nimmo, Ph.D. and published by the American Society of Health-System Pharmacists (ASHP). The text provides important tools for any hospital pharmacy department that is serious about increasing the provision of direct patient care by their pharmacists. It covers topics such as reframing the role of the pharmacist and how to train pharmacists for new roles.

A final helpful ASHP textbook that was heavily utilized in preparing this text is *Developing Clinical Practice Skills for Pharmacists*, by Kimberly Galt, Pharm.D. This text would be helpful for individual pharmacists who need a brush up on how to provide pharmaceutical care or for use in training and competence assessment. Helpful topics that are covered include developing a pharmaceutical care plan, interacting with patients, and care plan documentation. The text is very user-friendly with numerous case examples of important concepts discussed in the text.

The above listed texts are just examples of what can be found and used to prepare for and implement an inpatient service.

Conferences

Both the American College of Clinical Pharmacy and ASHP often cover numerous anticoagulation patient care topics at their meetings. The University of Wisconsin Extension Services in Pharmacy regularly has an all day conference the Saturday before the ASHP Midyear Meeting in the same city as the meeting. This is known as the Pharmacy Invitational Conference on Antithrombotic Therapy. This meeting is typically free of charge and interested pharmacist can sign up through their website, at: www.ce.pharmacy.wisc.edu/index.pl. The Anticoagulation Forum, a multidisplinary network of healthcare professionals interested in anticoagulation therapy, also holds an annual meeting every other year where both posters and presentations on anticoagulation related topics provide a excellent opportunity to keep current. If interested, registration information can be found at: www.acforum.org.

Credentials

The most widely recognized credential in this field is the Certified Anticoagulation Care Provider credential. This is a multi-disciplinary credential open to registered nurses, advance practice nurses, pharmacists, physicians, and certified physician assistants. To sit for the exam, the provider must document experience in caring for patients on anticoagulation therapy. Unfortunately, this experience requirement is largely focused on caring for anticoagulation patients in the outpatient arena, and it would be difficult to satisfy the requirements without working in an outpatient practice. For further information on this credential, please see www.ncbap.org.

Preparing for the Future

New Anticoagulants

The near approval of ximelagatran, which would have been the first new orally active anticoagulant since warfarin, is a good example of why pharmacists need to keep abreast of the anticoagulation medication pipeline.[10] Many predicted this could radically alter the role of all anticoagulation services (both inpatient and outpatient)[12] and numerous anticoagulant medications are currently in the pipeline. Approval of any agent that can largely displace the need for warfarin or heparin therapy has the potential to be a blockbuster and radically expand the thought process in utilizing anticoagulation therapy, broadening the role of an inpatient anticoagulation pharmacist.

Table 13-1, as of the publication of this text, is an up-to-date listing of the current anticoagulation medications in the pipeline. The medications in phase 3, the closest to approval, are listed first and then phase 2 medications.

The "Antithrombosis Service"

Due to the rapid changes coming in anticoagulation drug therapy, a popular concept is moving the terminology away from being an "anticoagulation service" and more toward an "antithrombosis service."[13] This type of service would focus more on caring for patients with thrombotic disorders from a range of antithrombotic options including more than just anticoagulants. This would likely be multidisciplinary in nature and the expertise of a pharmacist would be needed to help facilitate implementation of a successful medication management plan designed to meet the individual needs of each patient based on his or her clinical presentation and ability to complete the therapy. This may be especially critical as more treatment option and agents become available. Depending on the future evolution of therapy, future editions of this text may also be geared to follow this trend.

Conclusion

Both the inpatient anticoagulation pharmacist and the anticoagulation program manager will need a wealth of references (many of which were used heavily in preparing this text) to run an inpatient anticoagulation service. All pharmacists associated with these services should monitor investigational anticoagulants on the horizon that may change traditional therapies. Many of these changes may spur the development of more comprehensive antithrombosis services.

References

1. Schunemann HJ, Munger H, Brower S, et al. Methodology for guideline development for the Seventh American College of Chest Physicians Conference on Antithrombotic and Thrombolytic Therapy: the Seventh ACCP Conference on Antithrombotic and Thrombolytic Therapy. *Chest.* Sep 2004;126(3 Suppl):174S-8S.
2. Braunwald E, Antman EM, Beasley JW, et al. ACC/AHA 2002 guideline update for the management of patients with unstable angina and non-ST-segment elevation myocardial infarction—summary article: a report of the American College of Cardiology/American Heart Association task force on practice guidelines (Committee on the Management of Patients With Unstable Angina). *J Am Coll Cardiol.* 2002;40(7):1366-74.
3. Antman EM, Anbe DT, Armstrong PW, et al. ACC/AHA guidelines for the management of patients with ST-elevation myocardial infarction: a report of the American College of Cardiology/American Heart Association Task Force on Practice Guidelines (Committee to Revise the 1999 Guidelines for the Management of Patients with Acute Myocardial Infarction). *Circulation.* 2004;110(9):e82-292.
4. Hirsch AT, Haskal ZJ, Hertzer NR, et al. ACC/AHA 2005 Practice Guidelines for the management of patients with peripheral arterial disease (lower extremity, renal, mesenteric, and abdominal aortic): a collaborative report from the American Association for Vascular Surgery/Society for Vascular Surgery, Society for Cardiovascular Angiography and Interventions, Society for Vascular Medicine and Biology, Society of Interventional Radiology, and the ACC/AHA Task Force on Practice Guidelines (Writing Committee to Develop Guidelines for the Management of Patients With Peripheral Arterial Disease). Endorsed by the American Association of Cardiovascular and Pulmonary Rehabilitation; National Heart, Lung, and Blood Institute; Society for Vascular Nursing; TransAtlantic Inter-Society Consensus; and Vascular Disease Foundation. *Circulation.* 2006;113(11):e463-654.
5. Hirsh J, Fuster V, Ansell J, Halperin JL. American Heart Association/American College of Cardiology Foundation guide to warfarin therapy. *J Am Coll Cardiol.* May 7 2003;41(9):1633-52.
6. Ansell J, Hirsh J, Poller L, et al. The pharmacology and management of the vitamin K antagonists: the Seventh ACCP Conference on Antithrombotic and Thrombolytic Therapy. *Chest.* 2004;126(3 Suppl):204S-33S.
7. Bond CA, Raehl CL. Pharmacist-provided anticoagu-

Table 13-1.
Anticoagulants in the Pipeline*

Medication	Administration Route	Pharmacologic Effect	Phase	Manufacturer	Targeted Indications	Comments
Idraparinux (SR-34006)[14]	Injectable	Indirect Xa inhibitor	III	Sanofi-Aventis	Deep vein thrombosis (DVT) and pulmonary embolism (PE) treatment, stroke prevention for atrial fibrillation, extended treatment after a DVT or PE	Similar in pharmacology to fondaparinux, but longer acting; once a week subcutaneous injection; reversibility is a concern
Biotinylated idraparinux (SSR-126517E)	Injectable	Indirect Xa inhibitor	III	Sanofi-Aventis	DVT and PE treatment	Updated potentially reversible version of idraparinux; once a week subcutaneous injection
Dabigatran etexilate (BIBR-1048)[15,16]	Oral	Direct thrombin inhibitor	III	Boehringer Ingelheim Pharmaceuticals	DVT prevention after knee and hip replacement surgery, DVT and PE treatment, extended treatment after a DVT/PE, stroke prevention for atrial fibrillation	Prodrug that is rapidly converted to active dabigatran; closest oral anticoagulant to the market; must avoid liver problems seen with ximelagatran
Apixaban	Oral	Direct Xa inhibitor	II and III	Bristol-Myers Squibb	DVT prevention after knee replacement surgery and cancer, DVT treatment, treatment of acute coronary syndrome	No current trials to prevent stroke due to atrial fibrillation
Rivaroxaban (BAY 59-7939)	Oral	Direct Xa inhibitor	III	Bayer/Johnson & Johnson	DVT prevention after hip and knee replacement surgery (including extended therapy in hip replacement), DVT treatment	No current trials to prevent stroke due to atrial fibrillation

Continued

Table 13-1. (cont'd)
Anticoagulants in the Pipeline*

Medication	Administration Route	Pharmacologic Effect	Phase	Manufacturer	Targeted Indications	Comments
LY-517717	Oral	Direct Xa inhibitor	II	Eli Lilly and Company	DVT prevention after hip or knee replacement surgery	
YM-150	Oral	Direct Xa inhibitor	II	Astellas Pharma	DVT prevention after hip replacement surgery	
DU-176b	Oral	Direct Xa inhibitor	II	Daiichi Sankyo	DVT prevention after hip replacement surgery	
PRT-054021	Oral	Direct Xa inhibitor	II	Portola Pharmaceuticals	DVT prevention after knee replacement surgery	
Tifacogen[17]	Intravenous	Recombinant tissue factor pathway inhibitor	III	Novartis/Chiron Corporation	Severe community-acquired pneumonia	Previously failed to improve severe sepsis mortality
ART-123[18]	Subcutaneous	Recombinant soluble thrombomodulin; binds to thrombin to activate protein C	II	Asahi Kasei	DVT prevention after hip replacement surgery	Sepsis studies are planned in the future
Otamixaban	Intravenous	Direct Xa inhibitor	II	Sanofi-Aventis	Acute coronary syndromes	
DX-9065a[19,20]	Intravenous	Direct Xa inhibitor	II	Daiichi Pharmaceuticals	Acute coronary syndromes	
rNAPc2[21,22]	Subcutaneous	Inhibitor of the tissue factor/factor VIIa complex	II	Nuvelo	Acute coronary syndromes, DVT prevention after knee replacement surgery	Recombinant form of a protein isolated from the hemophagocytic hookworm *Ancylostoma caninum*
Ancrod[23]	Intravenous	Cleaves fibrinogen	III	Neurobiological Technologies	Ischemic stroke	Purified fraction of the Malaysian pit viper (*Calloselasma rhodostoma*)
TPP-889	Oral	Factor IXa	II	TransTech Pharma	Prevention of DVT after hip repair surgery	
BMS-562247	Oral	Direct Xa inhibitor	II	Bristol-Myers Squibb	DVT prevention after knee replacement surgery	

*The clinicaltrial.gov website was searched extensively in preparing this table. Other references are noted with each drug.

lation management in United States hospitals: death rates, length of stay, Medicare charges, bleeding complications, and transfusions. *Pharmacotherapy.* 2004;24(8):953-63.
8. Dager WE, Branch JM, King JH, et al. Optimization of inpatient warfarin therapy: impact of daily consultation by a pharmacist-managed anticoagulation service. *Ann Pharmacother.* 2000;34(5):567-72.
9. Dager WE. Initiating warfarin therapy. *Ann Pharmacother.* 2003;37(6):905-8.
10. Gulseth MP. Ximelagatran: an orally active direct thrombin inhibitor. *Am J Health-Syst Pharm.* 2005;62(14):1451-67.
11. Schneider BL, Gulseth MP, Cusick MA, et al. Computer program to assist pharmacy management of an inpatient warfarin dosing service. *Am J Health-Syst Pharm.* 2005;62(22):2393-6.
12. Nutescu EA, Pickard AS, Blackburn JC, et al. Impact of oral direct thrombin inhibitors on anticoagulation clinics. *Pharmacotherapy.* 2004;24(9):1204-12.
13. Nutescu EA. The future of anticoagulation clinics. *J Thromb Thrombolysis.* 2003;16(1-2):61-3.
14. PERSIST Investigators. A novel long-acting synthetic factor Xa inhibitor (SanOrg34006) to replace warfarin for secondary prevention in deep vein thrombosis. A Phase II evaluation. *J Thromb Haemost.* 2004;2(1):47-53.
15. Eriksson BI, Dahl OE, Ahnfelt L, et al. Dose escalating safety study of a new oral direct thrombin inhibitor, dabigatran etexilate, in patients undergoing total hip replacement: BISTRO I. *J Thromb Haemost.* 2004;2(9):1573-80.
16. Eriksson BI, Dahl OE, Buller HR, et al. A new oral direct thrombin inhibitor, dabigatran etexilate, compared with enoxaparin for prevention of thromboembolic events following total hip or knee replacement: the BISTRO II randomized trial. *J Thromb Haemost.* 2005;3(1):103-11.
17. Abraham E, Reinhart K, Opal S, et al. Efficacy and safety of tifacogin (recombinant tissue factor pathway inhibitor) in severe sepsis: a randomized controlled trial. *JAMA.* 2003;290(2):238-47.
18. Kearon C, Comp P, Douketis J, et al. Dose-response study of recombinant human soluble thrombomodulin (ART-123) in the prevention of venous thromboembolism after total hip replacement. *J Thromb Haemost.* 2005;3(5):962-8.
19. Alexander JH, Dyke CK, Yang H, et al. Initial experience with factor-Xa inhibition in percutaneous coronary intervention: the XaNADU-PCI Pilot. *J Thromb Haemost.* 2004;2(2):234-41.
20. Alexander JH, Yang H, Becker RC, et al. First experience with direct, selective factor Xa inhibition in patients with non-ST-elevation acute coronary syndromes: results of the XaNADU-ACS Trial. *J Thromb Haemost.* 2005;3(3):439-47.
21. Lee A, Agnelli G, Buller H, et al. Dose-response study of recombinant factor VIIa/tissue factor inhibitor recombinant nematode anticoagulant protein c2 in prevention of postoperative venous thromboembolism in patients undergoing total knee replacement. *Circulation.* 2001;104(1):74-8.
22. Moons AH, Peters RJ, Bijsterveld NR, et al. Recombinant nematode anticoagulant protein c2, an inhibitor of the tissue factor/factor VIIa complex, in patients undergoing elective coronary angioplasty. *J Am Coll Cardiol.* 2003;41(12):2147-53.
23. Sherman DG, Atkinson RP, Chippendale T, et al. Intravenous ancrod for treatment of acute ischemic stroke: the STAT study: a randomized controlled trial. Stroke Treatment with Ancrod Trial. *JAMA.* 2000;283(18):2395-403.

Index

A

Abbreviations, do not use, 19-20
Acarbose, 138
Acetaminophen, 137
Acetylsalicylic acid, 137
Action plan, implementation, 89, 90
Adverse drug events, 19, 81, 84
    fishbone diagram, 22
    review of, 40
    warfarin, 158
Advisory organizations, 18
Agency for Healthcare Research and Quality, 143
Agent selection, 14-15
Alcohol, 137
American Academy of Neurology, 146
American College of Cardiology, 216
American College of Chest Physicians Consensus Conference on Antithrombotic Therapy, 3, 44, 143, 189, 215-16
American College of Clinical Pharmacy, 216
American Heart Association, 146, 216
American Journal of Health-System Pharmacy, 216
American Journal of Pharmaceutical Education, 102
American Society of Gastrointestinal Endoscopy, 156
American Society of Health-System Pharmacists, 216
Amiodarone, 136, 137
Amiodarone-induced toxicosis, 137
Amoxicillin, 137
Amoxicillin/clavulanate, 137
Amoxicillin/tranexamic rinse, 137
Anabolic steroids, 138
Angina, unstable, 163
Annals of Pharmacotherapy, The, 216
Ansell, Jack, 3
Anticoagulant
    antithrombin, 178
    developing, 217, 218-19
    response, 43
    safety, 17-22
Anticoagulation Forum, The, 216
Antihistamines, 185
Antiphospholipid antibodies (APLAs), 147-48
Antiphospholipid antibody syndrome (APS), 147-48
Antithrombosis service, 217
Antithrombotic Gap Analysis Tool, 20-21
Appropriate therapy, 42
Argatroban, 191, 210-11
    contraindications, precautions, 206-7
    dosing guidelines, monitoring form, 66-67
    indications, 205-6
    monitoring, 208-9
    orders 63
    pharmacokinetics, pharmacodynamics, 204-5
    policy and procedure, 64-65
Aspirin, 136, 142, 146, 156, 163
Atrial fibrillation, 163
Automated dispensing cabinet, 17
Avocado, 138
Azathioprine, 137
Azithromycin, 137

B

Barbiturates, 137
Benchmarking, 14, 128, 129
Bezafibrate, 137
Bioprosthetic valves, 146
Birth control, 164
Bivalirudin, 203
    contraindications, precautions, 206-7
    monitoring, 208-9
    reversal, 210
Blood testing, follow up, 43
Bloom's levels of cognitive learning, 95
Bloom's taxonomy of learning, 94
Body weight extremes, 196-97
Boldo-fenugreek, 138
Bosentan, 137
Bridge therapy, 4, 5, 191
    guidelines, 44, 48-50
    plan, 156
Budget considerations, 78
Business description, 80, 84-85, 87
Business plan, 83-90
Business plan development, 80
Business proposal presentation, 82

221

C

Carbamazepine, 137
Cardiac dysfunction, 207
Cardioversion, 163
Carvedilol, 163
Case presentations, 95
Cefamandole, 137
Cefazolin, 137
Celecoxib, 137
Centers for Medicare and Medicaid Services, 14
Certified Anticoagulation Care Provider, 216-17
Chart documentation, 27-28
Chelation therapy, 138
Chloramphenicol, 137
Chlordiazepoxide, 137
Cholestyramine, 137
Choral hydrate, 137
Cimetidine, 136, 138
Ciprofloxacin, 137
Citalopram, 137
Clarithromycin, 137
Clofibrate, 137
Clopidogrel, 136
Cloxacillin, 137
CMF, 138
Coagulation cascade, 135
Cognitive tests, 97
Communication essentials, 40-44
Competencies, 41
Competency assessment, 96-97
Complications reduction, 77
Conferences, 216
Conjugated estrogens, 161
Consensus guidelines, 41-44
Continuous quality improvement, 123-24
Conversion, 181
Coordinated, systematic care, 3-4, 5
Cost-benefit analysis, 78, 79, 83
Costs
    of care, 88
    fixed and variable, 79
Cotrimoxazole, 137
Coumadin, patient education, 103, 109-13
Cranberry juice, 138
Credentials, 216-17
Curbicin, 138
Cyclophosphamide/methotrexate/fluorouracil, 138
Cyclosporine, 138

D

Dager, William, 7-16, 177-202, 203-13
Dalteparin, 20, 196
Dalteparin
    calendar, 122
    check-off list, 121
    patient education, 103, 119-20
Danazol, 138
Danshen, 138
Danshen/methyl salicylate, 138
Data tracking, 30, 32
Deep venous thrombosis (DVT), 143-45, 198-99
Delivery systems, 4
Developing Clinical Practice Skills for Pharmacists, 216

Dextropropoxyphene, 137
Dicloxacillin, 137
Diet, 140
Digitalis, 185
Digoxin, 161, 163
Diltiazem, 137, 163
Dipyridamole, 136
Direct observations, 97
Direct thrombin inhibitor (DTI), 13, 14, 203-4
    contraindications/precautions, 206-7
    dosing guidelines, 66-67
    indications, 205-6
    initiating, 205
    monitoring, 66-67, 205, 207-9
    orders, 63
    pharmacokinetics, pharmacodynamics, 204-5
    pharmacology, 203-4
    policy and procedure, 64-65
    reversal, 210, 211
    transitioning to warfarin, 209-10
Discharge follow-up orders, 55
Disopyramide, 137
Dispensing, 19
Disulfiram, 137
Dong quai, 138
Doxycycline, 161, 163
Drug Competition and Patent Term Restoration Act, 159
Drug concentrations, 20
Drug interactions, 136
Drug interactions, 4, 136
DTI. *See* Direct thrombin inhibitor

E

ECMO. *See* Extracorporeal membrane oxygenation
Economic assessment, 78-80
Economic evaluation, 83
Education
    program, 93-94, 96, 98-99
    techniques, 94-95
Endoscopic procedures, 156
Enoxaparin, 3, 5, 10, 192, 196
    calendar, 122
    check-off list, 121
    dosing timeline and surgery, 51
    NPSG, 20
    patient education, 103, 116-18
Entacapone, 137
Enteral feeds, 138
Erythromycin, 137
Ethinyl estradiol/norethindrone, 164
Ethinyl estradiol/norgestimate, 164
Etoposide/carboplatin, 138
Etretinate, 138
Executive summary, 80, 84
Extracorporeal membrane oxygenation (ECMO), 13

F

Factor V Leiden gene mutation, 164
Facts and Comparisons, 103
Failure mode and effects analysis (FMEA), 21, 22
Feedback, 97
Felbamate, 137
Fenofibrate, 137

Financial analysis, 80
Financial perspective, 77-78
  budget considerations, 78
  economic assessment, 78-80
  projections, 81, 87-89
Fish oils, 136, 138
Fluconazole, 136, 137
Fluorouracil, 138
Fluoxetine/diazepam, 137
Fluvastatin, 137
Fluvoxamine, 137
FMEA. *See* Failure mode and effects analysis
FMEAInfoCentre, 21
Folic acid, 198
Fondaparinux, 143, 203
  body weight, 197
  conversion to adjusted-dose SC UFH, 181
  conversion to IV UFH, 181
  dosing, administration, 188, 193-94
  indications, 188, 193
  mechanism of action, 178
  monitoring, 194
  neuroaxial procedures, 192
  NPSG, 20
  pediatric patients, 197-98
  pharmacokinetics/pharmacodynamics, 191, 193
  pharmacologic, clinical properties, 179
  pharmacology, 191
  pharmacy management of, 10, 13
  pregnancy, 197
  renal impairment, 195-96
  reversal of, 195
  side effects, precautions, contraindications, 194
Fresh frozen plasma, 153
Furosemide, 137, 161, 163

G

Galt, Kimberly, 216
Garlic, 136
Gatifloxacin, 137
Gemcitabine, 138
Gemfibrozil, 137
Generic warfarin, 159-61, 162
Genetic issues, 139-40
Ginger, 136
Gingko biloba, 136
Ginseng, 136, 138
Grapefruit juice, 138
Green tea, 138
Griseofulvin, 137
Gulseth, Michael, 3-6, 39-75, 77-91, 93-99, 101-22, 123-29, 215-20

H

Health literacy evaluation, 101-2
Heart failure, 139, 161, 163
Hemorrhage risk, 156-58
Heparin, 4, 5-6, 84, 137, 143, 164, 206
  bag concentration standardization, 183
  error, 17
  infusion standardization, 18
  ISMP, 19
  pharmacist-provided management, 11-12
  pharmacy management of, 8-9
  protocol, 68-75
  resistance, 183
Heparin/coumadin monitoring, 32-33
Heparin-associated thrombocytopenia (HAT), 185
Heparin-induced thrombocytopenia (HIT), 13, 14, 159, 185, 191, 197, 204-6, 209, 210-11
Hepatic dysfunction, 207
Herbal supplements, 136
High reliability organizations (HRO), 18
High-risk/high-alert medications, 19
HIT. *See* Heparin-induced thrombocytopenia
Hospital administration, inpatient anticoagulation service, 45
Hospital savings, 88-89
HRO. *See* High reliability organizations
Hypersensitivity reactions, 185, 207-8
Hypertension, 161, 163

I

Ifosphamide, 138
Implementation action plan, 81-82
Indomethacin, 137
Inflation rate, 80
Influenza vaccine, 138
Inpatient anticoagulation care, 4-5
Inpatient policies and procedures, 41-44
INR, 5, 8
  daily, policy and procedure, 57
  elevations, 152-54
  range, 42
  use, 42
Institute for Healthcare Improvement, 4, 21
Institute for Safe Medication Practices (ISMP), 4, 17, 19, 20-21, 84
Institute of Medicine (IOM), 4, 18, 102
Interactive sessions, 97
Interferon, 137
International unit, 19-20
Internet, patient education resources, 103, 104-5
Intracranial hemorrhage, 153
Intravenous argatroban, 63
Invasive procedures, warfarin, 155-56, 158
IOM. *See* Institute of Medicine
Ischemic stroke, 146-47
ISMP. *See* Institute for Safe Medication Practices
Isoniazid, 137
Itraconazole, 137
IV warfarin, 135

J

Joint Commission®, 4, 5, 14, 40, 143
  medication management standards, 18-19
  RCA, 21
Just culture, 17-18, 21-22
Justification, 40

L

Language barriers, 102
Leadership essentials, 39-40
Learning pyramid, 96
Lectures, 97
Leflunomide, 137

223

Lepirudin, 191, 203
    contraindications, precautions, 206-7
    indications, 205-6
    monitoring, 208-9
    pharmacokinetics, pharmacodynamics, 204
    reversal, 210
Levamisole, 137
Levamisole/fluorouracil, 138
Levofloxacin, 137, 163
Levonorgestrel, 138
Liability issues, 82
Lisinopril, 163
Literature generalization, 79-80, 83
Literature review, 7-16
Liver dysfunction, 138
LMWHs. *See* Low molecular weight heparins
Losartan, 161
Low molecular weight heparins (LMWHs), 3, 4, 84, 143, 164, 203
    body weight, 196
    conversion to adjusted-dose SC UFH, 181
    conversion to IV UFH, 181
    dosing, administration, 187-89
    indications, 187, 188
    ISMP, 19
    mechanism of action, 178
    monitoring, 189-90, 198
    neuroaxial procedures, 192
    NPSG, 20
    pharmacologic, clinical properties, 179
    pharmacology, 186
    pharmacy management of, 9, 10, 13, 14
    pediatric dosing nomogram, 190
    pediatric patients, 197-98
    pharmacokinetics/pharmacodynamics, 187
    pregnancy, 197, 199
    renal impairment, 195-96
    reversal of, 195
    side effects, precautions, contraindications, 190-91
Low molecular weight heparin-enoxaparin, 189
Lycium barbarum, 138

M

Macrolides, 136
Malpractice claims, warfarin, 82
Managing Oral Anticoagulation Therapy, 81, 103, 216
Mango, 138
Market analysis, 81, 87
Medical staff champion, 24
Medicare
    Part B, 77
    Part D, 77
    patients, 10, 11-12, 88-89
Medication
    administration, 17, 19
    dispensing, 19
    effects, 19
    order review, 18
    preparation, 18-19
    reconciliation, 20
    storage, 18
Medication error, 4, 19
Medication Error Reporting Program (MERP), 20, 40

Medication Management Standards, 18-19
Medication Teaching Manual, The, 103
Medication Therapy Management Services, 77
Medication use evaluation (MUE), 40
Meoprolol, 161
Mercaptopurine, 138
Mesalamine, 137
Methylprednisolone, 137
Metolazone, 137
Metronidazole, 136, 137
Micronazole, 137
Micronazole topical, 137
Multidisciplinary approach, 14
Multivitamin supplement, 138

N

Nabumetone, 137
Nafcillin, 137
Nafcillin/dicloxacillin, 137
Nalidixic acid, 137
Naproxen, 28
National Clinical Pharmacy Services Database, 10
National Patient Safety Goals (NPSG), 5, 18, 19-20
National Quality Forum, 14, 18
Neel, Scott, 133-75
Neuroaxial procedures, 192
Nicotine, 185
Nimmo, Christine M., 216
Nitroglycerin, 163
Nonsteroidal anti-inflammatories (NSAIDs), 136, 156
Norfloxacin, 137
Nutescu, Edith, 177-202

O

Ofloxacin, 137
Omeprazole, 136, 138
Operational structure, processes, 81, 87
Orlistat, 138
Outcomes
    measurement, 79, 83
    pharmacist-provided drug management, 11-12
Outpatient anticoagulation
    care, 3-4
    consensus guidelines, 41-44
    flow sheet, 30
Overanticoagulation management
    in bleeding patient, 61
    in patient without bleeding, 60
    in surgical preparation, 61-62

P

Paclitaxel, 138
Pairing, 98
Patient
    assessment, 42
    care plan input, 27-28
    information, 18
    monitoring, 43
    outcomes, 77
    profile, 31
Patient-care unit, 27
Patient education
    Coumadin, 109-13

Index

cultural considerations, 102
general tips, 102-3
handouts, 103
health literacy evaluation, 101-2
injectable anticoagulants check-off list, 121
Internet resources, 103, 104-5
warfarin, 106-8
warfarin calendar, 115
warfarin check-off list, 114
Pay for performance, 14
PC-SPES, 138
Pediatric patients, 197-98
Penicillin, 136
Personal data assistants (PDAs), 78
Pharmacists
hiring, 26-27
making more efficient, 27
Pharmacodynamics, 134-40
Pharmacokinetics, 134-40
Pharmacology, 133-34
Pharmacotherapy, 216
Pharmacy manager/director, 78
Pharmacy and Therapeutics Committee, 44-45
Phenylbutazone, 137
Phenytoin, 137
Philosophical basis, 39
Pilot service flowchart, 37
Piroxicam, 137
Plan, Do, Study, Act (PDSA)
act on results, repeat cycle, 126, 129
implementing, 124, 127
methodology, planning, 124, 127
study changes effect, 124, 126, 127-28
Policies and procedures, 34, 41-42, 43-44
daily INR, 57
direct thrombin inhibitors, 64-65
pharmacist-managed warfarin dosing, 52-54
Vitamin K use, 58
Practice guidelines, 215-16
Precepting, 95-96
Pregnancy, 159, 160, 197, 198-99
Pre-natal vitamin, 198
Process measure data collection form, 125
Program
background, 80
barriers and solutions, 25-27
manager, identification, 23-24
Progress note, pharmacist, 29
Propafenone, 137
Propofol, 137
Propoxyphene, 137
Prosthetic heart valves, 145-46, 148, 157
Protamine sulfate, 194
Protamine, 195
Prothrombin-complex concentrate, 153
Protocols, 41, 68-75
Purple toe syndrome, 158

Q

Quality of patient care, 4
Quasiexperimental trials, 79
Quetiapine, 137
Quilinggao, 138

Quinidine, 137
Quinolones, 136

R

RAID analysis, 24-25, 35-36
Raloxifene hydrochloride, 138
Randomized trial, 79
RCA. *See* Root cause analysis
Reading materials, 97
Recombinant activated factor VIIa (rFVIIa), 14, 44, 47, 153-54, 195, 210
Regulatory organizations, 18
Renal impairment, 207, 195-96
Residency program, 27
Resource measurement, 79, 83
Reversal therapy, 13-14
Ribavirin, 137
Rifampin, 137
Risk-benefit analysis, 42
Risk management, 77, 89, 142
Ritonavir, 136, 137
Rofecoxib, 137
Root cause analysis (RCA), 21, 22
Ropinirole, 137

S

Saquinavir, 137
Sensitivity analysis, 80, 83
Sensitization factors, 150
Sertraline, 137
Service design flowchart, 25
Side effects, 43
Simulations, 97
Simvastatin, 137
Six Sigma, 123
Skills, 98
Skin necrosis, 158
SOAP notes, 27-28
Software needs, 30, 32
Sound-alike/look-alike medications, 19
Soy milk, 138
Special patient populations, 195-98
St. Mary's Medical Center (Duluth, MN), 26, 31, 78
Staff Development for Pharmacy Practice, 216
Staffing, 26, 88
Statistical analysis, 80
Stroke prevention, 141-43
Strykowski, Jill, 17-22
Study
design selection, 79-80
perspective, 78-79
Sucralfate, 138
Sulfamethoxazole/trimethoprim, 5
Sulfasalazine, 137
Sulfinpyrazone, 136, 137
Sulfisoxazole, 137
Sulindac, 137
Surgery
dosing schedules, 50-51
patient management, 61-62
Sushi with seaweed, 138
SWOT analysis, 24-25, 36-37
Systemic lupus erythematosus, 147

225

T

Tamoxifen, 138
Team planning, 24-25
Teicoplanin, 137
Telmisartan, 137
Terbinafine, 137
Testing, 98
Tetracycline, 137
Textbooks, 216
Thromboembolism risk, 155
Thyroid status, 139
Tinzaparin, 196
To Err is Human, 4, 18
Tolmetin, 137
Tolterodine, 138
Topical salicylates, 137
Training, 34, 97-98
Tramadol, 137
Transitional care, 28, 30, 181
Trastuzumab, 138
Trimethoprim-sulfamethoxazole, 28, 136

U

Ubidicarenone, 138
Unfractionated heparin (UFH), 3, 177, 203
    administration, 179
    dosing, monitoring nomogram, 179
    indications, 179
    mechanism of action, 178
    monitoring, 183-85
    monitoring nomogram, 182
    neuroaxial procedures, 192
    pediatric patients, 197-98
    pharmacokinetics/pharmacodynamics, 179-80
    pharmacology, 178-79
    pharmacy management of, 8-9, 10
    pregnancy, 197, 199
    renal impairment, 195-96
    reversal of, 194
    side effects, precautions, contraindications, 185-86
    use of, 7
    weight-based dosing nomogram in acute thrombosis, 182
University of Wisconsin Extension Services in Pharmacy, 216

V

Valvular heart disease, 145-46. 149
Venous thromboembolism (VTE), 5, 7, 40, 144-45, 146, 147, 155, 187, 193
Vitamin C, 134
Vitamin E, 136
Vitamin K, 5, 8, 13-14, 138, 140, 216
    cycle, 134
    -dependent clotting factor, 135
    injectable, 154
    reversal guidelines, 154

use, policy and procedures, 58
Voriconazole, 137
VTE. *See* Venous thromboembolism

W

Warfarin, 3-4, 199, 216
    adverse effects, 158
    business plan, 84-90
    business process, 85
    cases, 161-64
    direct thrombin inhibitors and, 67
    discharge work checklist, 56
    disease interactions with, 136, 138-39
    dose initiation nomogram, 54
    dose management, 148, 150-52
    dosing timeline and surgery, 51
    education program, 42
    generic vs. brand, 159-61
    genetic issues, 139-40
    hemorrhage risk, 156-58
    high dose vs. low dose initiation nomograms, 151
    high dose vs. modified high dose initiation nomograms, 152
    HIT, 211
    indications, 140-46
    initiation algorithm, 54
    INR elevation management, 152-54
    INR results review, 40
    INR use, 42
    invasive procedures and, 155-56
    ISMP, 19
    laboratory monitoring, 152
    malpractice claims, 82
    NPSG, 20
    outpatient clinics, 4
    patient calendar, 115
    patient education, 102, 103, 106-8
    patient education check-off list, 114
    pharmacokinetics/pharmacodynamics, 134-40
    pharmacology, 133-34
    pharmacy management of, 7-10, 11-12, 52-54
    precautions, contraindications, 158-59
    responsiveness, 42-43
    restarting, 28
    reversal, 44, 59
    transitioning from direct thrombin inhibitor, 209-10
    use of, 7
Warfarin dosing service
    pilot flowchart, 37
    RAID analysis, 35-36
    SWOT analysis, 36-37
Weight-based dosing, 182-83

X-Z

Ximelagatran, 217
Zileuton, 138
Zweber, Ann, 102